YO-BDF-486

A DIGNIFIED ENDING

A DIGNIFIED ENDING

Taking Control Over How We Die

Lewis Mitchel Cohen, MD

ROWMAN & LITTLEFIELD
Lanham • Boulder • New York • London

Published by Rowman & Littlefield
An imprint of The Rowman & Littlefield Publishing Group, Inc.
4501 Forbes Boulevard, Suite 200, Lanham, Maryland 20706
www.rowman.com

6 Tinworth Street, London SE11 5AL, United Kingdom

British Library Cataloguing in Publication Information Available

Library of Congress Cataloging-in-Publication Data Is Available

978-1-5381-1574-9 (cloth: alk. paper)
978-1-5381-1575-6 (electronic)

∞™ The paper used in this publication meets the minimum require-
ments of American National Standard for Information Sciences—
Permanence of Paper for Printed Library Materials, ANSI/NISO
Z39.48-1992.

Printed in the United States of America

CONTENTS

∾

Part I
1

Part II
111

Part III
229

Part IV
293

PART I

"Do you know how Hercules died?" Dr. Paul Spiers asked.

We were sitting at a restaurant a block away from the courthouse in Worcester, Massachusetts. Paul was wolfing down a late lunch and talking between mouthfuls. I was taken aback by his question—a beauty of a non sequitur that hardly seemed germane to why we had gotten together.

Paul is a forensic psychologist who had just testified in court that morning as an expert witness. Back in the day, Paul was a leader of the Hemlock Society.

Paul could not know that before deciding on becoming a psychiatrist, I seriously considered the field of archeology and still recalled a few facts from mythology. As a child, I had excitedly read about the twelve Labors of Hercules (or Heracles as he was known to the ancient Greeks) in a juvenile version of *Bulfinch's Mythology*. However, even if I hadn't done my reading, just about everyone has heard of Hercules, the son of Zeus and mankind's mightiest hero.

"I'd be interested because?" I replied.

"We're talking about the original big guy," said Paul. "Arguably the world's greatest champion! And nobody remembers how he died." When Paul got agitated he squirmed around in his wheelchair. The tires squeaked under the table.

Paul began to expound: "Hercules was not only a major deal in Greek and Roman times, but in the 1950s and 1960s there were literally nineteen Hercules movies produced. He single-handedly employed most of Hollywood's musclemen! Before Arnold Schwarzenegger hit it big and governed California, he starred in the improbably named picture, *Hercules in New York*. Lou Ferrigno, who became better known as television's Hulk, was featured in two movies, and Dwayne Johnson, The Rock, had his turn in 2014. Who could forget *Hercules against Karate*, the 1973 saga set in Hong Kong? Or how about the 2012 soft-porn film with the titillating title, *Hercules Unbound*, promoted as being "sexier than *Game of Thrones*! Meaner than *Spartacus*! Hercules is back!' And for the kiddies, I can personally attest to the exceeding popularity of the Disney animated movie!"

Paul took a drink, wiped his mouth, and returned to what was obviously a soliloquy.

"But they were all eclipsed by the TV series, *Hercules: The Legendary Journeys* that paved the way for the even more popular, *Xena: Warrior Princess*."

I thought to myself, *Spiers has been watching too much television and spending way too much time memorizing Wikipedia.*

As he briefly rested from his own labors, Paul took a couple of self-satisfied bites.

"So, how did Hercules die?" I inquired.

"Funny you should ask," he said, and wriggled his eyebrows like Groucho Marx.

"None of the movies or TV series dealt with Hercules's death," Paul began. "Nowadays, not a lot of people recall Ovid's poem, *Metamorphoses*, or Sophocles's two plays, *The Women of Trachis* and *Philoctetes*, but all of them relate versions of the same strange tale. Hercules's wife innocently gave him a tunic infused with a dreadful poison. Upon draping the garment over his torso, the toxin caused Hercules's skin to begin melting. His blood hissed and boiled and the poison tore through his body like acid."

I remarked, "It sounds not unlike the flesh-eating bacteria that some unlucky people pick up in hospitals nowadays."

Ignoring my comment as if I were an audience member who coughed during a performance, Paul pulled out a scrap of paper from his backpack and began dramatically reading aloud Ovid's words: "He tries at once to tear off the fatal clothing: where it is pulled away, it pulls skin away with it, and, revolting to tell, it either sticks to the limbs from which he tries in vain to remove it, or reveals the lacerated limbs and his massive bones. . . . He raises his hands to the heavens, crying: 'Death would be a gift to me.'"[1]

Putting aside the paper, he continued: "Hercules was a demigod and therefore practically immortal. That is a sizeable problem when your skin is grotesquely sloughing off. Seeking the counsel of the Delphic oracle, he learned that the only way to stop the agony was by dying in fire. Hercules persuaded Hyllus, his son, to construct a pyre of oak and olive wood, and to place his tortured body upon it. But he could not convince his son to set it ablaze."

Taking another look at his notes, Paul quoted from Sophocles: "Hyllus said, 'Father, father, how can you? You are asking me to be your murderer, polluted with your blood.' Hercules replied to him, 'No, I am not. I ask you to be my healer, or healer of my sufferings, sole physician of my pain.'"[2]

Paul glanced at me and said, "When it was apparent that Hyllus had done as much as he was willing, Hercules requested that another of his companions ignite the pyre."

The men who gathered around Hercules were his dearest friends. They loved him, uniformly admired his fortitude and had faced many dangers together. They heard his words and saw the torment but, like Hyllus, none was willing to comply with the request. Hercules implored them for help. Again, no one responded. Finally, Philoctetes, whom Homer describes as being the captain of seven ships and 350 oarsmen, brought out a burning torch and placed it upon the oil-soaked wood. As the smoke arose, Hercules declared his gratitude to Philoctetes and pronounced him to be the recipient of a magic bow and quiver of arrows."

"And as the flames consumed Hercules, the demigod underwent an apotheosis—while the shell of his body descended into the underground, he ascended to Mt. Olympus and took his rightful place among the other gods of the pantheon."

"Who knew?" I said. "Assisted suicide in Greek mythology!"

This book challenges the dogma that prolonging life through every means possible is the only reasonable response to a dire diagnosis and that it is unacceptable to embrace and shape our deaths. These views are predicated on a long-held misconception about our capacity to grasp the act of dying.

In an ancient Sanskrit epic, a youth asked Yudhishthira, "What is the most wondrous thing on earth?" The sage replied, "Every day people die, but those who are living keep on believing that they are immortal. What can be more wondrous?"[3]

Freud, too, maintained that we cannot face our own mortality as evidenced by the fact that we never die in dreams. Our unconscious rejects the reality that we will eventually cease living.

La Rochefoucauld expressed this same opinion, stating, "One can no more look steadily at death than at the sun."[4]

In my experience, however, such views are flawed. Sure, many people may hope and pretend that it will all get better—right up until the moment of their last breath. Some can't imagine that the world will go on without them. But plenty of others know damn well they are dying. They can clearly see that their lives or at least the lives they have known are ending. In our era of longer life expectancies, we commonly experience and get to see firsthand the deaths of parents, siblings, acquaintances, colleagues, and occasionally children. There are those who do not want to be compelled to linger in old age or when physical and mental decrepitude begin to conflict with long-standing ideals of personhood. Many people know they have a cancer or are dying from a dire disease well before their physician imparts the diagnosis.

In Paul's retelling of the myth, Hercules accepted his demise. While renowned for overcoming seemingly impossible obstacles, Hercules decided to fearlessly die while surrounded by friends. I think that he chose for himself a more dignified ending.

This book is built around the accounts of men and women who similarly grasped what lay ahead. A few of them could be described as having been larger than life. But what they all had in common was a determination to be larger than death. Rather than passively accept cruel fate, these individuals wanted to shape how, when, and where they were going to die. Paradoxically, faced with the imminence of death, they became intensely alive, and they often reached out to involve loved ones.[5] Upon embarking on the preparation of this book, I wanted to both explore all the death-hastening options and to grasp more fully what these friends and family members experienced. I also was intensely curious about the activists—including Dr. Jack Kevorkian, Derek Humphry from the Hemlock Society, and Brittany Maynard—who had become leaders in a sociopolitical movement to promote and legalize assisted dying.

We have all made glib declarations about our future preferences ("I would rather die than suffer with . . . [fill in the blank]" and "If . . . happens, then kill me."). We have also seen movies or shows touching on these themes. But we have had—for better or worse—minimal real-life experience dealing with this subject and its practical, ethical, emotional, and legal issues. The narratives in A Dignified Ending are intended to redress that situation. Like the title of recent New York Times article "The Last Thing Mom Asked," the book's stories are stirring, gritty, and sometimes conflictual.[6] Most important, they are unabashedly truthful. When I conducted the preparatory interviews, I felt as if I were receiving death-bed confessions consistent with the observation of one of my favorite authors, Andrew Solomon, who wrote, "Euthanasia offers a remarkable liberation, for, once it is fully acknowledged, the imminence of death can be the basis for a stripped and pure honesty that is not possible under ordinary circumstances."[7]

As a physician, I've been privileged to participate in many meaningful conversations. I've also grown accustomed to encountering people's tendency to exaggerate, distort, and lie. I had enjoyed Paul's exuberant account of the myth concerning Hercules's death, but the fictional tale was surpassed by the "stripped and pure honesty" of the many narratives that I was privileged to hear during this project. Unvarnished truths—where people put aside their public personas and candidly recount intimacies—are a special treasure. I'm grateful for the opportunity to share them in this book.

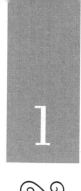

THE ADMIRAL
AND HIS WIFE

On New Year's Day in 2002, three generations of the Nimitz clan assembled for an unusual holiday lunch.[1] Rear Admiral Chester W. Nimitz Jr. and his wife, Joan, presided at their residence in a retirement community outside of Boston. They were obviously both pleased and proud the family had gathered. Their home was tastefully decorated with comfortable, older furniture and memorabilia from around the world. Like everything about the admiral and his wife, the place was clean and orderly.

Although the luncheon conversation included an energetic discussion of holiday football games, the overall atmosphere was subdued. This was not a typical raucous New Year's celebration, and the assembled sipped their wine thoughtfully. Chester Jr. and Joan were, by nature, reserved individuals, and they did not encourage effusive displays of emotion. Despite this, their daughter, Sarah Smith, explained, "We hugged them and gave them kisses, and my sister, Betsy, said something like, 'You've been wonderful parents.'"[2]

The family members were confident the matriarch's and patriarch's decisions were entirely consistent with long-held beliefs.

No one engaged in last-minute attempts to persuade them to change their minds. The family knew any such efforts would be fruitless and resented. You don't question or challenge a superior officer's decision. Everyone felt solemn as goodbyes were said. Children and grandchildren stepped across the threshold on that crisp New England day. The door was firmly closed behind them.

Earlier throughout that fall and winter, Betsy Nimitz Van Dorn and her youngest sister, Sarah, repeatedly visited their parents and inquired, "Why do you have to do it?"

Daily confronted with increasing frailty and growing dependency needs, Chester Jr. told his daughters, "It is the one last thing I have to do for your mother."

A *New York Times* article would later quote an aunt, "They didn't want to think in any way that their final days would be controlled by some whippersnapper internist at the hospital."[3]

"Nothing was left to chance," said Sarah, who lived in a nearby suburb. "He made sure everything worked the way he wanted." After all, Chester Jr. was a military man who conducted his affairs with the precision of a commanding officer. And Joan was the quintessential admiral's wife.

Joan had been born in England, educated as a dentist, and came to America for specialty training in orthodontia. Like many women of her generation, after meeting and falling in love with her future husband, she had little opportunity to practice her profession and instead devoted herself to furthering his career and raising their three daughters. As a Navy wife, she led a peripatetic existence, moving the family every year to a new base in a strange city, often located in a foreign country. She single-handedly oversaw the children's upbringing during the extended periods her husband was at sea.

Chester Jr. graduated from the Naval Academy and served as a submariner on the USS *Sturgeon* during World War II. He was awarded the Silver Star, which was presented to him by his father, Chester Sr., at a ceremony held at Pearl Harbor. It was one of three Silver Stars he would receive for valor. Chester Jr. was transferred to the command of another submarine, the USS *Haddo*, and later awarded the Navy Cross and a Letter of Commendation with Ribbon.

The official citation reads in part: "For outstanding heroism in action during her Seventh War Patrol in restricted enemy waters off the West Coast of Luzon and Mindoro in the Philippines. . . . Valiantly defiant of the enemy's overpowering strength during this period just prior to our invasion of the Philippines, the USS *Haddo* skillfully pierced the strongest hostile escort screens and launched her devastating attacks to send two valuable freighters and a transport to the bottom. . . . The *Haddo* out-maneuvered and out-fought the enemy at every turn launching her torpedoes with deadly accuracy despite the fury of battle and sending to the bottom two destroyers and a patrol vessel with another destroyer lying crippled in the water."[4]

Perhaps Chester Jr.'s most acclaimed exploit occurred when a Japanese destroyer steered directly at his submarine. Rather than resorting to the more common tactic of hugging the bottom and hoping to avoid depth charges, he sank the enemy ship by aiming three torpedoes at her bow.

The admiral was a plain-spoken man. In a recorded interview stored at the Naval War College he comes across as gruff and candid. He never minced words or shied away from tough issues or deviated from doing what he believed was the right thing. Asked about the awards, he replied simply, "Yes, the patrols were all deemed successful. We got a combat star. In other words, we sank something all the time."

In the wide-ranging interview, he displayed progressive ideals, touching on his satisfaction that the military had improved the lives of both American blacks and women. He strongly expressed indignation over the penurious salary that officers received while risking their lives at sea. Chester Jr. was irate that he couldn't afford private school tuitions or music lessons for his children.

After World War II, Chester Jr. fought in the Korean War. He served as the skipper of the destroyer *O'Brien* during the "Siege of Wonsan." But after completing twenty-three years of military service, he had enough. That he chose to resign and enter civilian life displeased his father.

Chester W. Nimitz Sr. is even more renowned in the chronicles of U.S. naval warfare than his son.[5] One week after the Pearl Harbor disaster, Navy Secretary Frank Knox gave Chester Sr.

command of the Pacific Fleet. Throughout World War II, he was Commander-in-Chief of Pacific Forces for the United States and the Allies. In the Battle of Midway, Chester Sr.'s fighter-bombers caught the Japanese fleet off guard as the carrier aircraft were being refueled. The Allied pilots sank four of the Japanese carriers. Part of what made this exquisitely sweet was that each vessel had originally attacked Pearl Harbor.

The Battle of Midway shattered Japanese naval power, and along with the Battle of the Coral Sea and the Solomon Islands campaign, the Admiral's leadership led to the defeat of the Japanese navy. On September 2, 1945, when Japan formally surrendered on board the USS *Missouri* in Tokyo Bay, Chester Sr. was given the honor of representing the United States.

While Chester Sr. remained in the military, Chester Jr. became a highly regarded business executive. Recruited by Texas Instruments, he later was president of the Perkin-Elmer Corporation. According to Betsy, he took considerable satisfaction in paying a larger amount in income tax during his first year in Dallas than he had cumulatively earned during two decades in the Navy.

Chester Jr. and Joan did not lead especially lavish lifestyles, but they were extraordinarily generous to all of their progeny. The couple's credo was: "We are not the kind of people who would ever want to leave any of our children a trust fund. We have given you decent educations and you are fine on your own. We want the pleasure of watching our grandchildren go to great schools and summer camps, take trips, and have adventures. That is the pleasure money can bring—not stockpiling it so some spoiled offspring can have it when he or she turns twenty-one."

In a photograph taken outside of their house on Cape Cod, the Admiral and his wife are a well-matched, gray-haired couple. In military parlance, they stand *at ease* with their hands behind their backs, casually dressed in slacks, slender and smiling with self-confidence.

Chester Jr. and Joan were longtime members of the Hemlock Society. The organization's philosophy—that people should be in charge of their deaths as well as their lives—appealed to them as meticulous managers. The couple freely discussed these beliefs with their children, and Betsy said, "They always proclaimed when they got sick and tired of feeling sick and tired that they would do themselves in."

Betsy is confident her parents also expressed these same opinions about end-of-life matters to Chester Sr. and his wife. "My grandparents were quite liberal and open-minded and not a bit religious—so that wasn't in the way. I would say while it never would have occurred to my grandparents to do anything like that for themselves, they would've heartily agreed it was a civil right, and they were big supporters of civil rights."

Hemlock's principles did not call for Joan and Chester Jr. to refrain from taking full advantage of medical science. When the admiral developed coronary artery disease, he underwent the recommended and grueling quintuple cardiac bypass surgery. He successfully dealt with the pain, accepted the cardiac diet, and embraced the challenge of the physical therapy. After several years, however, Chester Jr.'s litany of health problems became lengthy. His vision deteriorated and he could no longer safely drive. He had frequent bouts of congestive heart failure, experienced chronic back pain, repeatedly slipped and fell, suffered with gastrointestinal problems, lost thirty pounds, and, to his great shame, became incontinent. Extensive evaluations and treatment at the best Boston teaching hospitals proved ineffective at controlling the symptoms.

By age eighty-nine, Joan was suffering from severe osteoporosis, bone fractures, and the constant pain of peripheral neuropathy. Although she and her husband loved golf, this pursuit was no longer possible. Macular degeneration made it difficult for her to read.

Nurses were employed at their home to attend to Joan's worsening health problems, but the couple did not want to "squander all of their money on such care." They were both appalled at the vast sums spent at the end of life to sustain people who are frail and sick and unlikely to get better.

Joan's visual impairment became incapacitating. The admiral was eighty-six years old, and he worried his heart condition might suddenly worsen and that his wife would be unable to die by her own hand. She, too, was fearful that without her husband's help, she would not be in a position to make use of the pills they had accumulated. The couple openly talked about these concerns with their daughters.

According to Betsy, her father had a large file box labeled with a three-by-five-inch note card upon which he had written with a magic marker, "When CWN [Chester Williams Nimitz] Dies." In it were his important documents: the insurance policies, bank statements, and forms concerning his Navy pension. They were intended to save the family from scrambling around in search of his papers.

Throughout the last year, the Nimitz couple talked about their plan. It was to follow the suggestions in the book *Final Exit* written by Derek Humphry. Betsy said, "When ready, they intended to begin with an anti-nausea suppository, followed by barbiturate sleeping pills, chased with a little of their beloved Mount Gay Rum with a squeeze of lime and soda, and maybe a little peanut butter to settle their stomachs. The last step involved securing plastic bags over their heads as a precaution in case the medication was not sufficiently lethal. The admiral was going to let his wife take the pills first and make sure she was dead before he followed her example."

Betsy observed, "None of it was particularly pretty. But they were just so determined and upbeat about all of it."

The admiral and Joan wanted one more chance to write estate tax–exempt checks for the children, their husbands, and grandchildren; these were dated January 2, 2002, and left in the apartment. Death had been no stranger to this devoted couple, and it engendered no fear. She had experienced the deaths of siblings, including one of her brothers, a British Royal Air Force pilot shot down in combat. He had witnessed a surfeit of destruction in the wars.

After the family left their apartment on the evening of New Year's Day, Chester Jr. and Joan wrote a suicide note for the staff of the retirement home.[6] It read in part: "Do not resuscitate. Do not dial 911 in the event we are discovered unconscious but still alive. Our decision was made over a considerable period of time and was not carried out in acute desperation. Nor is it the expression of a mental illness. We have consciously, rationally, deliberately, and of our own free will taken measures to end our lives today because of the physical limitations on our quality of life."

The day after New Year's, Betsy was up early and waited impatiently by the phone for the call she knew was coming. After the police officially notified her of the deaths, she brought out the comprehensive list of people and telephone numbers that her father had compiled and left in the CWN file box in anticipation of this chore. She divvied it up with her sister, Sarah. Before any word had gotten into the newspapers, they called their parents' closest friends and told them what happened.

The almost universal response was, "Yup, that's your parents! They were extraordinary!"

But, as I will discuss in more detail, the deaths of the admiral and his wife would engender a great deal of both praise and condemnation. And, as I was to discover, some planned deaths are not nearly as orderly as the ones the Nimitzes had so carefully crafted.

|

2

A GERIATRIC ROMEO AND JULIET

One balmy Floridian morning in 1988, Dr. David Raft awoke in his room on the locked ward of the Palms of Sarasota psychiatric hospital. He was surprised to find himself there and was worried about his wife's welfare. David hoped his sons would arrive soon to arrange his release. He was also characteristically bemused by the situation and determined to smile and make the best of it.

The day before, two polite, uniformed Sarasota City police officers had rung the bell of David's condominium door.

"Can we come inside?" they inquired. David ushered them into his living room and they sat on the couch across from him. He anxiously offered them a cup of coffee, which they declined.

"What can I do for you?" David asked. "Is everything alright? Is my family okay?"

One of the policemen replied, "We have a warrant stating that you have been threatening to commit suicide and murder."

"Oh . . . ," said David.

"We need to bring you in," the police officer explained.

They escorted the eighty-five-year-old retired physician outside and proceeded to drive him in a squad car to the local psychiatric facility.

David had never previously been in psychotherapy, let alone involuntarily committed to an inpatient mental institution. He was a cheerful man, beloved in his community, where, over the past two decades, he had been providing free medical advice to his many friends and neighbors. He was known for having a wry sense of humor and an endless store of amusing anecdotes. Despite chronic back pain and a slow-growing bladder cancer, David's mind was unimpaired and he looked and acted much younger than his chronological age.

By contrast, Reba, his eighty-seven-year-old wife, had fared less well. She was troubled by heart disease, arthritis, and progressive deafness. Most important, her mind was failing. Although Reba still recognized friends and family and read the daily newspaper, she had trouble concentrating and was increasingly forgetful. A couple of times she accidentally left the frying pan on the burner and the baking pan in the oven. David responded by assuming greater responsibility for the household, and he rarely left her alone. Reba understood that she had Alzheimer's disease but overall remained in good spirits.

The Raffs were married for fifty-five years. Reba was an integral part of David's medical practice in Montreal and a splendid mother to their now-grown children, Anton and Martin. Although the profession of medicine totally consumes the lives of many physicians, throughout his career David had routinely taken off Wednesday afternoons—not to play golf with cronies, but to run around with his boys in the park adjacent to their home. He was always a very outgoing man and well liked; people constantly buttonholed his sons telling them, "You are so lucky to have such a wonderful father!"

When they were younger, David and Reba loved sports. He enjoyed ice-skating, swimming, canoeing, tennis, skiing, and sailing, while she was an accomplished golfer. In family portraits, the two have slender, athletic builds, wavy hair, prominent noses, and loving smiles. The camera is drawn to charismatic David, with his broad forehead, well-defined jaw line, and handsome cleft in his chin. In a photograph, Anton, the older son, stands upright and somewhat detached, while his parents warmly embrace Martin. Both sons would become doctors: Anton is now a well-regarded retired general practitioner and Martin is a neurologist, molecular cell biologist, and textbook coauthor with James Watson—the discoverer of DNA's double-helix structure and winner of the Nobel Prize.

Since moving to Florida, David and Reba had gradually settled into a quiet and self-contained existence in their fifth-floor condominium with picture windows overlooking the Gulf of Mexico. Sarasota is a city of powdery white sands, art museums, and botanical gardens containing dense mangroves and orchid-studded woods, not to mention a full complement of restaurants and shops frequented by retirees.

The Raffs' daily lives in Sarasota followed a simple routine. In the mornings, they drove together to a local coffee shop for brunch. In the afternoons, Reba napped while David answered mail and read the newspaper. In the evenings, they would go to a restaurant for dinner and then retire early to watch TV—much like Ronald and Nancy Reagan, who resided in the White House at the time (and were secretly dealing with the president's Alzheimer's disease). In winters, this pattern was occasionally enlivened by visits from old friends who would fly down from Montreal seeking warmth, sunshine, and the opportunity to reconnect with the Raffs. In 1982, Anton moved his medical practice to Sarasota and was then able to see his parents regularly. Martin continued to work as a professor at University College London, and popped over for a visit once or twice a year.

Physically, the Palms of Sarasota psychiatric hospital where the police had brought David was not entirely unpleasant, consisting of a large one-story building with spacious grounds and abundant tropical flora. Emotionally, however, it was a terrifying place. The lunatic asylums of the nineteenth century improved as they evolved into the psychiatric hospitals of the twentieth century, but they still mainly housed psychotic people who couldn't be managed outside of institutions. Economically, too, the place was in rough financial shape.

After being admitted, the retired physician was encouraged to change into pajamas and take a rest. Later that day he exchanged a few pleasantries with staff. Strolling around in his robe and slippers, he explored the facility and was given a supervised opportunity to venture into the gardens. All the while, David reflected on the circumstances that led him to being committed to this unit.

He couldn't help but think about his role in the death of his father over thirty years earlier. David had been extraordinarily close to him and was greatly upset when the elderly gentleman was hospitalized and diagnosed with meningitis. Following discharge, it was apparent that his father had undergone irreversible brain damage. David employed his considerable skills at managing his father's supportive care but experienced limited success controlling seizures and other symptoms.

Like many doctors of his generation, David had witnessed incredible medical advances: the discovery of antibiotics, development of ventilators and dialysis machines to compensate for failed lungs and kidneys, creation of surgical intensive care units to manage acute traumatic injuries, improved reliance on chemotherapy and radiation therapies to treat cancers, and the use of vaccines to prevent infectious diseases. For example, in 1953, there had been thirty-five thousand reported cases of polio; however, after mass inoculation began the next year using the Salk vaccine, the numbers dramatically dwindled.[1] By 1962, there were only 161 incident cases of the disease in the entire country.

Yes, David had seen miracles occur, but he did not delude himself that the sole goal of medicine was to save or prolong life. He recognized that an equally important goal remained the amelioration of suffering. When patients could not be restored to their previous state of function, then serious conversations needed to take place with them and their loved ones. It was David who concluded that his father's situation was hopeless, and it was David who then administered a lethal injection of morphine.

David's part in his father's death wasn't something to be shouted from the rooftops, but it also wasn't completely veiled in secrecy; he spoke about it on several occasions to his sons. Walking around the psychiatric unit, the complicated memory of euthanizing his father bubbled to the surface, and he thought, *Such an act leaves one feeling both guilty and righteous. It is a curse to have been present and it is a blessing to be able to bring an end to unendurable suffering.*

David and Reba were members of the Hemlock Society. The right-to-die organization, begun in 1980, attracted people like the Raffs who had seen firsthand the distinct limitations of modern medicine's marvels and emerged with a fervent desire to retain control over their destiny. The Society's membership roll was populated by individuals liberated from the societal delusion that they would live forever. Instead, each knew in a very personal way that *death is inevitable and it is natural*. David and Reba, like the Society's other members, did not believe in prolonging the process of dying; they wished to avoid medical death-delaying techniques; they wanted to choose how and when they would die.

The Raffs would have appreciated and intimately understood William Shakespeare's lines in Romeo and Juliet:

> Yet I should kill thee with much cherishing.
> Good night, good night! Parting is such sweet sorrow,
> That I shall say good night till it be morrow.

By nature, David was not a gloomy man, prone to brood, or quick to anger, but having now been abruptly ripped from his home and transported to the Palms of Sarasota, he experienced each of these emotions in quick succession. *By what right,* he thought to himself, *have they locked me up in this place?* David was no fool and he knew enough to conceal his outrage. The elderly man walked around the psychiatric hospital with a smile on his handsome face. Underneath, he fretted about his wife and was indignant that people who did not share their beliefs about autonomy at the end of life had locked him up.

In 2011, I sat alongside about a dozen others in a stunningly beautiful, modern conference center as part of a think tank organized by Dr. Martin Raff at the Cold Spring Harbor Laboratory in Huntington, Long Island. He entitled it, "Easeful Death: 21st Century

Perspectives on Assisted Suicide." The assembled included end-of-life researchers from Belgium and Switzerland, ethicists, palliative medicine physicians, and spiritual leaders. A few seats away from me was Adrienne Asch, director of the Center for Ethics at Yeshiva University in Manhattan (my alma mater).

Adrienne, who would die two years later from cancer, was a forceful advocate for people with disabilities, a scholar, and a public figure.[2] She was perhaps best known for her nuanced stance about abortion. A board member of the leading pro-choice organization, she firmly believed that women who did not want to be pregnant should have this option available. On the other hand, she forcefully opposed prenatal testing and the aborting of fetuses with abnormalities. She would argue that babies with Down syndrome have as much right to life as those without it, and it made little sense for people who shared this belief to undergo chromosomal testing of amniotic fluid. She was sensitive to the unavoidable clash of rights surrounding abortion—between the right of a woman to control her own body and the right of a fetus to survive.

At the Cold Spring Harbor Laboratory's elegant 1930s mansion, Adrienne and I sat together during most meals. We enjoyed each other's company and chatted about music and the damage wreaked by the eugenics movement in the first part of the twentieth century. The two of us sauntered arm-in-arm along the conference center's twisted pathways.

I should mention that Adrienne was blind. Her disability had likely contributed to the development of a personality that was determined and opinionated. Later, when I formally presented to the group, she surprised me with the vitriol of her critique. Adrienne was deeply suspicious of any arguments suggesting death might *ever* be preferable to a life with suffering or with disabilities. What were largely historical or theoretical topics to me were intensely personal ones for her, and she chewed my head off in front of the group. I can't recall her exact words, but they left me reeling. Upon reflection, I suspect her experience with me was akin to that of a black audience forced to listen to a white speaker offer his interpretation of the civil rights movement.

Adrienne taught me just how emotionally volcanic the subject of assisted dying can be. There is no way to address it without intentionally or unintentionally inflaming passions. Support or opposition may be framed as depending on logic, reason, history, and ethics, but it is actually propelled by exaggerated limbic factors and people's personal life experiences. Neuroanatomists might say that there is a primal part of the brain involved with survival that functions on an instinctual level and does not weigh such decisions in an orderly fashion.

The philosopher David Hume pointed out more than two hundred fifty years ago that we don't get up in the morning and think about whether we're going to first pull on our right or our left sock. We automatically slip into one or the other. I similarly don't believe that cognition plays much of a role as to whether we support or oppose assisted dying. But unlike one's choice of socks, there is a massive reservoir of feelings tied up in the topic.

Martin invited me to the event because I had recently published a book describing how doctors and nurses are occasionally accused of intentionally killing patients, when, from their professional perspective, they were merely providing sensible palliative care.[3] The book was prompted by my bafflement as to why some compassionate clinicians have ended up being subjected to criminal allegations by colleagues or otherwise considerate individuals. In *No Good Deed*, I strove to achieve nuance by conveying the opinions of the accusers, since their views differed drastically from my own. I wanted to explain the fervent opposition held by some religious leaders, politically conservative groups, nonwhites, and medical organizations to any clinical decisions that accelerate dying.

Since then I have come to appreciate that a similar phenomenon is evident in most societal conflicts over self-determination—from a woman's right to choose, to same-sex marriage, to bathrooms for transgendered children. Thoughtful debate about each of these issues is hindered by hyperbole, unrealistic fears, and unbridled anger.

As an author and palliative medicine researcher, I had long been curious about life-ending decisions. I arrived at Martin's conference knowing almost nothing about physician-assisted suicide/dying, which is illegal in Massachusetts. Adrienne's reaction to my brief presentation reminded me of Mark Twain's exasperation with Jane Austen, and his comment, "Every time I read *Pride and Prejudice* I want to dig her up and beat her over the skull with her own shin-bone." Consequently, I left the think tank with a realization that if I dared to write further about this topic, it would likely resonate emotionally with many readers but also infuriate many others.

Cold Spring Harbor Laboratory is situated on the shore of Long Island Sound, and you can smell the sea salt impelled by the blustery wind. From the shelter of the conference center we looked through enormous picture windows at swirling leaves of red and gold. But despite the beauty outside, everyone's attention remained tautly focused on the indoor conversations. Rain squalls punctuated the days and formed a suitable metaphor for our debates. We began by briefly introducing ourselves and later took turns broaching different aspects of the subject.

I exasperated Adrienne by openly speaking about the eugenics movement, which had been promulgated at the Cold Spring Harbor Laboratory a century ago. Mendellian genetics and the supposed improvement of the human species had been seized upon as a rationale for sterilizing and euthanizing "feeble minded," antisocial, and severely disabled populations. Pseudo-science was used as a basis for crafting immigration laws that were biased against non-Nordic or Aryan people. Rather than hiding the association, the current leadership of the Laboratory intentionally had exposed their shameful past and published several histories on the topic.[4]

Already irritated, Adrienne found it absolutely intolerable when I then brought up the subject of Terri Schiavo, whom I consider to be a Rosetta Stone for understanding our modern conflict with death-accelerating medical practices. Schiavo was a young woman who remained in an irreversible persistent vegetative state for fifteen years before her feeding tube was finally removed at a hospice in 2005. She became the object of a media frenzy, as parents and siblings noisily fought with her husband in a series of acrimonious court battles. These were accompanied by state and congressional legislative debates that attracted the attention of the Florida governor and eventually the president.

Schiavo's brother, Bobby Schindler Jr., told me during an interview, "Terri wasn't dying. She was cognitively disabled. It was needless. It was senseless. There was no reason to do this to my sister."[5]

I met Bobby in Toronto where he was the keynote speaker at an anti-euthanasia symposium. Accompanied by a companion, Brother Paul O'Donnell from the Franciscan Brothers of Peace, Bobby explained that Terri was neither terminally ill nor even calamitously sick. The two men nodded their heads in unison and agreed that she died from "euthanasia by omission."

"Life doesn't go back to normal after this," the Franciscan monk remarked. "There is a battle going on between the culture of life and the culture of death, and God has called upon our community to represent the culture of life."

Bobby continued,

> "It seems to be the premise of the other side that the acceptable alternative to human suffering is to kill . . . and I just don't go for that. I don't buy into the whole premise that killing is an acceptable alternative answer for someone who is suffering—whether emotionally or physically.
>
> "For those who believe in the whole autonomy thing— that we should be able to decide the manner and place of our death—I don't think it is for man to really decide when our deaths should occur. Obviously, I believe that we are all made in the image of God, we are children of God, and He is the one who decides when we should leave this earth. It doesn't change if we become disabled.
>
> "I look at it as a deliberate killing of a cognitively disabled person who had a family that was more than willing to care for her. I wholeheartedly believe that my sister was killed—killed by the system, killed by [her husband], killed by whomever. She was deliberately and purposely killed."[6]

Similar beliefs were expressed at the time by President George W. Bush, who declared, "I urge all those who honor Terri Schiavo to continue to work to build a culture of life where all Americans are welcomed and valued and protected."[7]

I told Adrienne and the other participants at the Cold Spring Harbor Laboratory meeting that the Schindler-Schiavo family feud was instructive because it spotlighted specific palliative care practices, such as the withdrawal and withholding of artificial nutrition and hydration (feeding tubes) and the proliferation of advance-care directives (living wills, health care proxies). The latter are tilted toward helping individuals avoid the initiation or continued use of life-extending therapies (ventilators, dialysis, etc.), although they also offer people who desire those treatments a better chance at receiving them.

I showed photographs taken at the hospice protest rally. In the pictures, one could see wheelchairs jumbled together, people sprawled on the ground, others marching around, a large home-made crucifix stretching above the protestors, and signs everywhere proclaiming: *Don't Devalue Our Lives*, *Thou Shalt Not Kill*, *It's Murder Not Mercy*, *Please Feed Terri*, and *Not Dead Yet*.

This may be a subtle point, but while activists in the anti-assisted-suicide coalition publicly claim to be supportive of hospice and palliative medicine and loudly praise its goals, I believe many of them choose not to express their true conviction that both the subspecialty and organized medicine as a whole have become seduced by death. They worry and proclaim, sometimes loudly, that there are new incentives—primarily financial—facilitating the denial of care. They are steadfastly opposed to all medical decisions that accelerate dying, including the withdrawal or withholding of medical technologies (especially feeding tubes), vigorous use of narcotics, and so forth. For most of the religiously motivated members of the coalition—and they are the chief financial contributors—the expression, pro-life, has now been expanded beyond abortion to encompass the terminus of life. It now includes the full range of practices that foreshorten existence.

Back in 1995, Andrew Solomon posited that there are six degrees of euthanasia under discussion in the United States.[8] The most basic is discontinuing life support—for example, ventilators—of patients in irreversible comas; followed by discontinuing feeding and hydration for comatose people; withholding therapies at the request of terminally ill patients; and giving pain medications to intractably suffering persons while knowing that the drugs might secondarily end their lives. All four of these practices are now widely considered to be ethical, legal, and acceptable to a degree Solomon could not have imagined at the time he wrote his piece.

The fifth practice Solomon discussed is giving a patient access to a lethal dose of medication they can use to kill themselves to escape from a severe or terminal illness. When Solomon's article was published, this was illegal throughout the nation; it is now available to one in five Americans—all those living in the geographical regions that have established lawful protocols to allow it.

The sixth practice—voluntary euthanasia—entails administering a lethal injection at the request of a dying patient. This has become an acceptable means of hastening death in Canada and several European countries, but it remains illegal throughout America and, at this time, no state is even considering making the practice lawful.

Solomon did not mention a seventh practice—involuntary euthanasia—to help someone to die who lacks the capacity to make such a request. David Raff made use of this method when he injected his neurologically impaired father with a fatal dose of morphine. While Raff's motivation may be understandable, involuntary euthanasia is now inextricably linked to the Nazi holocaust, which in turn was built on the eugenics movement.

I was stirred up emotionally and intellectually by the Cold Spring Harbor Laboratory gathering, and over the succeeding years, I tried to make sense of this subject. However, my opinions about assisted suicide/assisted dying—and its synonyms, which include medical aid in dying, death with dignity, assisted suicide, and self-deliverance—have been deepened and sometimes altered by my interviews. I have also concluded that the other death-hastening medical practices—withholding or withdrawal of life-support treatments, voluntary stopping eating and drinking (VSED), and terminal sedation—are more similar than different.

There is no simple and lucid argument to settle debates on these matters. There is no clear right and wrong, black and white. What's correct for me is not necessarily correct for you, and with different combinations of personal and societal circumstances, and with the passage of time, each of our opinions is likely subject to change.

Cognitive psychologists might argue otherwise, but one can't do a risk-benefit analysis—we can only conclude and act. The decisions to accelerate dying by individuals are mainly a product of automatic and unconscious calculations. Emotion, character, symptoms, functionality, the nature of relationships, spiritual and existential beliefs, communal values, and life experiences all factor into these life and death judgments, but either way, we are mainly unaware and unable to weigh the relative importance of each factor. These determinations either make sense to us or they don't. In cases such as the Nimitzes and Raffs, I believe people often arrive at the correct option for themselves, and it is usually consistent with long-held positions and values combined with emotionally evocative life experiences. But, of course, things don't always work out that way, and sometimes even clearly articulated plans go awry.

IT'S NOT LIKE SHE'S SUFFERING

Dr. Richard Epstein was a friend of a friend. I sat down in a booth with him to hear about his wife, Beth Weinstein. It was 2011, and we were meeting at a busy Connecticut diner. The place was jammed mainly with retired people taking their time finishing drawn-out breakfasts. A couple of harried waitresses scurried around leaving checks and occasionally clearing tables.

Richard married Beth in the late 1980s, and the couple had a lot more in common than the similarity of their last names. It began with their physical appearance. According to Richard, "When I looked at her, I would think that I was looking in the mirror." Both had adult children from previous marriages, and both were professionally involved with health care: Richard was an internal medicine specialist and Beth was Connecticut's director of the Preventable Disease Division and director of the AIDS Division. She was a Barnard College graduate who received an MPH on full scholarship from the Yale School of Public Health. The daughter of an ardent civil rights activist, she accompanied her mother and three younger sisters to the

Nevada State House and various protests. An accomplished linguist, she spoke Hebrew and Russian, and had delivered a speech in fluent French about AIDS legislation at a CDC conference in Paris. In 1992, Beth helped design and usher into law the country's first needle exchange program. Richard boasted that she was still greatly admired by the nation's AIDS community.

A few years before they met, Beth had started having memory problems. She had always suffered from anxiety, was employed in a highly stressful occupation, and had a staggering number of responsibilities at work. She consulted with a neurologist, who conducted a thorough physical examination that did not reveal any abnormalities. The doctor ordered a brain MRI that also proved to be normal, and he reassured her that she was probably suffering from mild depression.

In early 2000, Richard noticed the memory problems were worsening. Beth frequently forgot why she came into a room. Mid-sentence she would lose her train of thought. She was having trouble learning new things and at times got confused. "What's going on with me?" Beth asked Richard. She was forty-nine years old.

Beth underwent an extensive battery of neuropsychological tests. When this definitively documented the memory impairment, she was diagnosed as having an early dementia. The couple sought out additional consultants over the next two years. They saw nine specialists—who disagreed with each other—but the crucial thing was that Beth's memory continued to deteriorate. By assiduously delegating work, she managed to remain employed. Finally, in 2002, she took a temporary leave of absence, which then became permanent.

At the diner, Richard took a moment to butter some toast and compose himself. He then told me that in 2003, Beth sent a letter to her family about the dementia. He wanted me to better appreciate the woman he had married. Richard pulled out a piece of paper from his pocket and read Beth's words: "Don't worry about it. It's a shock, but I'm handling it. My urgent message to you is that I am well and well cared for. Get out the Kleenex box and cry. When you have stopped crying and are able to digest this letter, give me a call. I love you all, Beth.'"

Richard and Beth contacted Yale Medical Center to learn whether there were any promising dementia research studies. She enrolled in several clinical trials, but nothing altered the disease's progression. From the start, she never had any of the Alzheimer's risk factors and had always been and remained physically healthy.

Richard told me: "Beth and I decided to spend as much time as possible together traveling around the world. I cut back my medical practice to half time, and then I retired. *Life is too short* was the refrain we repeated to anyone who cared to listen."

Beth's father had died when she was quite young; her mother, three sisters, and she were exceptionally close to each other. There had been a family member who died after using the barbiturate regimen described in Derek Humphry's book *Final Exit*, and there was widespread agreement among the extended family that the individual had taken the appropriate action. Beth and Richard sat down with her loved ones to discuss assisted dying. She had formulated a simple mantra: *There is no way I am going to a nursing home!* Her family agreed.

According to Richard, "We had this naïve idea that this was a doable thing. We didn't really talk about specifics and how it would work. The family said, 'Oh, we've done it before and it shouldn't be a problem.' And somehow none of us talked about how we would be confident that the right time had arrived."

He had always considered himself to be adept at having end-of-life discussions with his patients. Richard looked at me from across the table and said, "I knew that Kevorkian's first client was a young nurse with early onset Alzheimer's. So I thought, *No problem!* All of us somehow believed that Beth would be the one to say, 'OK, let's do it now.'"

Several years ensued during which the couple traveled to exotic destinations. Occasionally, Richard checked in with Beth to discuss whether she was ready for the assisted dying. She always endorsed the idea in general but each time would tell her husband that she wasn't ready to implement it.

"When I broached the subject," Richard plaintively explained to me in the diner, "it was harder and harder to be sure that she was really understanding. The last time we talked about it, I thought to myself, *Oh yeah, Beth wants to go through with this.* But I waited and waited and she never took the initiative."

Beth's memory and functional abilities began to decline ever more rapidly. Richard and the family talked about the situation, and there was general agreement that "everybody was on board." The idea that they seized upon was that someone would travel with her to a kibbutz in Israel or to a clinic in the Netherlands. It seemed like there were plenty of possibilities. It also appeared that laws were being liberalized everywhere. However, according to Richard, neither he or any of the other family members fully grasped that there was no place in the world, not one single place, where it was legal to assist somebody to commit suicide who had become *non compos mentis*—not in one's right mind.

Another flaw in their thinking was predicated on the false belief that aid in dying could be triggered right before Beth needed to be placed in a nursing home. They didn't realize that there are many different thresholds to determine when people require the services of these facilities and they can be crossed in a nanosecond.

Then there were unresolved questions as to who would help her die and how would this be done? Richard thought it would be her mother or a sibling; they thought that he'd be the one taking charge.

Everyone agreed the intervention ought to be linked to when Beth's quality of life had sufficiently declined that she preferred being dead. But then they all struggled over defining the moment. Was it when she no longer recognized them, had become entirely incontinent, or was unable to conduct a conversation? Even when Richard and the family noticed that she was rapidly declining, they still deferred acting. They thought: *It's not like she is suffering. Is she?*

"It was around this time," he said to me, "that I decided I must have a life of my own. Beth and I had not had sexual relations for a long period of time, and she was sleeping in a different room. She was also wetting the bed." He was faced with the moral issue as to whether it counts as infidelity when a spouse no longer remembers your name.

Richard went to see a therapist who recommended obtaining an "emotional divorce." Richard attended a workshop where he met a woman, and shortly afterward the two of them began having an intimate relationship. He revealed this to Beth's family. They seemed understanding, but he was tormented by guilt.

Richard did not want to place Beth in a nursing home and explored various alternatives. He finally settled on an assisted-living facility situated a few miles from their house that offered a good patient-staffing ratio and a wide range of activities. She moved into the program in 2009.

Beth had always been an avid writer and reader. But one of the first things she lost from the dementia was the ability to identify objects or words. Beth often behaved as if she recognized people, including her husband, but she was feigning. Her main pleasure had been and remained music. Richard arranged to have a music therapist meet with her on a weekly basis. When people visited the assisted-living facility, she sang with them. She responded best to the music from childhood: Tony Bennett songs, Hebrew hymns, Broadway musicals, and Beatles hits.

After meeting with Richard at the diner, I called up Beth's mother, Dorothy, who told me, "I wake up in tears every morning."

These were not merely tears of sadness, because mixed into the anticipatory grief was great bitterness. There are a couple of lines that the radio host, Diane Rehm, wrote after her husband died from Parkinson's disease that captures the emotions. Rehm explained: "I rage at a system that would not allow John to be helped toward his own death. He was of rational mind, with no hope of recovery, knowing full well that the only way ahead was a slow downward slide, moving toward more incapacity and even greater indignity."[1]

Several times a year, Beth's eighty-three-year-old mother traveled to the East Coast from Nevada to see her at the assisted-living facility. Each visit was more agonizing than the previous, and she, too, raged at the system while ruminating about killing Beth. However, she told me, "Another of my daughters made it emphatically clear that I couldn't kill Beth at the nursing home. If I gave her an overdose, there probably wouldn't be sufficient unsupervised time for it to take effect and the police would be called."

Beth's mother thought about shooting her: "But I don't have a gun," she told me. "It would be too violent, anyway."

The fact that she was elderly or that her daughter was severely demented would not have been extenuating circumstances, as was apparent in several other cases.

For instance, in 2016, eighty-one-year-old Dr. Frank Kavanaugh faced a similar situation when his wife's dementia drastically worsened.[2] As a board member of Final Exit, a right-to-die organization, it is unclear why he refrained from using their recommended techniques to end life. Instead, he shot eighty-eight-year-old Barbara Kavanaugh and then turned the gun on himself.

A more recent case involved Philip M. Benight from Manor Township, Pennsylvania. In November 2017, Benight was sentenced to six to twenty-three months of home confinement with electronic monitoring to be followed by three years of probation after pleading guilty to the second-degree felony count of causing or aiding suicide.[3] In that state, the charge carries a maximum sentence of ten years in prison and a $25,000 fine, but sentencing guidelines considered the family's support of Benight's difficult decision, the district attorney's acknowledgment that Mrs. Benight had made multiple statements about not wanting to live in her condition, and the absence of a prior criminal record.

Benight had taken his seventy-three-year-old wife, Rebecca, out of a nursing home where she was receiving care for dementia, and the two of them got into their automobile and swallowed a prescription-drug cocktail mixed with vanilla pudding. When police officers were dispatched to check on Rebecca's welfare, the couple was discovered, unconscious, and parked in the driveway of their house. Both received treatment at a local hospital where Phillip recovered and his wife died eight days later.[4]

Rebecca had suffered with lifelong back pain due to a motor vehicle injury in childhood, was diagnosed as having throat cancer in 2003, had three strokes in 2005, followed by a heart attack and another stroke in 2015.

Longtime friend Marie Fouche said that Rebecca "wasn't ready to say goodbye," until September 2016 when she had another, more debilitating stroke.[5]

According to Fouche, the couple were "completely devoted to one another."

Following the conviction, Benight had to deal with the sentence, the expenses of the medical and nursing treatment, the notoriety, the cost of posting a $300,000 bail, the loss of his job, and assorted other psychosocial stressors—not to mention living with the memory of his wife's death and his own failed attempt to kill himself.

Rebecca's friend, Fouche, started a fundraiser on his behalf at GoGetFunding.com and posted: "What may or may not have happened leaves me with absolutely no doubt about the intent. It was all about their deep friendship, how much they cared for one another, and their deep love and respect for each other."[6]

In 2017, sixty-two-year-old Stephen Kruspe reportedly shot his wife, Pamela.[7] This occurred a couple of months after her admission to an assisted-living facility in Florida that specialized in dementia care.

After surrendering to police and being charged with homicide, he told them that they had been together for forty-two years and raised three children. Pamela had begged Kruspe to help her die.

A next-door neighbor explained, "They were crazy about each other. They'd run together, rode their bikes together. If one was at the mailbox, the other was at the end of the driveway, waiting."[8] During a court hearing, Kruspe was ordered to remain jailed without bond.

In a photograph of the handsome couple during happier times, both are smiling broadly and he is wearing a Marine dress uniform festooned with ribbons from his twenty-three years in the service.

However, even in situations like these that are so emotionally raw and give every appearance of being entirely justifiable, assisted dying is rarely straightforward. Back in 1985, in a case that is eerily like that of Stephen Kruspe, another South Florida man, Roswell Gilbert, also shot and killed his wife.[9]

Emily Gilbert, age seventy-three, had Alzheimer's disease and was suffering from excruciating osteoporosis that resulted in multiple fractures. Gilbert was seventy-five years old at the time, and he was subsequently convicted of murder. Gilbert received a life sentence and was incarcerated for more than five years before the former prosecutor wrote a letter on his behalf, arguing that he had served sufficient time and had health problems. He was then granted a pardon from the governor.[10]

Roswell Gilbert was interviewed in a poignant magazine piece at the state penitentiary in Avon Park, Florida.[11] This took place just before the broadcast of a made-for-TV movie, *Mercy or Murder*, that was based on his life.

Gilbert was a scientist—an electrical engineer—who frequently testified in court as an expert witness. At the murder trial, his dispassionate, and probably dissociated recitation of the facts, was poorly received. His daughter told the reporter, Linda Marx, "The jury felt his manner in court made him seem cold and insensitive. But that's just Daddy."[12]

However, he was perfectly able to convey to Marx the hell that led up to his wife's death. For months, their mornings began when he awoke at dawn, got two glasses of orange juice, and sat waiting for her eyes to open. Usually, she would neither recognize him nor recall where they were. Gilbert would carry Emily into the bathroom where he would bathe her and then brush her teeth. They would go to a local restaurant for lunch, but Emily had little appetite and in the final months her weight dropped below eighty pounds.

The last weekend was especially dreadful. The pain from new bone fractures was unmanageable at home, and she was brought to the hospital by her husband. In her confused and pain-ridden state, Emily couldn't tolerate an X-ray, and she yanked out the intravenous needle. Her clothing was already soiled, but now blood splattered everywhere.

Gilbert spent the night with his wife in the hospital. He must have fallen asleep when she snuck out of the room, pushed all the elevator buttons, and began to loudly shriek. The on-duty nurse told Gilbert, "We can't handle her; we're not used to this disease." Emily's agitation had previously led to her being turned away from three nursing homes.

Gilbert discharged Emily from the hospital and took her back to their condominium. When he briefly went down to the condo manager's office, she slipped out of the apartment, hobbled onto the elevator, and descended into the lobby. Dressed in the same bloody clothing, Emily was weeping uncontrollably. Gilbert and the office secretary looked at her and both of them also began crying.

Gilbert brought Emily back upstairs and placed her on the couch. Looking at his wife, he repeatedly asked, "What the hell can I do?"

According to his statement to the police, she turned to him and said, "Ros, I love you dearly. God, I want to die."

During the magazine interview, he explained:

> "It wasn't the first time she had said this. I even thought about killing her a year before. Had she not asked me in those last few hours, I wouldn't have gone through with it."
>
> "I walked into my lab and fetched the Luger. I shot her on the side of the head. Then I did something foolish. I felt the arteries in her neck. I realized she was still alive. So, I reloaded the gun. I was shaking like I'd never shaken. I shot her again. Her chin dropped. Her mouth just opened. Her right hand shook. No other movement. She was dead."
>
> "I felt grief. Not regret. I stood there and cried thinking my wife was dead. But the fact that she was no longer suffering gave me relief. The prosecuting attorney later said I got sick and tired of caring for her. He had no right to say that. Emily was terminal. . . . I did what I felt was right."
>
> "I do know this. If I get out of jail, I intend to work to legalize euthanasia. I may be helpful now that I'm well-known. I got caught in a bad law. Compassion has to be part of the defense."[13]

However, where the story gets especially complicated is five years later when he was granted clemency and pardoned by the governor. At that time, Gilbert told reporters that he no longer believed his behavior was justified. "I shouldn't have killed my wife; now I know that," he remarked. "I loved her dearly. I truly did."[14]

Gilbert said Emily's suffering "created just a complete state of desperation in my mind," and concluded, "It's a lousy excuse, but that's what it was."

It is unclear to me whether these statements represent a genuine retraction or whether they are the comments of a man who was fearful of being returned to prison. Either way, this story was not going to have a happy ending.

A year after Gilbert was released from the penitentiary, Barbara Walsh wrote a touching newspaper piece. The man was then eighty-two years old, had moved back to his tenth-floor condominium decorated with photographs of Emily, and there he became what Walsh called, "a prisoner of age, health and loneliness."[15]

Walsh explained that Gilbert was both a symbol of the tragedy that Alzheimer's disease can inflict on families, but also the cruel fate of numerous Floridians who spend their last years residing alone, trapped in high-rise buildings overlooking the sea.

While Gilbert may have expressed remorse at the time of his pardon, when he spoke to Walsh he appeared to have no further regrets about his actions. With the same measured tone that had contributed to his being convicted, he said, "I have no complications with what happened with my wife. She died where I'm sitting. I think about her a lot. I dream about her. She wanted to die. She said so. It was a rough go, though. I sure in hell miss her. I wish she could be back."[16]

A couple of years later, he would tell another reporter, "I think about it a lot, and I ask myself, what else could I have done? There was no honorable alternative. It was a straightforward solution to the problem, and the only one I could think of. Our life was just destitute."[17]

When he was eighty-five, Gilbert ceased being able to care for himself, moved to his daughter's home in Baltimore, and died shortly afterward in his sleep.[18]

When I spoke with Beth Weinstein's mother, she fully appreciated that killing her daughter would result in criminal charges like those faced by Gilbert, Benight, and Kruspe. She would not be shielded from legal consequences. The ensuing events could potentially destroy her entire family. Disconsolate, she told me, "It is an irreconcilable dilemma."

Clearly, the vexing issue of dementia added another level of complexity to an already fraught set of choices. How reasonable or fair was it to rely on Beth to signal the timing and manner of her death while hampered by the cognitive deficit of dementia? Could a family member judge the quality of life of a severely demented loved one? Once she or he has been admitted to a nursing facility, did that necessarily mark the end of accelerating dying? These were all questions that Beth's family struggled over.

SIGMUND FREUD'S DOCTOR

I was twelve years old when my mother walked into the living room of our New York City apartment overlooking the Hudson River and handed me a dog-eared copy of Sigmund Freud's *Interpretation of Dreams*.[1] By way of explanation, she said, "This is one of my favorite books, and I hope that you enjoy it, too."

I began reading and was suddenly oblivious to the view, the time of day, or my sisters happily playing with each other. Some years afterward, I would discover that my mother was about the same age as me when her family escaped the Nazis by fleeing Berlin. Reading about psychology was undoubtedly one of the principal activities that allowed her to accommodate to a dangerous and irrational world.

As I turned the pages of the book, I was bowled over by Freud's insights. He became my muse and instantly transformed my choice of careers. Archeology's goal of illuminating past civilizations had been important to me. Now, however, I wanted to comprehend people's behavior and elicit their background stories, listening not only to the manifest content of their words but also attending to the clues offered by slips of the tongue and dreams. Like Freud, I wanted to travel along "the royal road to the unconscious" and delve into complex emotions and contradictory motivations.

At age twenty-three, I was fortunate to spend the fourth year of medical school in London studying with Freud's daughter, Anna. During most of that time, I sat ensconced beneath Freud's marble bust in the Hampstead Child Therapy Clinic library.

"What should I read?" I asked Miss Freud.

"Anything you want!" she replied with her gentle Austrian accent.

I proceeded to immerse myself in the Standard Edition of her father's writings—all twenty-four volumes. Every so often, I needed a diversion and searched the bookshelves for something else. During one of those breaks, a book whose cover illustration depicted a photograph of Freud and his ever-present cigar caught my eye. *Freud: Living and Dying* was a firsthand account by his doctor, Max Schur, about how he died.[2]

When I first read about Freud's terminal illness in his daughter's library, I was too immature to understand what happened. But it touched me deeply nonetheless and I couldn't forget the story. This writing project and many of my forty years in medicine have been spent seeking to make greater sense of the circumstances of his death.[3] It made me appreciate the relationship I would like to establish not only with my patients but also with my own primary care physician. It offers a model I would want to follow in hastening my own death. I hope that I can summon Freud's forthrightness and courage, and that our nation's laws will change to facilitate such decisions for patients, their families, and the doctors who care for them.

In early 1923, sixty-seven-year-old Professor Sigmund Freud first noticed a small abnormal growth in his mouth.[4] Although he had become aware of a painful swelling on his palate several years before, he had reassured himself at the time that it was merely an insignificant sore or at worst, a benign tumor—neither would be unexpected after many years of heavy smoking.

During the next several months, Freud couldn't help but observe the lesion in his mouth was worsening, and in April he brought it to the attention of the doctor who was taking care of him at that time. He said to Felix Deutsch, "Be prepared to see something that you will not like."[5]

Freud's choice of words is intriguing to me because they suggest he not only recognized the severity of his condition but also anticipated Deutsch might have a deeply visceral reaction. Freud had discovered the concepts of transference and counter-transference—distortions that take place within relationships between clinicians and patients—and he must have been concerned whether his physician—who was also a devotee of the new field of psychoanalytic theory—could react with objectivity.

Fast forward to 1956 when Deutsch was invited to address the American Psychosomatic Society and offer reflections on what would have been Freud's one hundredth birthday.[6] Standing before the assembled medical specialists, physiologists, sociologists, anthropologists, and psychologists who convened in Boston, Deutsch recounted what happened after he looked into his famous patient's mouth. Deutsch's presentation was later published in a psychiatric journal.[7] It is a fascinating record of a proud, erudite, and accomplished man, but one who also knew that the seminal three-volume biography of Sigmund Freud written by Ernest Jones was about to be released. The last book of this tome would undoubtedly describe in stark detail Deutsch's treatment of the father of modern psychiatry, and he wanted to do his utmost to preemptively present this in the most favorable light. Ironically, Jones's account would recount the facts in a way that downplayed Deutsch's faults and magnified his virtues.[8]

The doctor was seventy-two years old when he stood at the podium facing the attentive audience, who knew him as one of the pillars of the field of psychosomatic medicine. Those present were unaware that his professional legacy hung in the balance. In retrospect, I think he was acutely aware that medical bioethics was in the midst of a sea change, and he had been cast ashore. While the science of medicine made incredible strides in the twentieth century, most people, including Deutsch, resisted the idea that the art of medicine, its ethical stance, and especially the relationship between physicians and their patients had also drastically changed. Deutsch was prepared to argue in his talk that the tradition expressed by the Hippocratic Oath, which states, "I will neither give a deadly drug to anybody who asked for it, nor will I make a suggestion to this effect," should remain static and inviolate.[9] If asked, he would have likely said, "The oath was good for twenty-five hundred years, and I see no reason at the present time to change it."

Deutsch and his wife, Helene, had fled war-torn, rabidly anti-Semitic Austria and immigrated to Massachusetts.[10] Helene was also a physician, as well as a highly praised acolyte of Freud, and she is acknowledged to be the first psychoanalyst to concern herself with the psychology of women. (Incidentally, this has proven to be a mixed blessing—as a subsequent generation of feminists has heaped scorn on Helene's obliviousness to the shortcomings of Freudian theory in her writings.) The couple applied psychoanalysis in novel ways and explored new techniques for conducting psychotherapy. They were highly respected, senior training analysts, and to their students and patients they represented a direct link in an unbroken chain to Freud. Some in the audience were aware that Deutsch had at one point been the great man's physician, but details of their treatment relationship were largely unknown.

At the start of Deutsch's presentation, the room was respectfully silent. He stood erect at the podium and asked his audience to consider the following question: "How much and when shall a patient be told about his condition, about the nature of his illness and the threat to his life he has to face?"[11]

Following a brief introduction, he described what happened the day he examined Freud's mouth, "At the very first glance," Deutsch said, "I had no doubt that it was an advanced cancer. To gain time I took a second look and decided to call it a bad case of leukoplakia, due to excessive smoking."

But it wasn't leukoplakia, the pre-cancerous condition that anyone would have preferred to have as a diagnosis. Deutsch knew instantly that it was a more dire malignancy, an epithelioma. Thirty-three years later, he tried to convince the assembled why he prevaricated. At no point during his talk did he admit that the lie effectively destroyed his doctor-patient relationship with Sigmund Freud. But nothing he told his Boston audience could change that fact.

At the American Psychosomatic Society meeting, Dr. Felix Deutsch tried to explain how physicians of his era feared doing more harm than good by using the dreaded word, *cancer*, and that concealment of "bad" diagnoses was commonplace.[12] Doctors routinely behaved in a paternalistic manner toward patients, and the notion of a professional behaving like a loving father was considered laudatory. Especially in Austria and throughout Europe, patient autonomy and shared decision-making were not valued. Instead, experienced, senior physicians made unilateral decisions as to how much to disclose and what course of treatment they would recommend.

Deutsch correctly identified the type of cancer, but he incorrectly sized up the man with the cancer. He was oblivious to Freud's powerful and demanding need to confront truth—no matter what the consequences. Instead, he was influenced by a number of different things, including having recently witnessed Freud's intense grief following the unexpected death of a beloved six-year-old grandson from tuberculosis.

Deutsch's concern as to how his patient would handle the unvarnished truth about the cancer was further exacerbated by Freud's admiration for the philosopher-physicist, Joseph Popper-Lynkeus. Deutsch read to his audience a few sentences from a Lynkeus book, *The Duty to Live and the Right to Die*, that he found highly questionable.[13] Lynkeus had written: "The knowledge of always being free to determine when or whether to give up one's life inspires me with the feeling of a new power and gives me a composure comparable to the consciousness of the soldier on the battlefield."

Deutsch worried that if he revealed the correct diagnosis then Freud might request assistance in dying. The biographer Peter Gay has written that Freud explicitly inquired about Deutsch's willingness to help him, if he should be condemned to prolonged suffering, to "disappear from this world with decency."[14] Deutsch denied that Freud was actively contemplating suicide, but understood he "wished only that I should spare him the suffering of a 'hopeless sickness' which cancer meant to him at that time. He apparently wanted to have the right of euthanasia. I at least understood it that way."[15]

In the Boston presentation, Deutsch doubled down by also suggesting that his patient wasn't really interested in learning the true diagnosis because he wanted to continue smoking his precious cigars. Freud had inherited a passion for cigars from his father, and he typically smoked twenty per day.[16] According to Deutsch, Freud repeatedly declaimed, "Smoking has rendered me such invaluable service during my life, that I can only be thankful. Without it I could not have worked as hard or as long as I did."[17] Although this was a rationalization, Deutsch's worry about getting into a losing battle with his patient over smoking cessation may not have been completely absurd. When, following a massive heart attack, Lyndon Johnson was advised by his doctor to henceforth refrain from smoking, the president remarked, "I'd rather have my pecker cut off."[18]

It was not until the 1960s and 1970s that Dr. Elizabeth Kübler-Ross would movingly write about the harm perpetrated on patients with cancer by medical staff unprepared to honestly address the severity of their disease.[19] Her insight was that patients often already know the extent of their condition and whether they are dying. Only by giving them a chance to speak about these matters can the greater harm—that of forcing them to deny reality and behave as if all is well—be avoided. The harm extends to their families, who enter into an awkward social contract to avoid the hard truth and are thereby stymied from expressing genuine feelings or properly taking leave.

As to Hippocrates, his oath has been modified numerous times. In 1964, it underwent one of the most significant revisions at the hands of Dr. Louis Lasagna.[20] That version deleted the prohibitions against euthanasia, abortion, refusing payment for services, and conducting surgical procedures, while also removing mention of slaves and the preamble's reference to Apollo, Asclepius, Hygieia, Panaceia, and all the other gods and goddesses. Lasagna's words have gained widespread acceptance and inspire graduating physicians to offer more compassion, nuance and humility in treating patients. His oath states: "Most especially must I tread with care in matters of life and death. If it is given me to save a life, all thanks. But it may also be within my power to take a life; this awesome responsibility must be faced with great humbleness and awareness of my own frailty. Above all, I must not play at God."[21]

In 2017, an updated version of the oath by the World Medical Association (they call it a "pledge" rather than an "oath") now emphasizes the responsibility of graduating physicians to "respect the autonomy and dignity of my patient."[22] It is apparent to me that the original Hippocratic Oath should be put aside as a weapon in the debates about assisted dying and abortion. It should be viewed solely as a lesson that ethics and morality, like gods and societies, change over time.

I don't fault Deutsch for being unable to see into the future. However, despite his words, the man knew full well that he had blundered with his most famous patient. However, he had no intention of acknowledging this to his audience.

To compound matters, Deutsch made another grievous error. Not only did he lie, but he also involved six of Freud's closest intimates in a conspiracy of silence. Ironically, this small group of analysts included Ernest Jones, who later wrote the official biography—the book that would prompt Deutsch to deliver his awkward speech. The men assembled at Freud's home to confer about psychoanalytic matters, and Deutsch confided to them the truth about the cancer. He then sought their counsel as to whether their mentor should be permitted to leave for a trip to Rome. In a letter, Jones wrote, "The chief news is that F. has a real cancer, slowly growing & may last years. He doesn't know . . . a most deadly secret."

Anton (Tony) Kris is presently a clinical professor of psychiatry at Harvard Medical School and one of the most highly respected training analysts in Cambridge. He is the son of Marianne and Ernst Kris, who were members of Freud's inner circle, and Tony knew the professor as a child. He also knew Deutsch as a playful older man, who was "the closest I had to a grandfather."

Tony has spent a lifetime devoted to studying and practicing psychoanalysis. He is considerate and reserved but, during our interview, his most spontaneous comment occurred while describing the above incident when he said, "What I know about

Freud is that he would have been pissed! He also would have been cordial and polite . . . but, I imagine Freud would have been truly pissed-off!"

Tony described to me how Jones eventually confessed to Freud the group's decision to refrain from revealing the diagnosis. Upon receiving this information, Freud literally shouted, "*Mit welchem Recht?*" (With what right did you do that? What was your authority?") Lying was anathema to Freud, and he could not bear that he had been patronized and the truth concealed.

At the Boston conference, Deutsch neglected to mention to the audience that upon discovering his true diagnosis, Freud immediately terminated their treatment relationship. Freud was so wounded by the experience that he was reluctant to seek medical care and did not have another doctor for the next five years. However, his friends and family recognized this was unwise, and through a concerted effort, they finally persuade the proud man to look for a new personal physician.

If nothing else, the story underscores the importance of providing dying patients with as much truthful information as possible to allow them to make informed choices.[23] But that doesn't mean the paths they choose will be readily acceptable to physicians or to their loved ones.

YOU DON'T
WANT CUSTER

I n the spring of 2002 when the ground had thawed, the Nimitz family convened in Cape Cod. It was a place filled with memories of summer barbecues and sailing expeditions and an appropriate homestead for a family of naval heroes. They stood by a small hole dug in sandy soil as the briny breeze blew on their faces. The ashes of Chester Jr. and Joan Nimitz were interred together. In a brief ceremony, the younger children placed small keepsakes, such as Lego blocks, into the grave. The adults spoke lovingly and respectfully of their forebears.

The *New York Times* wrote pieces about the deaths of Rear Admiral Chester W. Nimitz Jr. and his wife, Joan, that were admiring of their lives but strove for balance and offered the negative reactions of experts on aging.[1] They opined that the couple was highly unusual, as combinations of disease, depression, social isolation, and poverty lead to most suicides among the elderly. The authorities suggested that, with proper help, such deaths could be avoided.

A more contemporary version of this position has been expressed by some geriatricians and geriatric psychiatrists, who argue that "acceptance of the idea of rational suicide in older adults is in itself ageist. It implicitly endorses a view that loss is associated with aging resulting in a life that is not worth living."[2]

I am a great fan of the late surgeon and bestselling author, Dr. Sherwin B. Nuland. But Nuland sounded overly glib to me when he told a reporter, "In something like five out of six cases, if a physician is able to sit down and ask people why they really want to die, they can solve their problems with modern medicine or psychological help."[3]

Beginning around the time that Admiral and Mrs. Nimitz died, suicide rates have been climbing; between 1999 and 2016, they rose 28 percent.[4] According to the Centers for Disease Control and Prevention, more than eight thousand older adults committed suicide in 2016 and men over sixty-five are the group most likely to take their own lives. Three-quarters of the deaths among the elderly involve the use of firearms.

The fieriest critique of the Nimitzes came from Patrick J. Buchanan, the conservative political commentator and author, who wrote about the couple's lack of belief in religion or an afterlife.[5] Although in his commentary he acknowledged that one of Chester Jr.'s sisters was a Catholic nun and she had nevertheless remained sympathetic to her brother's decision to end his life, Buchanan labeled the deaths a moral tragedy. He warned that many observers might emulate the behavior and mistakenly view it as the reasonable decision of a brave man. But Buchanan declared the deaths of the admiral and his wife to be a victory for the "infamous Hemlock Society." He likened their action to that of misguided modern-day Greek Stoics or ironically—given the Nimitz family's war service—Japanese kamikaze pilots. He condemned the couple's conduct as being nothing less than a refutation of Christianity's cardinal belief in the sanctity of life.

Buchanan predicted: "With Christianity fading away in the West . . . involuntary euthanasia will be commonplace in Europe, and Gen-Xers' battles to stay alive into old age will be treated with the same cold contempt as they treated the silent screams of the unborn. Millions will be put to sleep like aged and incontinent household pets."[6]

And with a final rhetorical flourish, he concluded: "Since the 1960s, the radical young have pleaded for a world free of the strictures of the old Christian morality. They are close to getting what they have demanded . . . and my sense is that they will not like what they get. We are heading into Blade [R]unner Country."[7]

Although today's disability rights activists shun Buchanan's moralistic arguments, they would still roundly condemn the decision of the Nimitzes by pointing out that thousands of Americans endure pain, blindness, and other conditions while maintaining satisfying lives. They challenge the rationality of committing suicide simply because one has toileting accidents, requires adult diapers, or must rely on others for help with the basic activities of daily life. The activists claim such attitudes reflect societal bigotry and a false belief that one is "better dead than disabled." They angrily question whether parsimony or fiscal prudence should ever be a reason to die, and express fears that a day may come when America chooses to save money at the expense of the lives of the disabled. According to their view, "legalized assisted suicide and euthanasia is a loaded gun aimed directly at people with long-term disabilities."[8] Lastly, they point out that when couples die together it is frequently a murder-suicide, as most often the husband actively assists the wife before taking his own life.

The United States is deeply conflicted about whether to allow the terminally ill to shorten their lives, and we are an especially long way from accepting death-accelerating requests or decisions by the elderly, the frail, those troubled with chronic diseases, and the demented—basically, anyone who is not imminently dying.

There is a powerful and laudable American suicide prevention lobby devoted to saving the lives of people with psychiatric disorders and individuals who become transiently overwhelmed by life events. Many suicide prevention advocates understandably want to keep things simple and are not prepared to complicate the message; they would like to consistently affirm that under no circumstances should people be allowed to commit suicide. According to this position, a wish to hasten death is akin to suicide, which equates with mental illness. But it is difficult to build a case that people like the Nimitzes were psychiatrically ill or depressed when they ended their lives.

This represents a wake-up call for a psychiatrist like me who has spent nearly four decades trying to deter people from killing themselves. My mentors, Drs. Avery Weisman and Thomas Hackett, wisely recognized that although the medical profession is dedicated to survival and health, it cannot indefinitely postpone dying. Half a century ago they observed that "people's attitudes toward death correspond to their attitudes toward life; how each person dies is determined by how he has lived."[9] They were revolutionary in opining that it can be appropriate for the suffering and imminently dying to want to foreshorten life. In their writings, they took the progressive position that death is often a solution rather than a catastrophe, and they defined a good death as being "the type of death one would choose if there were a choice."[10] I imagine—but will never know—that they would have accepted how the Nimitzes died. I think Avery, a respected psychoanalyst and researcher, would have understood immediately, and despite his Catholic background, Tom, the chairman of psychiatry at Massachusetts General Hospital, might have shouted, "Huzzah!"

During the first half of my career, it would have been difficult for me to immediately grasp the decisiveness and courage required by the Nimitzes. But America has changed, the nation's mores are evolving, and I am older. Death no longer means failure, and I can recognize that improving the quality of dying is an admirable goal. Likewise, arriving at decisions shaped mainly by respect for patient preferences is a welcome development in the field of medicine. It is satisfying for me to know that there is a younger generation of Americans—both laymen and physicians—who instinctively feel these things to be true and proper.

In the ensuing years following the deaths of her parents, Betsy Nimitz Van Dorn joined the board of Compassion & Choices, the leading nonprofit in the country dedicated to improving care and expanding options at the end of life. I interviewed Betsy when a ballot campaign was underway in Massachusetts to legalize assisted dying. At the time, Compassion & Choices had asked Betsy to contribute to a newspaper piece in support of the referendum based on the circumstances of her parents' deaths.[11] In response, she remarked forthrightly: "You know they committed suicide? This wasn't aid in dying. Let's not muddy the waters here!"

After further consideration, though, she decided—and I agree—that her parents exemplify the personalities and attitudes of people who are most likely to appreciate such laws.

Betsy fully comprehends that none of the laws being considered in legislatures around the country would have directly helped her parents, as neither had a terminal disease. She understands, too, that a civil rights movement, such as aid in dying, takes incremental and politically expedient steps. She anticipates that the infirmities and chronic suffering of advanced age might by themselves qualify people to request this option in the future (as is presently true in Belgium, Switzerland, and the Netherlands). She looks forward to the day "when kids and their parents will regularly sit around the dining room table and talk about end-of-life issues the way you talk about college planning. Because, after all," as she puts it, "it is just another kind of planning."

She and the Nimitz family continue to admire the decision of the admiral and his wife. "I think it was very unselfish of my parents to do what they did," Betsy told me. "A great thing about my parents was their huge capacity to enjoy life. So, if you enjoyed life that much and you are eighty-nine and eighty-six it seems to me that it is logical to say, 'I have had my brimming cup and I am ready to go.'"

I often think about the following lines that Atul Gawande wrote in his bestselling book, *Being Mortal*:

> The simple view is that medicine exists to fight death and disease, and that is, of course, its most basic task. Death is the enemy. But the enemy has superior forces. Eventually, it wins. And, in a war that you cannot win, you don't want a general who fights to the point of total annihilation. You don't want Custer. You want Robert E. Lee, someone who knew how to fight for territory when he could and how to surrender when he couldn't, someone who understood that the damage is greatest if all you do is fight to the bitter end.[12]

HOW LIFE
TURNED OUT

At Cold Spring Harbor Laboratory, the presentation that moved me the most was the one offered by Martin Raff. He began with his professional biography—the man is a world-renowned neurobiologist and regular participant in the Laboratory's programs—and quickly turned to the circumstances of his family's story.

"I organized this think tank," he explained, "because of what happened to my parents. That experience made a tremendous impact on my own life."

As a psychiatrist, I was ashamed to hear Martin's tale of his father's psychiatric hospitalization and was deeply touched by the account. During a break, I approached him about meeting afterward to fill in the details. Beginning with his next trip from London to New York City for a scientific board meeting, I initiated a series of interviews that would take place over several years with him; his brother, Anton; and eventually with more than two hundred people from around the country involved with aid in dying. I was interested in learning about the circumstances that prompt individuals to seek death, the available methods, and the experiences of bereaved families. I also wanted to delve into why people became activists in this self-determination movement. In my previous book, I had paid insufficient attention to the members of the disability community who oppose this option. This time, I wanted to discover more about their perspective as well.

The Raff brothers are now in their seventies, and they—and others whom I interviewed—wanted me to use their real names. While sensitive to the highly unlikely possibility of future legal consequences, Martin and Anton remain proud of their roles.

"My parents had been planning it for decades—well before my mother showed signs of the Alzheimer's—and discussed it frequently with my brother and me," Martin said. "They did not use the word suicide, which to them connoted depression, and they were not at all depressed or tired of life."

"Why," I asked, "did your parents decide to die?"

Martin paused for only a second before responding: "They were financially secure. They were loved and respected by family and friends. They were devoted to each other and enjoyed each other's company. Paradoxically, their love and dependence on each other were major factors in the decision: neither wanted to live without the other. Dad believed that time was running out, as Mom would soon require more care than he could provide. His greatest fear was that he would die or become disabled before they could act on the 'exit plan.' Having seen too many of their friends end their days in a pitiful state in nursing homes with debilitating dementias, they did not want to lose control over their lives."

According to Martin, David couldn't conceive of continuing life without his beloved Reba. He had no interest in picking himself up afterward and finding new pursuits.

"The exit plan they came up with," said Martin, "was based on advice from brochures provided by the Hemlock Society of America." The Raffs had been interested in this organization for at least ten years, and the local branch, the Suncoast Hemlock Society, boasted of having 450 members.

Martin's brother, Anton, elaborated, "Dad originally accumulated the required drugs and brought them from Montreal to Sarasota. Nearly twenty years ensued, and he realized the medications had expired and newer ones would be preferable."

Martin resumed: "Mom was going to take as many barbiturate sleeping pills as she could, preceded by an anti-vomiting pill. Dad would then give her an injection of a mixture of sedatives and morphine, which would kill her within an hour or so. He did not want her to die before he was unconscious. He would next take an anti-vomiting pill, followed by many sleeping pills; he would quickly inject himself with the same mixture of sedatives and morphine. He intended to place plastic bags [as recommended by the Hemlock Society] over both their heads to ensure the outcome—the increasing carbon dioxide in the bag would kill them if the drugs failed."

Martin flew to Sarasota a week before the exit plan was to be put into effect. He and Anton preemptively consulted with a lawyer to discuss legalities and arrive at a suitably safe strategy. The attorney warned them it was crucial the arrangements not fail, as their father would be jailed for murder if their mother died and he survived. The lawyer also advised the sons to avoid being present when their parents carried out the plan. He suggested that Martin ought to be home in the United Kingdom.

Despite careful forethought and preparations, things took an unexpected turn. David and Reba decided to approach their local physicians and obtain a fresh supply of medications. The couple had a mutually agreeable meeting with their general practitioner, who wrote several prescriptions. However, David remained concerned that they had an insufficient quantity, and the elderly couple paid a visit to Dr. Irving Beychok, a general surgeon who had operated on Reba several years earlier. The Raffs naively assumed that he would share their philosophical beliefs. When David told Dr. Beychok of the plan, however, the surgeon became visibly upset and tried to dissuade the couple.

When I interviewed Dr. Beychok, he was long retired and in his eighties. He recalled David as having been a remarkably nice man, a fellow physician, and someone who suffered with chronic pain that was making it increasingly difficult for him to manage his wife's needs. He told me that the Raffs had requested a prescription for narcotics and sought his support for their suicide pact. He made it clear to them that he believed the action they were contemplating was illegal and immoral. He considered it to be an entirely unacceptable thing "for Jewish people."

Upon hearing from their parents about the encounter, Martin and Anton anticipated trouble. They made an appointment to see Dr. Beychok in the afternoon. At the meeting, Martin couldn't assuage the surgeon's concerns at having been put in what he felt to be a compromised position. Beychok was visibly angry when he said, "Your parents are depressed."

Martin thought, *This guy is a surgeon. How skillful could he be at diagnosing depression*? But he limited his rejoinder to, "I know them reasonably well and they are not depressed."

Anton also recalls Beychok as having been unsympathetic. "I said to him, 'Don't you see there is a certain romance to it? They love each other and don't want to survive each other.'"

But his reply was "Nonsense. It is absurd to think that way."

The brothers left the office convinced that Beychok was also apprehensive that he could get entangled in legal ramifications.

The following morning, the surgeon notified the police—but as a courtesy, he telephoned David and informed him what he had done. David promptly called his sons. Martin and Anton hurriedly conferred with one another. They met at their parent's condominium, removed the cache of pills that was concealed in the freezer, found a toy beach shovel, and then buried Reba and David's bag of medications in a nearby public beach.

Shortly afterward the police arrived and took their father to the psychiatric hospital.

Anton and Martin pulled into the parking lot of the Palms of Sarasota prepared to do battle on David's behalf.

"We were buzzed on to the locked unit to speak with the psychiatrist," said Martin. "It turns out that he had seen Dad for about ten minutes in total. He told us that Dad was clearly depressed and required antidepressants, which could take a month to have an effect. 'And if that doesn't work,' the psychiatrist said, 'then we will have to think about electroshock.'"

Martin continued, "The psychiatrist's evidence for depression was that Dad's eyes were watery. We pointed out this is a common eye condition in old people and that Dad had it for years. It was obvious to us Dad wasn't depressed. Despite the grim environment on the psychiatric ward, he remained in surprisingly good spirits, and we pointed out where he was sitting in the dayroom, cheerfully chatting with other patients."

Reba's situation was entirely different. In a matter of hours without her husband, Martin and Anton witnessed her mental state drastically decline. She became exceedingly confused and kept repeating, "How could Dr. Beychok do this to us?"

According to Martin, "My mother was well into the early stages of Alzheimer's. When you watch a personality fall apart, it is exceedingly difficult. They are not the same person anymore. My dad used to say my visits energized her but when I would leave she was no longer the same individual. I didn't understand this until he was yanked from his apartment and committed to the hospital. Suddenly she didn't recognize Anton or me. We had never seen her like that before. She was frantic."

In the apartment with her sons, Reba desperately wanted to know, 'Where is David? Why isn't he here?'"

Martin worried incessantly that if he fell asleep, she might let herself out of the apartment and wander the streets. Throughout the night, he was reduced to taking catnaps. David had told his sons that she was cognitively slipping, but for the first time they saw the progression of the dementia. While Martin and Anton had argued with their father that he should postpone ending their lives because it was too soon and life was still enjoyable, they now better understood David's position. When he had warned them that without his constant presence their mother would quickly regress, they hadn't appreciated the truth of his words.

David had told his sons, "It won't be long before I'm not able to look after her in this apartment. She leaves the kettle on. She puts her dress on backwards. It's serious. If I had a heart attack or stroke we wouldn't be able to do what we want to do. Your mother would be left alone. If anything happened to me, she would be brought to one of those nursing homes and tied to a chair."

Several weeks before David was committed to the psychiatric unit, Martin had a frank conversation with Reba about their plans. "Do you know what you're doing?" he asked her. "Do you appreciate what you're doing?"

"Of course, I know what I'm doing," she replied. "We have been talking about this for years."

"Do you have any fears?"

"I don't have any fears. Why would I have any fears?"

Martin pushed further, "Do you have any reservations? Are you going to miss anybody?"

She replied, "Naturally, I am going to miss my husband and I am going to miss your brother and you."

At the time he thought, *How demented could she be?*

However, the two sons now understood that they must immediately get David out of the hospital or their mother would need to be institutionalized. Anton and Martin accepted at last that their parents had decided unambiguously they did not want to live without each other, and following the frustrating meeting with the psychiatrist, they drove to the Sarasota library and photocopied the Florida State laws dealing with psychiatric commitment. They underlined the relevant material, took notes, and figured out the options. The brothers discovered that the police and hospital doctor had denied their dad several of his legal rights: they did not give him an opportunity to seek the opinion of a psychiatrist of his own choice before being committed; they did not tell him that he could apply for habeas corpus; and they did not give him a comprehensive psychiatric assessment within twenty-four hours of admission.

Armed with this knowledge, they revisited the hospital that evening. The psychiatrist was unavailable, and they asked to see David's medical record, which as next of kin and having been assigned a power of attorney was their legal right. The nurses resisted, but following several harried private meetings among the staff, Martin was permitted to speak to the psychiatrist on the phone.

The psychiatrist barely had a chance to say hello before Martin began shouting: "We are all physicians, and I want to see the records! If we don't have them in an hour all hell is going to break loose. Here are all the things that you have not done and what should have been done. If my dad is not out of here by tomorrow then we will close down this hospital."

David woke up the next morning in the psychiatric unit at the Palms of Sarasota Hospital, fearful that having fallen down the rabbit hole, he had been abandoned. But once again, he put a smile on his face and cooperated fully with the ward routines. Later that day, David received the welcome news that he would be permitted to sign himself out. He had been hospitalized for only forty-eight hours, but it seemed like weeks to his distraught family and to him. Anton and Martin promptly unearthed the hidden cache of medications and returned it to their parents.

With David's arrival back home, Reba immediately regained her old form. The elderly couple conferred with each other and told their sons that they had decided to postpone the exit plan for two months. There was agreement that this amount of time would allow everything to calm down.

The Raffs resumed their usual routines and settled back into their quiet lives. David continued to clean, shop, and do all the driving. They mostly ate out at local restaurants. The handsome man with the cleft in his chin continued to joyfully greet his neighbors, kibitz, and crack jokes.

When Martin returned to Sarasota for a final visit, they were in high spirits. From the family discussions, it was clear that neither David nor Reba feared death or believed in the existence of heaven or hell. The couple had no doubts that they were doing the correct thing and the time had arrived.

Martin explained, "It could not have been a better last visit. I was grateful to them for being so brave, open, and cheerful, but I was already missing them greatly as we embraced. They had always been there, always unconditionally supportive, but now they would be gone. There would no longer be an intervening generation separating me from my own death, which suddenly seemed more imminent. Even though I was prepared for their exit plan and had anticipated it for years, it still came as a shock that they were going to be dead and that's it. You lose both parents in one shot, and then there is nothing between you and your death."

Following the legal advice, Martin was outside of the country on the day his parents died. Anton could not sleep that night and tried to calm his nerves by listening to music with his headphones. The next day, he drove over to the condominium and let himself in with his key.

"I arrived that morning knowing what to expect," said Anton. "My parents were dead. I called emergency medical services.

They came. The only thing that I did before they arrived was I took the bag off my mother's head. She was in bed. My father, I think, had injected himself in the kitchen. It was strange how he practiced the same kind of immaculate medicine as always. He wiped his skin with an alcohol swab—for which there obviously was no need—before injecting himself. I think he had trouble getting back to bed. He made a mistake by injecting himself in the kitchen because he was half on and half off the bed when he passed out. He had also vomited slightly."

The police arrived and questioned Anton. They took samples from all parts of the bedroom. They looked at the note on the kitchen table. Initially labeled as a murder-suicide, the causes of death were later amended because Anton protested there was evidence David died before Reba. In the end, it was called a joint suicide.

"For several months," he said, "the police harassed my wife and me. When I was at work they would call her twice a day. They called repeatedly at my medical clinic and at home. They asked me to take a lie detector test, and my attorney told me to refuse."

"Why were they harassing us? I think the police hoped I would confess to providing my parents with the drugs. But the reality was they intentionally obtained them from other sources. The lawyer reassured me the police needed to investigate and everything would blow over because there is too much public opposition against this kind of intrusiveness."

Nevertheless, the recurring telephone calls troubled Anton's wife and the couple quarreled. "She questioned why I agreed to be the one to *discover* the bodies when it should have been anticipated that I would then become an *obvious* suspect."

Anton began to feel concerned he was being monitored by law enforcement. "I worried," he said, "whether the phone was tapped and my conversations with Martin were being recorded."

David and Reba had never wanted a funeral or service of remembrance, and they made arrangements for cremation. Anton and his wife scattered their ashes in a state park that is a bird sanctuary and an alligator habitat. It is a beautiful wild place with verdant foliage, a meandering river, and splendid shorebirds.

When Martin returned to Florida a couple of months later, the two brothers visited the park. They sat on a bench, listened to the lizards rustling about in the undergrowth, and talked about how much David and Reba loved nature. The elderly couple used to step out to the balcony of their condominium every evening and admire the sunset over the Gulf, as if it were the first one they had ever seen. Anton and Martin fondly recalled them walking along the beach in the mornings on the way to get coffee at a local café. They were always holding hands. Occasionally, they would stop and smile at each other, and it was apparent to any observer that this husband and wife were satisfied with how their lives had turned out.

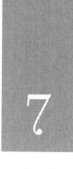

PUTTING THE "MENSCH" IN DEMENTIA

Beth Weinstein was sixty-one-years-old when she died in 2012. Her obituary concluded, "She will be remembered for her commitment, integrity and, finally, courage in the face of her disease. . . . Donations may be made in her name to the Alzheimer's Research and Prevention Foundation and/or the Alzheimer's Association."[1]

Six years after her death, I reconnected with Richard. That afternoon I had been listening to traditional Chinese instrumental music and the melancholy melody of "Chiang ho shui" formed a backdrop to our conversation. This piece is especially poignant because the composition depicts the grief of a young widow whose spouse suffered and died in a far-away place. According to the lyrics, she sits weeping alongside a river where the couple had originally bid each other goodbye. The erhu, a two-stringed violin-like instrument, plays a song for which there are no adequate words.

During our conversation, Richard filled in further details about the circumstances of Beth's death. The Alzheimer's unit at the assisted-living facility where she resided wisely had a policy of not rushing patients to the local hospital and not condoning the use of feeding tubes when they no longer were interested or able to swallow food. Beth had ceased eating and drinking, she was not transported to the community hospital, and she died at the facility. Family were present at her bedside, and others arrived from the West Coast on the following day.

Richard chuckled ruefully about the power of denial, stating, "It seems strange but I hadn't given any thought to funeral arrangements. We had to find someone quickly for a cremation, and after a discussion with her family the ashes were placed in a West Hartford cemetery."

When Beth died, Richard felt crushed by her absence from his life. Of course, given Beth's dementia, it had been a very long time since they had really been present for each other or had bid each other goodbye. Her death evoked and capped this earlier loss. As Richard talked to me about Beth, I couldn't help but think about a comment uttered at the funeral of columnist Thomas L. Friedman's mother: "She put the mensch in dementia."[2]

Beth was familiar with assisted dying primarily because of her family's earlier experience, but I am sure she also knew about the practice because of her involvement with the AIDS epidemic. For several decades, the disease she devoted her life to managing was a death sentence for the gay community and for the drug-abusing population. The predominantly young and articulate men who contracted the virus were doomed to suffer with hideous and disfiguring complications before dying. Within the AIDS community, considerable interest arose in death-hastening practices.

A *New York Times* article from 1993 describes a meeting held in a church in San Francisco, the epicenter of the AIDS epidemic, to talk about which drugs to use for suicide.[3] Derek Humphry was the chief participant, and he answered participants' questions, discussed how to avoid a botched attempt, and spoke about the potential legal consequences when involving loved ones. Derek told a journalist, "If people are revolted by what I'm saying and doing, then we must change the law."[4]

The seminar was advertised in Bay Area gay newspapers and attended by more than one hundred fifty people. Dr. Lonny Shavelson—who has just recently established an outpatient practice in the Bay Area of California to consult with people seeking assisted dying—explained that it was convened because AIDS sufferers "were taking the wrong medication at the wrong times and having bad outcomes. [These] included things like partial overdoses, where people would fall asleep for two days from an overdose of morphine that did not result in death, but resulted in brain damage. And they'd wake up two days later, sicker than they started and with even more suffering."[5]

Derek and other panelists warned against using cyanide, which would cause a violent death, or kitchen chemicals and random pills from the medicine cabinet that were more likely to result in the would-be suicide having his stomach pumped in the hospital. They discouraged participants from relying on automobile exhaust asphyxiation, which had become less effective following the institution of pollution controls and catalytic converters. They cautioned against using violent suicide methods, like hanging or self-inflicted gunshot wounds, which are always traumatizing to families and first responders.

The reporter wrote: "The most reliable method, short of a lethal injection administered by a doctor, Mr. Humphry said, is barbiturates, which require a prescription. Wash them down with alcohol after a light snack, and ingest them quickly to prevent falling asleep before the full dose is administered. Using a plastic bag as well, to cut off oxygen, will insure death."[6]

"This is a daily phenomenon in San Francisco, and people need to do their homework," said Steve Jamison, regional director of the Hemlock Society, who estimated that one of six AIDS deaths in San Francisco at that time was a suicide—although not necessarily classified as such by the coroner.

The seminar attendees were advised to "mix in circles that care about these things and you'll pick up information about people who are courageous, and leave nothing to chance. Do not skimp on the details. A well-planned self-deliverance almost always works."

A community organizer, Gerald Lenoir, later told me about his experiences as the executive director of the Black Coalition on AIDS in San Francisco during this era before retroviral treatments were developed. He said, "What happened in California and the AIDS community was a landmark series of events that changed a bunch of things. It was one of the greatest experiences of my life. People were dying every single day, but what I saw were people dying with dignity. Communities came together to take care of their loved ones, whether a partner, a friend, or a family member. On a personal level, my two brothers-in-law died of AIDS-related causes. My wife and her family and our friends helped them to die."

Gerald's eyes filled with tears as he said, "It was humbling."

"What happened to your family members?" I inquired.

"They were in such pain and in such dire straits," he responded, "that it made no sense to allow the suffering to go on. They decided they didn't want to live like that. One was hospitalized. The other was at home. In both instances a morphine drip allowed them to drift into death. Health care professionals let us to do that with a wink and a nod and without any opposition."

I asked him about "public suicides" and "living wakes," which I understood were taking place in San Francisco. Gerald explained, "That's absolutely true. There were multiple cases happening. We knew of occasions where people would say, 'Today's the day.' We would then all go and visit them and say our goodbyes. That was very, very common. There was no cure and people knew they were going to die. They planned way ahead of time. They informed their friends and loved ones that they wanted to celebrate life while they were still here. To me it is the most humane thing in the world when people choose to go out with such dignity and with such love. Yet it's still looked at [nowadays] as being criminal. That is insane."

"How was this accepted by the black churches?" I asked, knowing that African Americans are often skeptical of the concepts of hospice or advance care planning—let alone assisted dying/suicide—and their suspicions remain deep seated.[7] While almost half of today's white Medicare beneficiaries enroll in hospice before death, only a third of black patients do. Approximately 40 percent of whites aged seventy and over complete advance care planning, compared with only 16 percent of blacks.[8]

Varney has written that the racial divide is an understandable outgrowth of "toxic distrust of a health care system that once displayed 'No Negroes' signs at hospitals, performed involuntary sterilizations on black women and, in the infamous Tuskegee study, purposely left hundreds of black men untreated for syphilis."[9] Even in Boston, perhaps the Mecca of American medicine, segregation patterns are engrained; only 11 percent of residents admitted to Massachusetts General Hospital are black, while across town they account for half the population receiving care at Boston Medical Center.[10] When people have difficulty getting reliable access to the finest health care, then they are naturally going to become highly suspicious if a doctor broaches the possibility of ceasing life-prolonging therapies and transitioning to hospice and palliative care. This is compounded by the belief among many blacks that suffering is a test from God and can be redemptive.[11]

"Early on in the disease," Gerald said, "AIDS was always disproportionately African American. The news media never covered it. We were very conscious of that. When I came to direct the coalition in 1989, the disproportionality was already a known fact among black gay men. The white gay men viewed it as *their* disease. This led to battles around resources and treatment. White gay men felt like we were intruding on their turf. It was ugly. On the African American side, there was real disdain for the injection drug users and gay people."

American medicine first became aware of the AIDS epidemic in 1981 with publication of a CDC Morbidity and Mortality Weekly Report describing five cases of pneumocystis pneumonia found among previously healthy, white, homosexual men from Los Angeles.[12] Two additional documented cases of the unusual pneumonia that we now associate with AIDS were not mentioned because they came to the attention of the first author after the report was finalized. Interestingly, both were black. According to the report's author, if they had been included in the publication, "in retrospect, I think it might've made a difference among gay black men."

As a community organizer, Gerald found himself floundering to create ways to counter these biases. The racism in the white gay community and the homophobia and prejudice against drug abuse in the black community were taking place all the while people were helplessly dying every day. "The black churches were very hard to crack," he said.

Front-page stories began to appear about needle exchange (and Beth was, indeed, a pioneer in espousing the practice). According to Gerald, "99 and ¾ percent of the black leaders thought it was genocide. They believed the social policy was encouraging drug use in our community."

After he and his group were excoriated by black leaders, they reacted by launching a public relations campaign on radio and television. The only black newspaper was owned by a physician, and he understood it to be a medical issue and allowed them to publish articles reviewing European research data.

Gerald and his fellow activists approached the churches. They sought to identify church-going mothers whose sons had HIV or who had died of HIV-related complications. He explained:

> The church has always been the center of the African American community on a whole range of issues; it is our pillar. The church was rabidly against us because the ministers believed we were supporting homosexuality and supporting drug use, but we would arrange basement meetings within the churches and give those mothers opportunities to talk. It was a subversive strategy to not go to the preachers directly but to instead go to the congregations. We knew that the congregations would be empathetic and sympathetic to their own members, even if the church leaders remained opposed.

Over a three-year period, the public relations campaign and the church strategy "began to change hearts and minds." And as far as needle exchange, many of the church leaders came to understand that this was a public health intervention and not a means to increase drug use. Some of the more progressive churches also accepted the gay issue.

Gerald concluded:

> But suicide was never talked about publicly. It was a personal decision made in conjunction with partners or friends, and it was very private and holy. It was completely outside of the bounds of the traditional church. Except for those churches that happened to be gay churches—churches that were specifically organized by gay and transgender people—it was not spoken about or accepted.

It must have been traumatic when the Weinstein family viewed *Still Alice*, a 2014 film based on the novel by Lisa Genova.[13] The movie starred Julianne Moore as a linguist diagnosed with an early onset dementia, and it depicted how the disease took control of Alice's life. Any wish on her part to foreshorten life became impossible.

There is an especially heartbreaking scene where Alice's husband asks if she is ready to "leave." It made me think of Richard's efforts to ascertain whether Beth thought the time had come for assisted dying. In the movie, Alice is happily eating a treat at a local frozen yogurt store. She misunderstands the import of the question, demurs, and continues contentedly spooning down the desert.

In another scene, Alice discovers a video she had previously made for herself. Anticipating that the dementia would continue to progress, she had given simple instructions in the video how to take out a hidden bottle of sleeping pills from the drawer and to overdose. But by the time she watches it, Alice has become too cognitively impaired to carry out the directives. We watch as she gets distracted and the tablets spill all over the floor.

In 2018, I spoke with Beth's mother, who is now ninety years old, and she calmly concluded, "The film verified everything I felt."

Derek Humphry, the founder of the Hemlock Society, has carefully argued that aid in dying should be available to people with Alzheimer's disease. However, he related an anecdote to me about one of his best friends, an elderly woman who was living in San Francisco and declining from dementia. Although Derek has only rarely been present when people employed the techniques described in his books, he promised to promptly come if called. A substantial amount of time ensued before the summons. When it finally came, he quickly traveled to her home. However, when the door opened, she stood at the threshold looking perplexed and inquired, "Who are you?"

"Needless to say," Derek explained, "I did *not* help her and left the house shortly afterwards."

Gillian Bennett, an eighty-five-year-old Canadian, had her family post a four-page letter to be made public after her death on a website called Deadatnoon.com.[14] In the letter, Bennett offered an impassioned argument as to why medical aid in dying options should be available for the terminally ill, elderly, and those who, like herself, resolutely reject the indignities of dementia.

In 2014, Bennett was still in the early stages of the disease when she chose to end life with a drink of good whiskey, a hefty dose of Nembutal, and a last look at her favorite vista on Bowen Island, Vancouver.[15] Her husband, Jonathan, was present to witness the death, and he contacted the attending physician immediately afterward. Jonathan carefully explained the circumstances to the coroner and law enforcement authorities. There were no legal complications.

Gillian and Jonathan had been married for sixty years. She was a psychotherapist and he is a retired philosophy professor. Jonathan told a reporter, "I held her hand. I agreed with her choice."[16]

"She wouldn't let me help her, and I didn't wish to," he explained. "I don't know where she got the Nembutal or the instructions; she didn't tell me. . . . She was absolutely not frightened. Not even slightly. She was as calm and peaceful as you could imagine."

Bennett's daughter, Sara, fifty-six, and son, Guy, fifty-five, were invited to visit earlier in the weekend to say their goodbyes. Both understood and were supportive of her wishes.

With permission of the family, I have liberally excerpted Bennett's missive. Throughout the online letter, her ironic sense of humor and keen intellect are in evidence:

I will take my life today around noon. It is time. Dementia is taking its toll and I have nearly lost myself. I have nearly lost me.

There comes a time . . . when one is no longer competent to guide one's own affairs. I want out before the day when I can no longer assess my situation, or take action to bring my life to an end.

I have known that I have dementia, a progressive loss of memory and judgment, for three years. It is a stealthy, stubborn and oh-so reliable disease. I might have preferred an exotic ailment whose name came trippingly off the tongue, but no, what I have is entirely typical. I find it a boring disease, and despite the sweetness and politeness of my family I am bright enough to be aware of how boring they find it, too. It is so rough on my husband, Jonathan. I don't think my lovely cat has noticed, but I'm not sure.

Dementia gives no quarter and admits no bargaining. Research tells us that it's a "silent disease," one that can lurk for years or even decades before its symptoms become obvious. Ever so gradually at first, much faster now, I am turning into a vegetable. I find it hard to keep in my mind that my granddaughter is coming in three day's time and not today. "Where do we keep the X?" (coffee / milkshake-maker / backspace on my keyboard / the book I was just reading) happens all the time. I have constantly to monitor what I say in an attempt not to make some gross error of judgment.

Every day I lose bits of myself, and it's obvious that I am heading towards the state that all dementia patients eventually get to: not knowing who I am and requiring full-time care. I know as I write these words that within six months or nine months or twelve months, I, Gillian, will no longer be here. What is to be done with my carcass? It will be physically alive but there will be no one inside.

I can live or vegetate for perhaps ten years in hospital at Canada's expense, costing anywhere from $50,000 to $75,000 per year. That is only the beginning of the damage. Nurses, who thought they were embarked on a career that had great meaning, find themselves perpetually changing my diapers and reporting on the physical changes of an empty husk. It is ludicrous, wasteful and unfair. . . .

Three outsize institutions: the medical profession, the Law, and the Church will challenge and fight any transformative change. Yet we all hear of changes in each of these professions that suggest a broader approach, guided and informed by empathy. My hope is that all of these institutions will continue to transform themselves, and that the medical profession will mandate, through sensitive and appropriate protocols, the administration of a lethal dose to end the suffering of a terminally ill patient, in accordance with her Living Will. . .

Just in case anyone is tempted to think I must be brave to off myself, you should know that I am a big sookie. I am sorely fearful of being alone in the dark. I am scared something will get me. I do not want to die alone. If my cat were failing in the way that I am, I would mix some sleeping medication in with top-quality ground beef, and when she fell asleep, carry her lovingly to the garden and do the rest. Who wants to die surrounded by strangers, no matter how excellent their care and competence?

Gillian's family were very aware that during the last six months her memory impairment had worsened, and she ceased being able to play her beloved game of Scrabble. The family understood that the window was closing. As long as she talked about euthanasia, the window was open and her family were ready to support her wishes—while carefully observing the elements of criminal law. If Gillian ceased discussing euthanasia then that option was over.

Four years have transpired since the death, and Sara has had ample opportunity to consider the experience. She has dissected her mother's reasoning and cites several factors that contributed to the decision, beginning with the observation that Gillian was neither a whiner nor a complainer and abhorred physical suffering. Gillian understood that most discomfort comes in the last part of life, so that if you want to avoid it then you need to control your death. Gillian was also determined to not inflict upon her family the indignities that inevitably lay ahead. In addition, she had well-established political and ethical views. As mentioned in her letter, she believed it was morally repugnant for elderly people to consume large portions of the public funds. She weighed this against educating every single child in the country and never wavered in her resolve that protracted dying was wrong. Sara told me,

> My sons were in eleventh and twelfth grades in 2014. They knew the plan, but they didn't know the timing. None of us knew the timing, but we knew that it was going to have to be reasonably soon. When she was closing in on her day and I needed to tell my sons that it was going to happen pretty soon, I sat down in my living room and we had a talk about it. I said "You know how Gram has always said that she would make her own decision about when she died, and now she is getting close to possibly losing the capacity to make that decision. She will take her life sooner rather than later."
>
> My youngest son began to cry and his brother said, "I get it, Mom. We have to help her. *We have to help so that she sticks her landing.*" He completely understood it is not that we want Gram to be dead. It is that we want her to have the victory of sticking her landing.

Much like the Raffs, Sara and her family consider themselves to have been fortunate. Like Martin and his mother, she had asked Gillian, "Are you scared?"

"Don't be silly, darling," was the reply. "There is nothing to be scared of." And Gillian continued, "What's there to be scared of? I'm just going to stop existing!"

Two bioethicist friends of mine, Professors Paul Mentzel and Bonnie Steinbock, are interested in the moral aspects of dementia. The philosophers contend that if people carefully compose advance directives, then they no longer need to be competent at the point loved ones implement their wishes for a medically assisted death.[17]

Sara Bennett agrees with this stance and argues that not only should it be legal to assist people with Alzheimer's, but the support should be allowed to occur even when they are in the more advanced stages of the disease. "If someone could have helped her," Sarah said shortly after her mother's death, "she wouldn't have had to die *yesterday*. She could have waited. If the law was different so that she could have had help, she would not have had to choose to end her life as soon as she did. Even though my mom died painlessly in exactly the way she chose, at the time she chose, knowing that she left the legacy she chose, it's still unbelievably painful."[18]

This position was also put forward by another Canadian, Ron Posno, who said, "I want my death to occur at the beginning of the severe stage of Alzheimer's, and not the end."[19] Posno explained that he wanted to die "when I am unable to recognize, and/or cognitively and/or adequately respond with appropriate emotion and thought to family members, care providers or friends . . .or when I am unable to eat, clean or dress myself without assistance." Having been diagnosed with an early dementia, Posno filled out an application for an assisted death, rewrote his will, reconfirmed his Do Not Resuscitate form, and amended his advance directive. He intentionally articulated his wishes in a series of conversations with his lawyer, health care proxies, family doctor, and a physician who provides medical assistance in dying.

However, the Alzheimer Society of Canada opposes the use of advanced directives for medical assistance in dying. CEO Pauline Tardif maintains that many of the people her organization serves have different concerns than Posno. They want to know: "How will you protect us? How will you defend our interests to make sure that we're not vulnerable to decision-makers?"[20]

Other defenders of the current Canadian law point out that people can be transformed by dementia, and the "new" individual may have a greater tolerance for incapacity and an entirely different definition of what constitutes a meaningful life. Those who rush in and accelerate dying are ignoring that changed reality and the moral ambiguity.

In 2001, The Netherlands was aware of these issues when it passed the Termination of Life Request and Assisted Suicide Act.[21] In 2015, a Code of Practice was instituted that better defines the circumstances and offers more detailed guidance.[22] The act makes it legally possible for patients in that country who are incapable of verbally expressing their will, including those with severe dementia, to receive assisted dying *if they have an "advance euthanasia directive."*[23]

Norman L. Cantor, distinguished professor of law emeritus at Rutgers, has argued that when we become demented the same individual then has two personas: an earlier competent self and a demented self; they share the body and have in common the same property, the same religion, and the same moral principles.[24] He contends that the self-determination prerogative has been earned by the competent person who nurtured and developed the body, character, and relationships.

While Cantor does not specifically address assisted dying, he covers the balance of the death-hastening practices with the following statement in his version of a model advance directive:

> My determination not to prolong my life at the described point of debilitation includes rejection of any and all life-sustaining means. This includes simplistic medical interventions such as antibiotics, blood transfusions, and antiarrythmics, as well as more complex interventions like CPR, mechanical ventilation, dialysis, and artificial nutrition and hydration. Indeed, if my dementia or any other affliction has produced inability or unwillingness to feed myself—for example, because of swallowing difficulties, or other eating disorders, or just indifference to eating—I instruct that my caregivers refrain from hand feeding unless I appear receptive to eating and drinking (show signs of enjoyment or positive anticipation). If I am indifferent or resistant to hand feeding, I do not want to be cajoled, harassed, or in any way impelled to eat or drink.

America's Alzheimer's Association has also addressed the questionable wisdom of initiating artificial nutrition and hydration. The organization points out that in comparison with careful hand feeding, tube feeding neither significantly improves nutritional status nor prevents or lowers the incidence of aspiration complications (like pneumonia) among people with dementias.[25]

"We support the idea of comfort feeding [by hand], offering it to the patient as long as he or she is able to swallow and tolerate it," said Beth Kallmyer, vice president of constituent services for the Alzheimer's Association.[26] "At some point they're unable to swallow, and . . . at that point you move to comfort measures and keeping their mouths moist. Typically, that's in the last week or two of life."

Judith Schwarz, clinical director of End of Life Choices New York, has written that "While it was once common to surgically implant feeding tubes into severely demented patients who could no longer safely swallow food or fluids by mouth, mercifully, that is no longer routinely done."[27]

But she goes on to make a cautionary point, "Individuals with advanced dementia are instead spoon fed, often for months or years, until they no longer know what to do with what is put into their mouths, or they begin to cough and aspirate liquids into their lungs. Only then will efforts to provide assisted oral feedings be stopped."

Judith warns that even when family members attempt to advocate on behalf of their loved one, such feedings may continue unless clear and convincing evidence opposing this is provided. Her group has developed an advance directive that permits decisionally capable individuals to make choices about receiving oral food and fluids at a future specified time of severe dementia.[28] They also recommend completion of supplemental forms, such as a MOLST form (Medical Orders for Life Sustaining Treatment) and the designation of a health care proxy.

The New York organization's directive (which can be found online) has two options.[29] The first states that oral assisted feedings should cease once the person is in an advanced stage of dementia and incapable of self-feeding and participating in decisions. The second option requests that oral assisted feedings be discontinued at the point the person has become disinterested or unwilling to be fed—the position that Cantor takes.

Such written advance directives could be further augmented by brief videotape recordings in which people explain their preferences. The Italian Parliament's 2017 end-of-life bill allows patients who are incapable of writing to express binding preferences for care through a video. The legislature does not specifically apply to euthanasia or assisted dying,[30] but does address other life-shortening practices, including the suspension or rejection of artificial nutrition and hydration.

There are several organizations, including MyDirectives, Life Messages Media of Wisconsin, and In My Own Words, which are assisting people to create video memoirs, ethical wills, and digital advance directives. For a fee, the Institute on Health-Care Directives offers a consultation with a physician followed by production of a carefully scripted videotape, usually lasting forty-five to ninety seconds, as well as follow-ups.[31] The institute's website states their process will "ensure that your voice will be heard & will do so by offering a customized MIDEO[TM] (My Informed Decision on VidEO) Safety Statement that is quickly and easily retrievable by medical personnel any time, day or night." Both cards and jewelry containing the links are available. These allow the online video segment to be viewed by hospital personnel with smart phones or other devices.

Maya Salam has written about technological approaches to "the concept of affirmative consent—the act of giving verbal permission clearly and often during intimate encounters."[32] Her article relates to apps that have been created for people, and especially college students, who are trying to establish boundaries before engaging in sex. Yes, sex—not dying. But take a step back and one can imagine how a similar strategy might be applied to end-of-life behaviors.

We-Consent is an app created in 2015 for students to enable them to adhere to affirmative consent rules.[33] It was inspired by California's decision that such matters should be accepted as the standard in disciplinary determinations, and it involves the recording of a short video of two people explaining their affirmative consent. Facial recognition technology is employed and the recording is encrypted. A legal petition is required before it could ever be accessed. There are currently over one hundred thousand We-Consent files, and only two formal requests have been made to retrieve videos. The availability of recordings and the fact that details are spelled out in advance serve to lessen the likelihood for meaningful disagreements occurring afterward.

LegalFling is a recently developed app that similarly makes agreed-upon sexual behaviors explicit.[34] Salam explains that,

"Condom use, bondage, dirty talk, sexting: the app lets users set their boundaries before an encounter—boundaries that can be adjusted at any time with a tap and shared with potential partner." One forges a dynamic document that users can alter and update.

Andrew D. Cherkasky, a former special victims prosecutor and now a criminal defense attorney, maintains that such agreements can hold up in court. While not technically contracts, he describes them as being documentation of intent.[35]

I can well see a future where variations of the above approaches will be constructed to better inform and ensure that we receive our terminal care treatment preferences in the digital age. Israeli citizens already have their advance directives on an online server that is available to medical and hospital staff throughout the country.[36] A LegalFling or We-Consent type of app could be developed that supplements written documents and spells out such things for one's health care proxy, power of attorney, and physician.

I would maintain that there is no way to entirely avoid the moral residue of death-hastening events or to negate the emotional conflicts they engender. However, I believe that these can be mitigated or at least lessened if we not only complete formal advance directive documents but also make a concerted effort to have regular conversations about such matters. In a recent column, Paula Span tackled this dicey subject, and she observed that many elderly people and an increasing number of medical professionals and ethicists are actively discussing the logic of planned deaths to forestall dementia and whether suicides can be rational.[37]

YOU WON'T
LET ME SUFFER
UNNECESSARILY

uch of what is known about Dr. Max Schur, Freud's personal physician, has been compiled in the Jones and other biographies.[1] But in 1994, additional information was presented before the Vienna Psychoanalytic Association by his son, Dr. Peter Schur.[2]

Max Schur was born in the town of Stanislaw, now part of the Ukraine. As the Russian armies approached in 1914, his family moved to Vienna. Schur completed gymnasium (high school) and enrolled in the University of Vienna to study medicine. As a student, he attended Freud's Introductory Lectures on Psychoanalysis, which were delivered in 1916 and 1917. They made a tremendous impact on the young man.

Despite encountering considerable anti-Semitism, Schur graduated in 1920 and specialized in internal medicine. He underwent psychoanalytic training with Dr. Ruth Brunswick, who had been analyzed by Freud. In 1932, he became a member of the Vienna Psychoanalytic Society, which had evolved from the Wednesday Psychological Society. The Wednesday group originally consisted of Freud and five of his followers, who met weekly at the professor's apartment to eat cake, drink coffee, smoke numerous cigarettes and cigars, and then heatedly argue about psychology and neuropathology.[3] This humble coffee klatch would become the seed for the worldwide psychoanalytic movement.

In 1926, while covering for a colleague, Schur provided medical care to Princess Marie Bonaparte, a great-grandniece of Emperor Napoleon I of France and the wife of Prince George of Greece and Denmark.[4] At the time, she was in Vienna undergoing an analysis with Freud. Marie Bonaparte had inherited great wealth from her grandfather, a real estate developer, and her royal connections proved invaluable in the diplomacy and finances required to eventually help Freud leave Austria. It was Marie Bonaparte who would pay Freud's exit ransom or "refugee tax" (more than 31,000 Reichsmarks) demanded by the Nazis.[5]

After Freud became incensed with his original doctor, Felix Deutsch, he asked his colleagues for recommendations to replace him. Marie Bonaparte was pleased with the care she had received from Schur and was quick to suggest that Freud consider him for the position. Schur later wrote in detail about his interview.[6]

During the encounter, the young internist (he was thirty-two years old and his patient was forty years his senior) heard about two foundational elements that the professor insisted were necessary for their doctor-patient relationship. According to Schur's account: "Before telling me his history or his present complaints, [Freud] expressed the expectation that he would always be told the truth and nothing but the truth. My response must have reassured him that I meant to keep such a promise. He then added, looking searchingly at me: 'Promise me one more thing; that when the time comes, you won't let me suffer unnecessarily.' All this was said with the utmost simplicity, without a trace of pathos, but also with complete determination. We shook hands at this point."[7]

Over the next few years, Schur supervised the medical care and arranged for Freud's various surgeries. He cautioned Freud about his smoking habit and offered the literature of the time about the dangers of nicotine dependence. Freud was willing to discuss his habit, but he also continued to smoke. On one occasion, he presented Schur with a cigar, which the internist felt constrained to accept and light up. Freud quickly recognized that Schur was not enjoying himself and made a good-humored comment about the outlandish expense of fine Havana cigars. He never offered his doctor another.

Schur usually made house calls to examine the psychoanalyst. He frequently encountered family members and provided medical care for several of Freud's children and nephews. In 1932 alone, Freud saw his surgeon for ninety-two visits and required five separate operations.

The doctor and his patient spoke often about the international financial depression and the rise of Nazism in Germany. Freud was aghast to see what was happening to "the home of Goethe and Kant"—his two greatest heroes. Shortly after Hitler came to power in March 1933, all Jewish analysts, including Freud's sons, had to flee Germany with their families or face extermination. Tensions began to rise in Austria that the Nazis would take over the country.

On May 6, Schur examined Freud as usual. That day was special because not only was it his patient's birthday but also because the doctor's wife, Helen, was pregnant and past her due date for their first child. Freud urged him to hasten back home, and in a contemplative tone remarked, "You are going from a man who doesn't want to leave the world to a child who doesn't want to come into it."[8]

Three days later, Peter Schur was born; he was given several gold Austrian coins by Freud (which he has safely kept until this day) in honor of his birth. On May 10, the newspapers reported widespread burning of Freud's works by crowds that were agitated by the Nazis. As the books were fed into fiery pyres the mob chanted, "Against the soul-destroying overestimation of the sex life, and on behalf of the nobility of the human soul, we offer the flames the writings of Sigmund Freud."[9]

Following the February 1934 Austrian civil war—precipitated by the Nazis murdering Chancellor Dollfus—Freud conceded for the first time that he was considering leaving the country.

Despite the increasing violence, few Jews grasped what was happening and were ready to abandon their communities.

It was around then that my own maternal grandfather was encouraged by his Socialist colleagues to flee Germany. My grandfather packed his possessions and moved his family from Berlin to New York.

Back in Vienna, Schur began leading a boycott of German pharmaceuticals, and his patient proudly reported to a colleague, "My personal physician . . . a very able doctor, is so deeply indignant about the events in Germany that he is no longer prescribing German medicines." Schur also began to seriously consider emigration.

The following years were punctuated by the appearance of new malignant tumors that spread on Freud's palate and required more extensive surgical procedures. In 1938, his surgeon determined that part of the cancer was no longer accessible.

In February 1938, Hitler summoned Austrian chancellor Schuschnigg to Berchtesgaden and issued an ultimatum to capitulate or be invaded. Schur went to the U.S. embassy and applied for a visa. He urged Freud to leave the country immediately. Freud considered and then rejected the advice; either way, it was too late. On March 11, the German army invaded and rapidly annexed Austria. Nazi flags fluttered in front of many residential homes. Joyous Viennese paraded in the streets.

Marauding hooligans in brown shirts with swastika armbands attacked Jewish stores, synagogues and homes; a wave of assaults and murders ensued. This was followed by a virtual epidemic of suicides.[10] During the spring, some five hundred Austrian Jews committed suicide to avoid further brutality and humiliation.

Shortly following the Nazi occupation of Austria, Anna asked her father, "Wouldn't it be better if we all killed ourselves?" Freud pugnaciously replied, "Why? Because they would like us to?" She understood his position, but feared being arrested.

Anna and her brother, Martin, did not tell their father about a meeting they arranged with Schur. In it, they requested and then received from the doctor a lethal amount of barbiturates. If faced with torture or internment in a concentration camp, the

Freud children could choose to commit suicide. Schur promised that in their absence he would take care of their father.

The Nazis appeared at the Schur household, confiscated an automobile, and took other valuables. Knowing about the extermination of the Jews, gypsies, and others that was taking place in Germany, the Schurs considered themselves thankful that nothing worse happened.

The circumstances at the Freud household were considerably more worrisome. On the day following the annexation, Freud's son, Martin, went to the office of their psychoanalytic publishing company and began destroying sensitive documents, including correspondence related to private bank accounts. While shredding the papers, a gang of ruffians arrived; one man pressed a gun to Martin's head and threatened to shoot. The standoff was only interrupted by the appearance of a Nazi officer. Immediately afterward, hurrying to his parent's apartment, Martin found the Gestapo had just departed. Freud commented that the "gentleman of the SS" left with a substantial sum of cash, and he wryly remarked, "Dear me, I have never taken so much for a single visit."[11]

Ominously, Freud's "guests" departed only after confiscating everyone's passports. The loss of identification papers was not insignificant in a city where at any moment and for any reason a person could be stopped and forced to prove his identity. The absence of documents was sufficient to result in arrest and confinement.

Schur wrote: "It is hard to describe our state of mind during that period. A great deal has been written about the cruelties of the concentration and extermination camps. But less is known about the condition of suddenly being outside the protection of common law. Not to be afraid of a knock on the door would have been abnormal. Friends and relatives were disappearing. The Gestapo had moved in and established its headquarters, and the first news about torture was beginning to circulate."[12]

On March 22, the Gestapo returned to the Freud home, banged on the door, and resumed searching. The SS rummaged through the family's belongings, pulling out the contents of drawers and closets. This continued until Mrs. Freud indignantly confronted one of the men and ordered him to stop. The intruders left the house with money, but more importantly they took Freud's daughter, Anna.[13] She was escorted outside to a big black touring car with two heavily armed officers in front and two in the back. The automobile headed directly to Gestapo headquarters. Her brother, Martin, vividly recalled, "Far from showing fear, or even much interest, she sat in the car as a woman might sit in a taxi on her way to enjoy a shopping expedition." Concealed in her clothing was the barbiturate she had obtained from Schur.

It was noon when the Gestapo drove away. While Anna was gone, Freud and Schur fretfully paced from room to room. In the parlor, the radio softly played while the two men nervously talked. During those "endless" hours, Freud smoked cigar after cigar. The eighty-two-year-old father was by nature emotionally controlled and stoical—but not now.

Night had fallen over the city of Vienna when Anna safely walked into the house. It was seven hours after she had been taken away by the Nazis. She returned, shaken but unharmed, and fell into the arms of her father. "At Gestapo headquarters," Anna explained, "they mostly ignored me. I mainly sat by myself. I don't think they knew what they wanted to do once I was there. After a while, I simply left the office where they had deposited me, stepped outside, and came home."[14]

Relieved, the old man began to loudly weep. Abruptly, his mood changed to indignation and he declared his intention to leave Austria immediately.

9

∾

MY WAY

Like the Raffs, many modern proponents of assisted suicide are uncomfortable with the pejorative connotations of the word "suicide" and have been seeking a more palatable nomenclature. In 2006, the Oregon Department of Human Services went so far as to adopt a policy banning the expression "physician-assisted suicide" in favor of "aid in dying," or alternatively, "death with dignity."[1] Similarly, the American Public Health Association concluded: "Medical and legal experts have recognized that the term 'suicide' or 'assisted suicide' is inappropriate when discussing the choice of a mentally competent terminally ill patient to seek medications that he or she could consume to bring about a peaceful and dignified death."[2]

In 2017, the American Association of Suicidology, a suicide prevention and medical research organization, issued a statement concluding that medical aid in dying "is distinct from the behavior that has been traditionally and ordinarily described as 'suicide.'"[3] They pointed out that in suicide, a life that could have continued indefinitely is abruptly shortened, while assisted dying usually involves a foreseeable death that occurs a little sooner but in an easier way, in accordance with the person's preferences

and values. Other differences include the unrelenting psychological despair of suicides, who cannot enjoy life or see that things
may change in the future, versus the desire of people who seek
assisted dying to live while also accepting that they have a terminal condition; the isolation, loneliness, and loss of meaning of
individuals who commit suicide versus the intensified emotional
bonds with loved ones that often precedes assisted dying; and
the physical self-violence of suicide methods versus the physically peaceful forms of death sought by people who are already
dying or suffering from irremediable symptoms.

Especially if people are already fatally ill, it seems incorrect
to label actions to shorten the dying process with the same word
as that applied to physically healthy people with psychiatric disorders who choose to die by their own hands. The families of
my palliative care patients who die after decisions to withhold
or withdraw dialysis would take umbrage if these actions were
labeled as suicide.

However, I use all the various synonyms, including suicide.
For the most part, "suicide" is a potent word that describes a
behavior some people consider to be a sin, others a crime, and
still others the ultimate expression of psychopathology. But
there are many individuals like my iconoclastic friend the late
Dr. Thomas Szasz who regard some suicides in a positive light
and as nothing less than a "fatal freedom."[4] By 1989, with publication of the second in a series of articles on physicians' responsibility toward hopelessly ill patients, a shift in societal attitudes
has become apparent; there is growing recognition by medical
professionals that the terminally ill may rationally desire or seek
death as a means to end suffering.[5]

Szasz summarized the legal history of suicide in Western
Europe and America, pointing out that after Rome became Christian, the Catholic Church adopted the Jewish ban on self-murder
as a sin against God. Suicides were punished according to the
Council of Braga in 563 by denying them burial in consecrated
ground, and in medieval times their bodies were interred at
the crossroads so that people would intentionally step on the
graves. The property of suicides was legally forfeited to the king
and nobles. Around the eighteenth and nineteenth centuries, the

self-killers were considered, ipso facto, as insane, while in the past century the rabbinic and church authorities classified them as non compos mentis, and only then began allowing them normal religious burial services. However, laws punishing suicide remained in effect throughout many American states until the middle of the twentieth century. These were gradually removed from the criminal code, although the act of assisting suicide continues to carry penalties of up to ten years in prison. As suicide shifted from being a sin to being a criminal act to being the behavior of the mentally ill, the specialty of psychiatry assumed responsibility for coercive suicide prevention.

Szasz ardently maintained in several of his books that suicide should not be constrained by religion, law, or organized medicine.[6] He always opposed the commitment of people to psychiatric facilities and especially felt that way about the suicidal. Szasz was predictably outraged when I told him about how David Raff was forcefully brought to the Palms of Sarasota.

Whatever it is called—physician-assisted suicide, death with dignity, assisted dying, self-deliverance, medical aid in dying, deliberate life completion, planned death, or voluntary euthanasia—the U.S. Supreme Court has, since 1997, encouraged individual states to wrestle with the issue.[7] In a ruling involving combined cases from Washington State and New York, Chief Justice William H. Rehnquist wrote that the court's decision "permits this debate to continue, as it should in a democratic society."[8] Eight jurisdictions have currently legalized aid in dying through court challenges, legislation, and voter ballot initiatives, including Oregon (1994 and 1997), Washington (2008), Montana (2009), Vermont (2013), California (2015), Colorado (2016), the District of Columbia (2016), and Hawaii (2018). They encompass 18 percent of the nation's population.[9]

The appointment of Neil Gorsuch to the Supreme Court heralded the arrival of an ardent judicial opponent, who has articulated his ideas in a book developed during his time attending Oxford University. "All human beings are intrinsically valuable," he wrote, "and the intentional taking of human life by private persons is always wrong. . . . We seek to protect and preserve life for life's own sake in everything from our most fundamental laws of homicide to our road traffic regulations to our largest governmental programs for health and social security."[10]

Gorsuch suggested that jurists like Judge Richard Posner of the U.S. Court of Appeals for the Seventh Circuit who have argued in favor of assisted dying, "tend toward, if not require, the legalization not only of assisted suicide and euthanasia, but of any act of consensual homicide."[11] Posner's position, Gorsuch melodramatically asserted, would allow for legal duels, illicit drug use, organ sales, sadomasochist killings, mass suicide pacts and the "sale of one's own life."[12]

While the issue has instantly become more contentious in the Supreme Court, I believe that more death-with-dignity laws will be approved across the country for three primary reasons: (1) America is built upon the fundamental values of autonomy and self-determination; (2) as the baby boomer generation ages and actively deals with their own or their parents' deterioration, they are likely to continue to insist on having assisted dying as an option; and (3) support among gray-haired celebrities is likely to grow and help sway public opinion that this should be an end-of-life option.

Desmond Tutu, archbishop emeritus of Cape Town and a Nobel Peace laureate, offers an interesting example of the last reason. In the week leading up to his eighty-fifth birthday, Tutu spoke with dismay over the way his friend Nelson Mandela was artificially kept alive for photo opportunities with visiting dignitaries.[13] Witnessing Mandela's last days crystalized the archbishop's thinking, and he decided to try to influence a debate taking place in the United Kingdom's House of Lords about aid in dying.[14] Tutu wrote in the *Washington Post*: "Now . . . with my life closer to its end than its beginning, I wish to help give people dignity in dying. Just as I have argued firmly for compassion and fairness in life, I believe that terminally ill people should be treated with the same compassion and fairness when it comes to their deaths. Dying people should have the right to choose how and when they leave Mother Earth. I believe that, alongside the wonderful palliative care that exists, their choices should include a dignified assisted death."[15]

Tutu continued:

There have been promising developments as of late in California and Canada, where the law now allows assisted dying for terminally ill people, but there are still many thousands of dying people across the world who are denied their right to die with dignity. Two years ago, I announced the reversal of my lifelong opposition to assisted dying in an op-ed in the *Guardian*. But I was more ambiguous about whether I personally wanted the option, writing: "I would say I wouldn't mind." Today, I myself am even closer to the departures hall than arrivals, so to speak, and my thoughts turn to how I would like to be treated when the time comes. Now more than ever, I feel compelled to lend my voice to this cause.[16]

Public opinion polls demonstrate that although there is now popular support in the United States for death-with-dignity reform, this was not always the case, According to Eli Stutsman, an attorney from Oregon who is responsible for originally spearheading the nationwide campaign to legalize the practice, a 1947 Gallup survey asked, "When a person has a disease that cannot be cured, do you think doctors should be allowed by law to end a patient's life by some painless means if the patient and his family request it?"[17] At that time, only 37 percent of respondents were in favor, 54 percent answered "no," and 9 percent didn't answer or replied that they didn't know. Seventy years later, however, the numbers have been nearly reversed.[18] When the exact same question was asked in 2017, 73 percent were in favor of allowing a hastened death, 24 percent opposed, and 3 percent were unsure or unprepared to answer. Put another way, support for euthanasia has nearly doubled and two-thirds of respondents now favor physicians accelerating people's deaths when they have irreversible conditions.

Gallup had been conducting this survey on an annual basis, and the turning point was in 1990.[19] Since then, solid majorities of Americans have expressed support for euthanasia. Views differ according to religious and political persuasions; only 55 percent of weekly churchgoers responded affirmatively to the question, in contrast to 87 percent of those adults who described themselves as rarely attending church. When it comes to political parties, 67 percent of Republicans and Republican-leaners positively endorsed the question versus 81 percent of Democrats and Democratic-leaning independents.

A 2014 Harris poll found that an overwhelming 74 percent of American adults affirmed that terminally ill patients who are in great pain should have the right to end their lives; only 14 percent were opposed.[20] The survey also asked a slightly different question: "Do you think that the law should allow doctors to comply with the wishes of a dying patient in severe distress who asks to have his or her life ended, or not?" Sixty-six percent of respondents said doctors should be allowed to comply with the wishes of such patients, up from 58 percent in a similar poll conducted in 2011. Opposition decreased from 20 percent in 2011 to 15 percent from three years earlier. Humphrey Taylor, chairman of the Harris Poll, concluded, "Public opinion on these issues seems to be far ahead of political leadership and legislative actions."[21]

Physicians, meanwhile, have been more ambivalent about assisted suicide. In 2014, coinciding with the publicity surrounding Brittany Maynard, the young and appealing Californian woman with a brain cancer who spoke up forcefully for her right to have a medically assisted death, for the first time the majority of U.S. doctors—54 percent—backed the rights of patients with an "incurable illness" to seek "a dignified death."[22] The survey included seventeen thousand respondents. NBC News quoted Arthur Caplan, founding head of the division of bioethics at NYU Langone Medical Center, as observing, "It represents a remarkable shift. If physician opposition continues to weaken, it is likely that despite fierce resistance from some religious groups and some in the disability community, more states will follow Oregon, Washington and Vermont, and legalize."[23]

Demographic trends favor greater support for further legalization and an extension of assisted-dying practices. The aging boomer generation is actively encountering the nightmare of dementing illnesses. It is also facing a worsening social situation created by harsh economic realities and the absence of family members who are willing or able to provide personal care. Many of those boomers were the revolutionaries of the 1960s and 1970s, and they are accustomed to making changes.

Then there are the families. In an article entitled, "The Job to End All Others," Celia Watson wrote, "To work full-time and take care of a parent with dementia is a contradiction in terms—unless your full-time job is taking care of a parent with dementia."[24] She cites a study that concluded when the process of caregiving conflicts with work, seven in ten people report they have had to cut back on their hours of employment, shift jobs, take a leave of absence, stop work entirely, or make other such changes.[25]

However, it cannot be emphasized enough how many family caregivers find the role to be incredibly vital and fulfilling. One of my psychiatrist colleagues retired nightly to the assisted living facility where he slept alongside his demented wife. The fact that she rarely recognized him did not detract from his overriding conviction that he was fulfilling the most important duty of his married life. Another colleague dealing with a similar situation pointed out to me that even when a demented spouse cannot recall characters or follow a plot, it may still be mutually pleasurable to sit together and watch a television series at home.

But some caregivers experience this same scenario as terrifying, burdensome, and profoundly unfair. After decades of marriage, couples have become entwined, and like the Raffs, the misfortune of one spouse excruciatingly impacts the other. While the relatively healthy spouse may welcome the opportunity to assist his or her life partner, all the while there is an ominous background drumbeat reminding everyone that demands will eventually outweigh resources, finite savings are being expended, and institutionalization is likely to become a necessity. Furthermore, for a couple dealing with dementia there is a pervasive sadness as the spouse's personality slips away in an unpredictable manner—made more unbearable during those moments when the person seems to briefly return.

Susan Jacoby has aptly observed, "My generation's vision of an ageless old age bears about as much resemblance to real old age as our earlier idealization of painless childbirth without drugs did to real labor."[26]

Faced with inevitable decay and the possibility of unremitting suffering, it is reasonable to predict that our society is likely to reconceptualize suicide and rewrite our laws and policies about end-of-life care options. Americans are going to demand to be in control. They will insist on having options.

David and Reba's son, Martin, is a tall, skinny, seventy-three-year-old man who bears a startling resemblance to the actor Alan Alda. Martin is a neurologist/researcher who is best known for studying a process of suicide that occurs on a cellular level and is necessary for the prolongation of life in organisms. It is called apoptosis. Martin explained: "Cells die in huge numbers, not only in development but even as we speak. Hundreds of millions of cells are dying each minute in our bodies. The good news is that, if you are healthy, for every cell that dies, a cell divides to replace it. . . . So, the cell is committing suicide in a sense; it is making a decision and killing itself in a very special way so that the debris is eaten and cleared very quickly . . . and you really do need this cell death for lots of reasons in development."

For example, the way a fetus develops fingers is by means of the cells between the digits killing themselves off and leaving spaces or clefts. "I see suicides on a cellular level," he explained, "as being part of a necessary and natural process, like horticultural pruning."

"I feel like I have had a great life," Martin told me. "I have done everything I want to do. There is nothing big that I feel I need to do. I have had a good run and it wouldn't be a terrible thing if I kick the bucket in the near future."

Martin continued:

My wife has views that are like mine, and she will help me if the need arises and do it at whatever risk. She has provided me with great confidence that if I need her help, she will be there. And I will do the same for her. We are extremely lucky.

I always thought of the approach my parents took as being a magnificent thing. Number one, they didn't suffer at the end of their lives. They had a really good life and a good death. Second, it was a wonderful thing what they did for my brother and me (at this point his voice chokes up), because when I see what my friends have been going through with their parents . . . when they end up in intensive care units for months or in a nursing homes with Alzheimer's, it is almost always, always bad. And by discussing it [our parents] made it easy for us. Since that moment, I have been a proselytizer for assisted dying. There are very few things that I feel more strongly about.

His brother, Anton, who received a PhD in English literature before going to medical school, also believes strongly in self-determination, but, unlike Martin, he never became active in the assisted-dying movement. Anton chose to remain more private about his opinions because he views Florida as being a moderately conservative state that is unwelcoming of such opinions.

I asked Anton if he could foresee following in his parent's footsteps.

"Certainly!" he responded. "There is no question about it. I don't see myself doing it now, because I'm in good health. But when the time comes that I am not and can look forward to suffering and using resources my children could better use—" Anton solemnly gazed into my eyes. "Yes," he quietly said, "without any hesitation."

Listening to the two Raff brothers I was reminded of the conclusion of a *New York* magazine piece entitled, "A Life Worth Ending."[27] In it, Michael Wolff wrote:

I do not know how death panels ever got such a bad name. Perhaps they should have been called deliverance panels. What I would not do for a fair-minded body to whom I might plead for my mother's end.

The alternative is nuts: to look forward to paying trillions and to bankrupting the nation as well as our souls as we endure the suffering of our parents and our inability to help them get where they're going. The single greatest pressure on health care is the disproportionate resources devoted to the elderly, to not just the old, but to the *old* old, and yet no one says what all old children of old parents know: This is not just wrongheaded but steals the life from everyone involved.

And it seems all the more savage because there is such a simple fix: Give us the right to make provisions for when we want to go. Give families the ability to make a fair case of enough being enough, of the end's, de facto, having come.

While driving back home from my last meeting with Martin in New York City, I fiddled with the car radio and happened to land on Frank Sinatra crooning his signature song, "My Way." There is a stanza that begins, *"And now the end is near / And so I face the final curtain."* It is followed by the well-known chorus: *"I've lived a life that's full / I traveled each and every highway / And more, much more than this / I did it my way."*[28]

The lyrics were written by the pop singer, Paul Anka, for his buddy, Frank Sinatra, the Sultan of Swoon. There have been more than one hundred recorded versions, but the song is indelibly identified with Sinatra and Anka.[29] For seven years in a row in the United Kingdom (where they apparently keep count of such things), "My Way" was the most popular song played at funerals.[30]

Following the final interview with Martin, the song's lyrics felt especially poignant and personal. My head swirled with intense reactions to the Raff family story. I couldn't help but identify with the aged Jewish physician who sat at the heart of it. Like him, I have two sons and would hope that they, too, would support my end-of-life decisions. I have been married for four decades, and my wife and I are so intertwined that the thought of continuing without the other is difficult to grasp. According to the account of their sons, Reba and David were not clinically depressed or irrational and their deaths remain a justifiable source of pride. At the same time, I can empathize with both the surgeon and the hapless psychiatrist who were uncomfortably drawn into the double suicide.

This family's story reinforces that there are exceptional people who not only live life their way but who also want to bring things to a close in their own way—and, on a very gut level, this feels honorable to me. Yes, most everyone wants to survive for as long as possible, but ideally on their own terms. David and Reba were fortunate to have lived privileged and self-determined lives, and I fully agreed with Anton's assessment that they chose a romantic ending—a Romeo and Juliet ending.

So, as I drove down the Mass Pike, I flipped off the car radio and perhaps not surprisingly found myself humming, *"I did it my way. . . ."*

10

❧

NOTHING BUT
TORTURE

Following Anna's release from Gestapo headquarters, Freud prepared a list for the British Consul in Vienna of the sixteen people, including the four members of the Schur family and two maids, he wanted to accompany him to England.[1]

Through the combined efforts of Marie Bonaparte and others, exit visas and permit papers were secured for the Freuds, Schurs, and several psychoanalytic associates. As departure became imminent, government officials handed the psychoanalyst a document stating: "I, Prof. Freud, hereby confirm that after the Anschluss (annexation) of Austria to the German Reich I have been treated by the German authorities and particularly by the Gestapo with all the respect and consideration due to my scientific reputation, that I could live and work in full freedom, that I could continue to pursue my activities in every way I desired, that I found full support from all concerned in this respect, and that I have not the slightest reason for any complaint."[2]

Before signing his name, Freud added one additional line, *"Ich kann die Gestapo jedermann auf das beste empfehlen"* ("I can most highly recommend the Gestapo to everyone").[3]

Early in the morning of June 4, the refugees embarked on the Orient Express. Anna handed their passports and exit visas to the officials. After the Nazis marched down the corridor to check the occupants of the next carriage, the conductor surreptitiously came to see the Freuds. "I wish I could come with you," he whispered.[4]

The group of immigrants departed Austria without Schur, who had developed acute appendicitis, requiring an emergency appendectomy at the Sanatorium Loeb. Jewish patients were not normally admitted to the medical facility, and this unfortunate event prompted a series of tense encounters with the Gestapo. Still bandaged and with a surgical drain in his abdomen, Schur was finally brought to the train station. On June 10, he was carefully helped on board the locomotive. The following day, he and his family were met in Paris by Marie Bonaparte and escorted to her palace. Schur convalesced until he was sufficiently well healed to proceed to London and rejoin the Freuds.

The regular routine between Schur and Freud resumed with more house calls and further attention to the cancer. The British government allowed Schur to act as Freud's physician even before he passed the required medical examinations. They arranged for Freud's regular surgeon to come from Austria for procedures. In February 1939, another malignant lesion was deemed inoperable and more radiation therapy instituted.[5]

Freud's condition deteriorated. He developed an ulcer on his right cheek, and became largely bed-bound. During the final six months, Anna attended him constantly, arising several times during the night to apply a local anesthetic.[6]

The psychoanalyst had a much-loved pet, a chow named Lün. But now the smell of necrotic bone from his jaw was so repulsive that the dog howled and refused to stay in the same room as the master.[7] Freud was distraught over this development.

It was not until 1972 that Schur's in-depth, first-person account—a copy of which I would find in Anna's library—was posthumously published.[8] This was intentional, as Freud's personal physician was interested in both protecting patient-physician confidentiality and avoiding the need to publicly defend his actions.

In the book, he described how over a span of sixteen years, his patient had undergone some thirty painful operations and several courses of radiation therapy. During much of the time, Freud was reduced to wearing a hideous, denture-like prosthesis to keep his oral and nasal cavities separated, and this device unfortunately prevented him from eating and speaking normally. Following the original series of surgeries in 1923, Freud became deaf in his right ear and the analytic couch was shifted from one wall to the other so that he could listen with his left ear.[9]

Nevertheless, Freud persevered in seeing patients. Even in London, he had four analysands in treatment and his clinical practice was only disbanded two months prior to his demise. During the final days, Freud requested that his bed be brought down to the study so that he could be near his books, his desk, and his prized antiquities (which were assembled in London to replicate their positions in his Viennese office).

According to Schur's account, on September 21, the frail and pain wracked man reached out, grasped him by the hand, and said, "My dear Schur, you certainly remember our first talk. You promised me then not to forsake me when my time comes. Now it's nothing but torture and makes no sense any more."[10]

Schur indicated that he had not forgotten his earlier commitment. He wrote that Freud "sighed with relief, held my hand for a moment longer, and said 'I thank you,' and after a moment of hesitation he added: 'Tell Anna about this.' All this was said without a trace of emotionality or self-pity, and with full consciousness of reality."

Schur continued, "I informed Anna of our conversation, as Freud had asked." She reluctantly agreed, thankful her father had remained lucid and able to make this final decision.

Schur wrote, "When he was again in agony, I gave him a hypodermic of two centigrams of morphine. He soon felt relief and fell into a peaceful sleep. The expression of pain and suffering was gone. I repeated this dose after about twelve hours.

Freud was obviously so close to the end of his reserves that he lapsed into a coma and did not wake up again."

There is some dispute about the completeness of Schur's account, and it has been suggested that a third dose of morphine was quietly administered by Dr. Josephine Stross.[11] This occurred when Schur was no longer present at the bedside. Dr. Stross was an intimate friend and colleague of Anna Freud.

Whether we call this voluntary euthanasia or palliative sedation, there is no question that Schur complied with his patient's request to accelerate his death. Jones wrote, "For someone at such a point of exhaustion as Freud then was, and so complete a stranger to opiates, that small dose sufficed. . . . He was evidently close to the end of his reserves."[12] Freud quietly died on the morning of September 23. Three days later, his body was cremated. The ashes were later placed in an ancient Greek urn that he had received as a gift from Marie Bonaparte and that sat for many years in his Viennese study. Freud bequeathed to Schur his pocket watch, which in turn was passed along to Schur's children and their children in perpetuity.

Four of Freud's elderly sisters remained behind in Vienna, where despite repeated efforts, Marie Bonaparte was unable to secure their passage to Britain.[13] The women were eventually detained by the Gestapo and transported to concentration camps. Mitzi Freud (eighty-one) and Paula Winternitz (seventy-eight) were brought to Theresienstadt and taken from there to the Maly Trostinets extermination camp, where they were killed. Dolfi Freud died in Theresienstadt of internal bleeding, which is presumed to have been caused by starvation. Rosa Graf (eighty-two) was deported to Treblinka. Accounts differ, but according to an eyewitness, Rosa approached SS Untersturmfuhrer Kurt Franz, identified herself as being the sister of the famous Sigmund Freud, and told him that she was not feeling well.

Franz "assured her that her arrival in Treblinka was a mistake, in view of her poor health and that as soon as she had had her bath, she would be put on the first available train back to Vienna."[14]

About his famous patient, Schur stated, "I saw him suffer pain and sorrow. I saw him show scorn and contempt for brutality and stupidity as well as tender love and concern for those close to him. He was always a deeply human and noble man, in the fullest meaning of the word. And I saw him face dying and death as nobly as he had faced living."[15]

In one of the last letters that Princess Marie Bonaparte sent to her aged teacher, she wrote, "Perhaps you yourself . . . do not perceive your full greatness. You belong to the history of human thought, like Plato . . . or Goethe."[16]

After Freud's death, Schur would write the biography that I found in the clinic library. Years later, I interviewed his son, Dr. Peter Schur, who told me, "I have never met anybody before you who actually read my father's book. I have encountered people who were familiar with it, but I don't think they actually read it."

When I met Peter, he was seventy-eight years old, a professor of medicine at Harvard Medical School, and a senior physician at Brigham & Women's Hospital in medicine and rheumatology. Each year he would take part in a European bicycle trip where, he told me with some pride, "I'm the oldest man in the group, but not the slowest man in the group."

It is startling how closely Peter resembles photographs of his father, and I quickly ascertained that they shared a similar work ethic—despite his age, he is a full-time member of the rheumatology department and arrives each day to the hospital at 7 a.m. and leaves at 6 p.m. "I love what I do," he enthusiastically exclaimed.

Peter speaks softly and deliberately. Any tendency toward somberness is lightened by a smile, and this was evident when he talked about death. "I am proud of how my father cared for Freud," he said to me. "I am also proud about the way my parents died."

"Oh?" I asked. "Tell me more?"

We were quietly chatting in the Ether Dome, an old-fashioned surgical operating amphitheater at Massachusetts General Hospital where anesthesia was first publicly demonstrated in 1846. I had just delivered a talk about Freud's final illness that was largely based on Max Schur's book. During a fellowship at that Harvard teaching hospital, I had sat many times in the amphitheater, often after climbing to the top to pay my respects to Padihershef, an Egyptian mummy that resides in an oak and glass display case. This was my first opportunity to give a grand rounds presentation, and I invited Peter to attend.

Following the talk, we sat down together in a conference room and Peter handed me a sheath of papers. He said, "This is a copy of a speech I delivered several years ago on the same subject to the Vienna Psychoanalytic Association."[17]

I thanked him for the gift and asked, "So what did you mean about Freud and your parents' deaths?"

"As you know," he said, "both of my parents were physicians, and they knew full well that we are all going to die. Back then nobody openly talked about euthanasia any more than they talked about abortions before these were legalized. But doctors knew which of their colleagues were performing them. . . . My father didn't ever discuss Freud's death with me and I learned about it like everyone else when I read Jones's biography and my father's manuscript."

Peter continued, "My father gave Freud sufficient morphine to put him to sleep and relieve his pain. There is no way to know whether all the psychological factors that keep you alive got turned off or whether the morphine was sufficient in an elderly gentleman to shut down the respiratory center of his brain. In any case, Freud had decided his time had come and my father did the right thing."

"To the best of your knowledge," I asked, "did your father assist anyone else similarly?"

"No, but I don't really know."

"If a patient asked you to do for him what your father did for Freud, what would you say?"

"I'd say, Yes! People should have choices when it comes to such things. Doctors also have responsibilities to alleviate pain and to make one's breathing more comfortable."

I asked, "So what were the circumstances around your parents' deaths?"

"My father," he said, "was home with a mild case of the flu when he got chest pains. He had cardiac problems many years before, so he knew what was happening. During the original heart attack, he insisted on being taken care of at home and eventually had a full recovery. This time my father once again refused to be admitted to the hospital, and he died in his own bed in the house."

"My mother had a living will appointing me her proxy and making it clear that if her chances of a meaningful recovery were poor, then she, too, did not want to receive aggressive care, such as artificial feedings or even antibiotics. When she had a massive stroke, I had her admitted to my hospital and would visit her. . . . I spoke up on her behalf to prevent nursing staff from starting intravenous fluids and was at the bedside when she died."

Anton (Tony) Kris, a Cambridge psychoanalyst and childhood friend of Peter, was raised with him in the small, tight-knit Jewish, Viennese medical community that revolved around Freud. The two men remember the previous generation as having been "realists" who had no illusions about the role of physicians in helping people to die. Tony is completely comfortable about how Freud died, and he maintains, "I was taught that cancer deaths are morphine deaths, and sooner or later the pain medication does the job." Tony believes, "The most important thing is to stay out of the hospital so it can be done. . . . There was nothing unusual about what Schur was doing. . . . It was unusual only because he was a young man treating one of the giants of history. But to be the one who actually gives the final dose is always daunting."

Peter solemnly offered his opinion: "Freud, my father, and my mother each had what they wanted: peaceful and quiet deaths. That is all anyone could desire."

But there were two other things that Freud insisted upon that should be spotlighted: truthfulness in the doctor-patient relationship and respect for autonomy.[18] More than a half century later there is general agreement in North American and Western European medical practice that it is obligatory to honestly disclose diagnoses and to elucidate the benefits and risks of treatment. The involvement of patients in medical decision-making has become mandatory.[19]

A colleague and I have written about Freud's medical care: "Although he could probably have self-administered a lethal dose of morphine, Schur's account of his final years indicate that

Freud relied on the knowledge and sensitivity that one's personal physician can bring to the moment of death. He trusted his doctor not to abandon him at that most vulnerable moment."[20] In a moment of despair Freud had once asked, "How long must I continue to suffer such intolerable pain? When will I be permitted to accept 'sweet peace' or even to ask for it?"[21] Perhaps it was feeling confident that Schur would intervene when life became unbearable was what permitted him to continue his productive professional life during almost two decades of disfiguring surgical procedures and nearly unendurable pain.

In Freud's funeral oration, Ernest Jones declared, "It was hard to wish that he would live a day longer when his life was reduced to a pin point of personal agony. . . . Thus one can say of him that as never man loved life more, so never man feared death less. . . . He had warmed both hands at the fire of life, and life had nothing left to offer."[22]

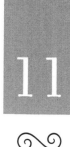

FATE WORSE
THAN DEATH?

How common is dementia and how likely is it that a situation akin to the ones faced by Dell Weinstein, Reba Raff, or Gillian Bennett will befall you or your loved ones?

Alzheimer's disease is the most frequent type of dementia. According to the Alzheimer's Association, 5.4 million Americans have this disorder.[1] The condition affects one in eight older adults and the numbers are expected to spike significantly as baby boomers age. In our society, dementia is not a boogey man—it is a genuinely terrifying epidemic that most of us choose to deny and ignore.

There are several different types of dementia, including those following strokes, chronic alcoholism, and neurological disease like Parkinson's, and while they can begin at any age, the numbers rise dramatically among the elderly. One in five people over age sixty-five have mild cognitive impairment (the earliest stage of dementia), and approximately one-third will be diagnosed with Alzheimer's disease within five years.[2] The Alzheimer's Association estimates that 10 percent of people over sixty-five have that disease, and in 2018, the direct costs to American society will total an estimated $277 billion.[3] Hurd and colleagues concluded in a *New England Journal of Medicine* article that Alzheimer's disease is the most expensive illness in the United States.[4] Unfortunately, they also found that in recent years the National Institutes of Health has decreased research spending on the disease and expends five times as much for cancer and heart disease, respectively. While there are five FDA-approved Alzheimer's drugs that treat the symptoms of Alzheimer's by temporarily helping memory and cognition, none of these medications treats the underlying causes of the dementia.[5] The first large clinical trial to show positive results for an anti-amyloid agent in patients with early-stage Alzheimer's disease looks promising, but experts are calling for caution.[6]

America is longing for drugs that will slow down or reverse the progression of dementing illnesses. We can't help but get excited when preliminary research involving a brain implant that electronically boosts memory is reported.[7] Gray-haired people quickly pull out their credit cards after being bombarded with radio and television commercials touting the purported benefits of brain-exercise products. It's a real stretch to say that such developments or commercialized technologies will do anything meaningful for cognitive impairments. Furthermore, there is little evidence that the drugs used to treat symptoms are effective beyond a year, while the majority of older adults diagnosed with dementia are routinely prescribed these costly medications for up to a decade.[8]

Unlike AIDS or breast cancer, Alzheimer's has yet to spawn a vigorous public health movement to combat the disease. Physicians talk about the other disorders and therapeutic approaches, but medical scientists are mainly silent about dementing illnesses. So far there has been no general acceptance of the need for a shared mission to face dementia, prevent it or slow it down when possible, and to minimize the associated suffering as it inexorably shifts into the final stage. The presence of even severe dementia, "failure to thrive," or debility are insufficient to qualify people for hospice services unless they have a prognosis of less than six months to live.[9] Unfortunately, there are no scans, blood tests, or empirical instruments to arrive at such a prediction, and individuals can linger in late-stage dementia for years. The baby boomers and their parents have hitherto been unable to break through society's denial of the prevalence, progression, and horrors of the disease. One recent and notable exception has been the announcement by Bill Gates that he is personally investing $100 million to fight Alzheimer's disease.[10]

Seventy-eight million Americans were born in the postwar birth explosion from 1946 to 1964, and ten thousand turn sixty-five years old every day, many of whom would like to imagine they are healthier than their forebears.[11] Accordingly, they revel in their youthful tastes for Bruce Springsteen or Mick Jagger or Tina Turner, watching these musicians still belting it out on the stage. But the reality is that while baby boomers have the longest life expectancy of any previous generation, they have higher rates of obesity, hypertension, diabetes, and elevated cholesterol levels than members of the previous generation.

In a study published in *JAMA Internal Medicine*, researchers found that only 13 percent of a sample of baby boomers rated their health as "excellent," while nearly three times as many, 32 percent, of those in the sample from the previous generation, considered themselves to be in excellent health.[12] Seven percent use a cane or other device to help them walk, compared to 3 percent in the earlier cohort; and 13 percent of boomers have some limitations in their ability to perform everyday tasks, such as walking up a flight of stairs or mowing the lawn, as compared to 8.8 percent of those from the previous generational cohort.

The boomers' fantasy is that after leading a healthy and productive life, death will come suddenly and without discomfort from an accident or a massive stroke. However, the reality is that for the great majority of Americans, the last years will be challenging. They will hopefully continue to find meaning and pleasure in their daily lives, but they are also likely to confront cognitive and physical disabilities and medical conditions that make it impossible to remain independent.

A provocative piece in the *Economist* makes the point that most everyone believes there are fates worse than death, and the article describes how a group of investigators from the University of Pennsylvania set out to identify those conditions.[13] Rubin and associates interviewed 180 patients over age sixty who were hospitalized and suffering from serious illnesses, including cancer and lung and heart disease. The sample did not have any documented preference for life-support treatment limitations. The patients were asked by medical staff to hypothesize whether they would prefer to die rather than continue living in different debilitated states, with dependencies on various forms of life support and reliance on others to perform different activities. Patients rated each situation on a five-point scale indicating whether they considered the state to be worse than death, neither better nor worse than death, a little better than death, somewhat better than death, or much better than death. The researchers discovered that most of their sample considered bowel and bladder incontinence, requiring a breathing tube, and being confused all the time to be fates that are worse than death. More than a third of the sample similarly named being unable to get out of bed, relying on a feeding tube for nourishment, and requiring care from others all the time as the same or worse than death. Most of these scenarios are commonly found in severe dementia.

For my part, I suspect I am hardly alone in being far more frightened of living a long life with a dementing illness than of dying from cancer, heart disease, or other rapidly terminal illnesses. I am equally terrified of witnessing a loved one become demented. I agree with Anna Freud, who wrote, "I believe there is nothing worse than to see the people nearest to one lose the very qualities for which one loves them."[14]

Likewise, I imagine that many others share my dread of bumping along into old age, gradually accommodating to multiple chronic medical disorders, and becoming increasingly dependent on an array of medications, therapies, supportive services, and whichever family members are kind enough to come along for at least part of the ride. It was shocking to read in the *JAMA* article that only one in eight boomers consider their health to be excellent, and that one out of every four people living in the United States will die in a nursing home.[15]

There is a cartoon series called *Futurama* that sometimes depicts the heads—and I literally mean the heads—of wealthy celebrities being kept alive in fluid-filled bell jars where they chat, complain, and crack jokes. In my opinion these are animated Hieronymus Bosch paintings of pure, unadulterated hell.

As a romantic, I am attracted to the conceit that David and Reba Raff were geriatric incarnations of Romeo and Juliet. As a psychiatrist, I am appalled at the inappropriateness of the elderly retired physician being committed to a hospital and distressed at how his spouse would have found most nursing facilities.

Like Chester and Joan Nimitz, I also resent the idea of becoming increasingly dependent on others while watching my assets steadily dwindle. No one—and I mean not a single person who isn't in the top 1 percent—has sufficient insurance or savings to comfortably cover all the exigencies of old age.

Nevertheless, I believe that the Weinstein story came to an understandable, if tragic, conclusion. Yes, it was heartrending. But, despite her early protestations and those of her family, the opportunity for doing something passed. Human beings have a remarkable gift for both adapting to trying circumstances and procrastinating. It appears to me that, at least superficially, Beth accommodated to her cognitive deficits and institutionalization while continuing to find enjoyment in the most basic of activities. All the while, her family found reasons to delay acting, and to their credit, they regularly visited her at the assisted-living facility.

Beth's story is hardly unique in warning that even if one knows exactly what lies ahead and is determined to hasten one's death, there are still myriad shoals upon which to founder. The *Guardian* columnist, Polly Toynbee, wrote recently about an eighty-year-old colleague, Katharine Whitehorn, who was a fervent advocate of the assisted dying.[16] She now resides in an English nursing home,

> suffering from Alzheimer's, with little understanding left, no knowledge of where she is or why. She often doesn't recognise people, can no longer read and curiously sometimes talks in French, not a language she knew particularly well: she will never read or understand this article. In other words, she is not herself. Her old self would not recognise herself in this other being who sits in the care home dayroom. What or who she has become is a difficult

philosophical question, but she is no longer Katharine Whitehorn as was.

Toynbee concludes with the following thoughts:

> How many times have I sat with friends, promising one another that we won't let this happen to us. Yes, we'll find the pills to do the deed, find the willing purveyor on the dark web. (No, none of us knows how to access the dark web.) We will know the right day, just before losing our minds. But that's a comforting delusion. Chances are, we will not be in charge of our fate. Under current tyrannical law, a living will can't save us from dementia. Mostly, Katharine Whitehorn is placid, but in rare flashes of depressed lucidity, her sons say she asks for it to end, to stop now.

Presently, anyone who lives in Britain or the United States and is intent on dying in the early stages of dementia not only needs to communicate preferences, but also must formulate a highly detailed plan with designated loved ones assigned to help implement and oversee it. A timeline is difficult to formulate but essential. The afflicted person, like the remarkable Gillian Bennett, must ideally take the leading role and shouldn't count on others to assume responsibility. One's family must be brought on board and be prepared for all considerations.

In Oregon, a new organization is attempting to change America's "tyrannical" laws and add dementia to the permissible situations for death with dignity.[17] Spearheaded by the indefatigable Derek Humphry, the small group has tentatively settled on the following statement:

> Dementia and Alzheimer's Disease are . . . included . . . [if] the patient has signed an Advance Directive to this effect, and . . . family members (spouse, sibling, offspring; or in the complete absence of family the patient's two closest friends) agree that this form of medical assisted dying was known to be the patient's clear wish before the onset of dementia.

The nonprofit End-of-Life Options in Oregon is preparing for a heated debate when it puts forward this controversial amendment at the State Legislature's meeting in 2019.

In Canada, one of the political parties running in the 2018 election, the Coalition Avenir Quebec, has proposed to both increase provincial funding into Alzheimer's research by $5 million a year and to host public discussions on the use of advance consent for medically assisted deaths for people with neurodegenerative disorders.[18] Quebec's current law on end-of-life care stipulates that an eligible person who is in agony and suffering from an incurable disease must be sufficiently clear-headed to provide consent for obtaining medical assistance in dying. Thus, people suffering from various forms of dementia, including Alzheimer's disease, are presently excluded. Officials would examine the possibility of extending the application of the law to persons who had given prior consent through a living will. A 2017 survey of Quebec caregivers found 91 percent were in favor of medical aid in dying with prior consent, and 72 percent endorsed the use of assisted dying for Alzheimer's patients who signed a written directive before the onset of their illness.

Upon beginning this writing project, I knew almost nothing about quick and effective means to end life; this subject was certainly not covered in medical school. As a psychiatrist, I had been taught that there was nothing worse than suicide—which was automatically equated with prematurely hastening death for mentally ill people. I had not seriously thought about modifying present and future medical aid-in-dying laws to include neurodegenerative disorders. But the stories I uncovered changed me and reconfigured my beliefs. The complexity of the situations and the interplay of values and family relationships combined to suggest that a nuanced and humane approach is sorely needed. Dying people should be afforded more dignity and more choice at the end of life. My next step was to seek out assisted-dying activists—particularly the supporters, but also the disabled opponents—and examine their stories for further insights.

PART II

⟲

When Paul Spiers told me about the death of Hercules during our meeting in Worcester, I was left with the impression that there was more to the mythological saga. After a suitable pause, I inquired, "So, what happened after Hercules died?"

"Funny you should ask," Paul said, and he reprised his eyebrow-twitching Groucho imitation. Brandishing a breadstick like a cigar, he gave me a mischievous smile of delight.

"A few years later and still in possession of the demigod's miraculously accurate bow and arrows, bold Philoctetes joined the Achaean troops who were assembling to wage the Trojan War. His company was led by wily Odysseus (also known as Ulysses), who had them stop for provisions by a sacred island in the Aegean Sea."

"It turns out that one should not disembark on a sacred island unless invited by the deity," said Paul. "This is not only impolite but dangerous. Philoctetes was foraging for food when he was bitten on the foot by a viper. The poisonous snakebite caused him to scream with unbearable pain and to collapse on the ground. In short order, the wound began to emit a repulsive smell."

"Tissue necrosis and gangrene," I interjected.

"Either way," Paul said, lightly dismissing my medical commentary, "the troopers brought the suffering man aboard the ship, set the sails, and resumed their voyage to Troy. But after a while, Philoctetes's companions could no longer bear his tortured cries or the stench. Who knows if they also resented him for having been the one to ignite Hercules's funeral pyre? One could say that there is a steep cost for participating in an assisted suicide, even when it is at the request of a demigod. In any case, the band of warriors were sailing by a desert island when Odysseus decided to drop anchor and abandon Philoctetes on the sandy shore. The boat then resumed its voyage, leaving the poor man to his fate."

GOODBYE, MY LOVE

I went to Oregon expressly to see Derek Humphry, whom Paul Spiers called the "guru" of the Hemlock Society. Peg Sandeen, executive director of the Death with Dignity National Center, had made it clear to me that a respectful pilgrimage to meet Derek was required of anyone seriously exploring the subject of assisted dying.

Joined by my twenty-one-year-old son, Jake, I sat down with Derek in his home office situated within the tiny farming community of Junction City, Oregon. Located in an outbuilding are a couple of sofas, a few photos on the walls, and some exercise equipment pushed to the side. The office looks out over lush countryside and neatly plowed fields.

Derek did not resemble my preconception of what a guru might look like but rather bore a striking resemblance to a Hobbit straight out of a J. R. R. Tolkien book: short, stocky, and clean shaven, his well-rounded facial features accented by prominent white sideburns and impressive eyebrows.

Later, after the meeting, though, Jake and I agreed that, in more important ways, Derek reminded us of another Tolkien character altogether: the wizard, Gandalf the Gray. For one thing, as we came under the influence of Derek's charisma, he seemed to grow in size. He is an enchanting man, quick to laugh and disinclined to take himself too seriously. An octogenarian with many of the usual aches and pains of the elderly—hence the exercise machines—he clearly enjoyed the distraction of an audience. But like Gandalf, Derek has long committed himself to trying to save the world. His cause centered around the idea of giving people the right to end their life at a time, place, and manner of their own choosing. Through his tenacious efforts, he had become the steward of America's death-with-dignity movement. Derek either created or helped fund the Hemlock Society, Caring Friends, the Final Exit Network, NuTech, the Federation of World Right to Die Societies, the Euthanasia Research and Guidance Organization, and the Death with Dignity National Center. Like Gandalf, he traveled constantly, was an inspirational figure who sought to catalyze change, and was decidedly unafraid to engage in conflict—whether at the ballot box, in the courts, at town hall meetings, or within people's homes.

My son and I spent the day listening to the triumphs and tragedies of a life story recounted with panache and passion. We fell into the thrall of a born raconteur, a classic Englishman, master journalist, and revolutionary. Unlike Gandalf the Gray, who only hints at his backstory, Derek was willing to recount in detail how he first came to help a loved one die, as well as the travails that ensued afterward.

Derek was born on April 29, 1930, in Bath, England.[1] He was quite young when his parents acrimoniously divorced. His brother and he were then sent to live with various family members in Somerset. On his fifteenth birthday, Derek fled his devout Anglican aunts and uncles and boarded a train to London. Determined to become a newspaperman, he secured a job as a messenger boy in the London office of the *Yorkshire Post*. Just as World War II was winding down, Derek was drafted into the army. The fighting ceased before he completed basic training, and his military service was uneventfully spent in occupied Germany and Austria.

Upon returning to Britain, the young man achieved his dream by securing a position as a reporter and then moving to the north of England. He worked for the *Manchester Evening News* before meeting and marrying a local girl, Jean Crane. The Humphrys had two children, and in 1960 they adopted a biracial child. By 1967, he was writing feature stories for the prestigious *London Sunday Times* and had also been employed by the *Daily Mail*, the first British newspaper to sell a million copies a day. Derek's investigative reports examined immigration, race relations, police brutality, and the war in Northern Ireland. Despite the lack of a formal education, he authored several topical books, including the award-winning *Because They're Black*, which discussed racial issues in the UK. However, in 1973, Derek's world exploded. Jean was forty-one years old when she noticed a lump in her breast.

The discovery of the tumor was terrifying but hardly a complete surprise. Breast cancer was rampant in Jean's family: four of her aunts had died from the malignancy. Jean promptly underwent a radical mastectomy and afterward was informed that the disease had spread to the lymph nodes. She had a team of skilled doctors and underwent courses of radiation and chemotherapy. Derek decided to move the family away from the bustle of the capital, and he purchased an old house in a tiny Wiltshire village. Jean was in partial remission for nearly a year before the cancer metastasized to her bones and she became progressively more infirm.

A few years earlier, Jean's mother had died of lung cancer. It was a brutal death. Jean had nursed her mother while Derek assumed primary responsibility for their children. "No one ever told the poor woman that she was dying," Derek said to Jake and me. "They didn't have the guts."

To be fair, though, in those days, people rarely had honest, freewheeling discussions about prognosis or terminal care preferences. Derek said his mother-in-law was in constant and agonizing pain and "suffered spiritually and physically." Jean was more traumatized by the experience than her husband realized, but they overcame the worst of the horrors and did not dwell on them until 1974, when Jean, herself, was dying.

One afternoon, Derek went into the Oxford hospital to visit his wife. Jean had just gone through a bad bout during which she almost died. Throughout the illness, Derek continued to hold on to the image of her as being a young and physically strong woman. He was unprepared when she looked up at him from her hospital bed and calmly stated, "I want you to do something for me."

"What's that?"

"I want you to go to a doctor and get an overdose of drugs with which I can take my life when I am ready to go."

This was the first time the couple had ever discussed euthanasia or suicide. Derek knew nothing about the right to die. If you had said to him the word, *euthanasia*, he would have had to pull out a dictionary to look it up. It wasn't commonly spoken except in the context of the Nazi Holocaust.

Jean continued, "I want an agreement now so that when I ask to die, there will be no argument. Nothing. Just get me the drugs. And when I decide, I will take my life."

"What do you want me to do?"

"Go to a doctor and ask him. Store the drugs at home, and when I'm ready to die—and if you agree there is no hope—hand them to me, and I'll die."

"Alright," said Derek. "If our positions were reversed, I would be asking you to help me."

Jean had clearly considered different scenarios, and in the event painkillers might cloud her cognitive faculties she expected Derek to intervene.

He explained, "In other words, if I thought she was under the influence of morphine, I could refuse to give her the lethal drugs." Otherwise, she was insisting on both having the means and being in control of her death.

Jean finished their conversation by announcing she intended to undergo her third course of chemotherapy.

The treatment helped, and Jean carried on and appeared to be doing well for another eight or nine months. She and the family celebrated Christmas and New Year's. However, by February, "She was going down, and the pain was tremendous." The morphine and other analgesics provided only temporary relief. By March, it was apparent that the cancer had spread to the liver and kidneys.

Derek understood but was still denying that she was termi-nally ill. He explained, "It was hard to realize she was dying, because you couldn't see it. But she knew what was going on, on account of the pain."

On the Saturday morning of March 29, 1975, Jean awoke in agony and couldn't raise her head without first taking the pain-killers. Ten minutes later she was finally able to prop herself up in bed and ask her husband, "Is this the day?"

It was a monumental question, and Derek didn't realize that it was also rhetorical. He hemmed and hawed before finally say-ing, "Well, things are getting worse. You are going to have to go back into hospital for more pain control."

Jean answered her own question by stating: "I will die at one o'clock today."

Her spouse was stunned but said, "Okay."

During Derek's career as a journalist, he occasionally reported on health issues in London and had cultivated a relationship with a doctor who, he said, "was my private 'Deep Throat.'"[2] The two men would meet at exclusive restaurants in the city, where the investigative reporter used his expense account to pay for fancy dinners during which "Dr. Joe" would provide colorful details and analyses of medical advances, changes in practice, and current controversies. Several weeks earlier, Derek had begun to accept that his wife's health was rapidly failing and he needed to fulfill her request to acquire medications. He had thought about going to her general practitioner or to a physician from the Oxford medical team and decided instead to consult Dr. Joe. Derek went to his office on Harley Street.

"Jean's dying," he said. "She wants help to die."

Dr. Joe quizzed him at length about the situation. He con-cluded that "Jean had no quality of life left," picked up the phone, and called the Charing Cross Hospital. As the physician spoke with the chief pharmacist, Derek listened to one side of the tele-phone conversation. The two medical professionals had obviously worked together for many years and trusted each other.

"Ideally, what should a person take to end their life?" Dr. Joe inquired into the phone.

Derek couldn't hear the response, but after a minute or two, the physician hung up the receiver and went to his medicine cabinet. He didn't need to write a prescription. Instead, he poured out two types of capsules from large containers and handed over a packet while saying, "Here it is. You will never ever tell that I did this for you."

Derek brought the medication home and carefully hid it away until that March morning when Jean said, "at one o'clock." And even then, he thought: *If one o'clock comes and she doesn't say anything, I'm not going to say anything either.*

While telling this story to Jake and me, a look of admiration settled on his face, and he exclaimed, "But blow me! At one o'clock she said, 'Look at the time. Go and get it!' She was that type of woman, a North countrywoman, blunt spoken, no playing around with her."

Derek left the room, got the packet, and tears were streaming down his face as he mixed its contents in a cup of coffee with some sugar. He brought it back and put it down next to the bed on the nightstand.

"Is that it?" she asked.

"Yes. If you drink this you'll die."

Derek got into bed alongside her.

Forty years later, he told Jake and me, "We had a last . . ."

I think he was going to say "snuggle," but at this point he interrupted his narrative, visibly distraught, and began to cry out, "It hurts! It hurts! Despite all these years! It hurts!" Derek not only began weeping, but he also started to loudly and repeatedly smack his forehead with his hand, again, and again, and again.

Although it seemed to go on for an eternity, it was probably less than a minute before Derek regained his composure and explained to Jake and me, "I can't stop it. I am an emotional person. . . . It just comes . . . and I want it to stop."

"What is the feeling?" I asked him.

"It is loss. I don't regret helping her to die at all. I'm proud that as a duty of love I helped her to die. . . . We had a good marriage for twenty-two years."

Calming down, Derek picked up the thread of his story: "She raised the cup and drank the contents. She just said, 'Goodbye, my love,' and she was gone." He resumed crying, but this time more softly, more tenderly. "I was amazed at her courage," he said. "She looked like the same woman . . . and then she was dead."

In Derek's memoir, he adds a bit more to this story relating that, after Jean passed out, she vomited and, worried that she might have expelled the medication, Derek readied himself to suffocate her with a pillow.[3] According to his account, however, she died without any further intervention.

Jean had told each of her three boys what she was going to do. They were together in the next room. Derek's father and his brother knew too, and understood. No one objected. They had all witnessed her suffering and her bravery.

Derek telephoned the family physician, who came to complete the death certificate. The widower intentionally took refuge in the garden. He was not prepared to lie. But the general practitioner did not ask any questions of him, remained unaware of the overdose, and wrote on the official form that the cause of death was metastatic carcinoma.

Jean's body was later cremated.

Derek returned to his assignments at the *Sunday Times*. He would eventually write, "Not once did the manner of Jean's death bother me. My conscience on that score was, and still is, clear."[4]

During the next year, he met and married an American woman, Ann Wickett. According to Richard Côté, Derek's chronicler, whom I later interviewed, "both were on the rebound from different marital disasters and brought substantial emotional baggage to their union."[5]

Wickett encouraged Derek to write a book, and she helped him to understand that, even if it was told from his perspective, it was basically a woman's story. Despite the vigorous efforts of one of the best agents in London, nobody wanted to publish *Jean's Way*. Derek's newspaper bought the rights, paid him the agreed-upon amount of money, and then decided not to run the series. The explanation? "It is too depressing," the editors told him. "It will make the readers cry."

Derek says he seriously doubts that this was the real reason. Rather, he believes it was, and remains, a radioactive topic for many people.

When Derek finally found a publisher, he was told, "Yes, I'll publish this, but you have to be prepared to accept the consequences. You will need to stand by this book." What the publisher understood better than Derek were the criminal ramifications of the story. Section Two of England's Suicide Act of 1961 listed a prison sentence of up to fourteen years for anyone found guilty of the felony of assisting suicide. Similar laws are still on the books in many American states.

Meanwhile, a few thousand copies were printed and placed in bookstores. They promptly sold out in a week and *Jean's Way* became the bestseller of the month. Suddenly, Derek was all over the newspapers and on television, where he debated various bishops, as well as Malcolm Muggeridge, the BBC media personality and moral campaigner of the day. The book received tremendous publicity, and Derek found himself articulating a philosophy that spoke to his new-found belief in the morality of assisted suicide. He had never previously considered these issues but acted reflexively in writing the book, much as he had instinctively responded to the love and duty he felt toward his wife.

Jean's Way was immensely popular in Australia, and Derek was invited on a speaking tour. Upon returning to London, Derek realized he and Wickett wanted to leave the UK and live elsewhere. So, he joined the reporting staff of the *Los Angeles Times* and prepared to move with his new partner to California.

As Derek recalls, "However, when the newspapers ran out of stories, they called the director of public prosecution." At that time, there was but one prosecutor for the whole of Britain, and no case, including violations of the Suicide Act, could be undertaken without his approval. The media approached his office about Derek's presumed criminal behavior, and the director issued a statement announcing that he would launch an investigation. The Wiltshire police had jurisdiction in the town where Jean had died, and he ordered them to begin conducting a formal inquiry.

When a reporter from the *Daily Mirror*, Britain's largest-circulation paper at the time, called Derek to ask what he was going to do, he said: "I'll plead guilty and throw myself on the mercy of the court." That statement produced big headlines. But, as Derek remembers it, he thought, *What else can I do? I am guilty as hell.*

Derek made an appointment with the Wiltshire police to meet him at his attorney's office. Having secured the help of an experienced civil liberties lawyer, Derek wrote out a two-paragraph confession in which he stated that everything he had written in his book was true. He had helped Jean to die. All he had said on radio or on television about the circumstances was factual. As the chief detective entered the room, the lawyer handed him the brief document. The police officer read it and was flabbergasted that he had come all the way to London to be given a confession that took one minute to read.

But the law enforcement official also wanted to know the name of the doctor who supplied the lethal medicines, and Derek refused to provide it. This is a confidence that he has continued to keep for the past forty years. He and the chief detective argued over the issue for twenty minutes. Derek felt that he had otherwise been entirely cooperative. He gave permission for the police to interview his extended family, as well as the various physicians who had managed Jean's cancer. The widower explained to the police how he had kept the general practitioner in the dark about the overdose. Only after reading the book had that worthy gentleman learned how Jean ended her life.

Although Derek must have had more than a few anxious moments, with a big grin he told Jake and me, "I was a hardnosed reporter for thirty years and used to public life and television. I had a good guess they would not prosecute. I knew that the prosecutor was a liberal-minded man. . . . In the pub one night, a group of us were drinking. . . . We were all drunk, and my attorney stood up and said, 'Members of the jury, if you convict Derek Humphry,' and the lawyer paused dramatically before continuing, 'You will make him a rich man!' All of us laughed! Nobody realistically thought I would be prosecuted."

Derek moved to California while the investigation was still taking place. Disembarking from his plane in San Francisco, he perused a copy of the *San Francisco Examiner* and spotted a small article with a headline that read: "Mercy Killer Goes Free." As he glanced at it, he thought to himself, *They've got the same problem here, too!* However, examining the newspaper more closely, he realized that the story was about him! *He* was the mercy killer. While in transit, his lawyer had tried repeatedly but unsuccessfully to contact him with the news that the case had been dropped.

The investigation had lasted about six months before Derek's lawyer heard from the director of public prosecution. The director privately told the lawyer that he admired Jean's courage. He said that Jean had made the decision and carried it out, concluding that the determination to die in this manner was obviously her responsibility and not Derek's.

But Derek's odyssey would continue.

ᘓᒻ

DR. DEATH

On a rainy evening in 2011, I finished giving an ethics lecture at the New York Academy of Medicine, grabbed a plate of food from the buffet, and made an extra sandwich that I handed to a homeless man who was lying wrapped in a sleeping bag outside the building's marble entrance on 103rd Street and Fifth Avenue. I thought of my sons, who routinely do such random acts of kindness. I am usually less inclined but needed something to counteract the opulence of the Academy meeting and to prepare for my next activity. I was going to the preview of an auction, and these can sometimes figuratively or literally entail rooting through a deceased person's underwear drawer. I had a premonition that the forthcoming experience was going to be disquieting.

Slipping along the windswept rainy streets, I searched for the location of the Dr. Jack Kevorkian auction at the New York Institute of Technology. The address brought me to the slick glass door of a place that appeared as if it had been a fashionable clothing boutique in a previous incarnation. There were no signs indicating that I had arrived at the correct destination.

"Hello? Hello?" I called. "Anyone here?"

My clothes were dripping as I carefully slid through the dark entranceway and left my umbrella propped up against a wall. Sitting at a dimly lit table with papers spread out in front of him was an older, heavy-set man in an expensively tailored suit.

My shoes made squeaking sounds on the tile floor as I approached. "I'm here for the auction preview," I said. "I'm Dr. Lew Cohen, and I've come from Massachusetts." I explained that I was doing research for a book about assisted suicide.

"And I'm Mayer Morganroth," he replied. "That's Jack's niece, Ava Janus, over there," pointing to a preoccupied-looking young woman huddled over another pile of papers. "You are welcome to walk around and see what's here."

Pausing for a moment and mistakenly assuming I knew what was going on, he continued, "Don't worry about the ridiculous lawsuit. It is just a delaying tactic and will get settled."

I was hardly shocked to hear that there was a conflict involving the estate. Having spoken to numerous people acquainted with Jack Kevorkian, no one ever suggested he was an easygoing individual. His biography is written by two close friends, Neal Nicol and Harry Wylie, but even they could not conceal his habitual pugnaciousness.[1] Kevorkian's personal attorney, Geoffrey Fieger, witnessed numerous diatribes when he was in the midst of his "real asshole" mode.[2] *Time* magazine called him a man "who has made defiance of the law a passion second only to suicide."[3] The word, *defiance*, is well chosen. Faye Girsh, the president of the World Societies for the Right to Die, maintains that Kevorkian consistently displayed moral courage and the will for self-sacrifice toward the greater good of humanity, but even she can't help but admit these attributes were matched by his penchant for being cantankerous.

According to multiple accounts, Kevorkian was a man who neither worked nor played well with others; he consistently refused to compromise or to cooperate with other leaders in the movement for death with dignity, insisting that *his* was the only rational approach. Derek Humphry recalled a visit from Kevorkian in the 1980s when he had proposed that all Hemlock Society members be referred to a suicide clinic.[4] When Derek tried to explain his belief that people should ideally end life in the privacy of their own homes and not in a medical facility, Kevorkian began to shout that it was in their best interest to do it *his* way under *his* supervision. At that point, Derek explained, "Jack stormed out of my office."

On the other hand, Kevorkian's biographers describe him as being "a shy, eccentric man who lived a monastic, ethical life, buying his clothes at the Salvation Army and subsisting on the plainest of food, particularly white bread."[5] They write that he was incapable of guile, and "when he played poker with his friends he never bluffed, and if he bet, everyone folded."[6] No one ever accused him of being self-indulgent or of trying to financially capitalize on his fame. He resided for much of his adult life in a one-room apartment above a store, and he never charged anyone for assisting in their deaths.

Love or hate him, though, there is no getting around the fact that Kevorkian was the brash face of the American right-to-die movement for almost a decade. Although he arrived on the scene ten years after Derek had founded the Hemlock Society, it was the antics of Kevorkian—or "Dr. Death" as he came to be known—that repeatedly brought the issue of the right to die to breakfast table conversations all over the world. During an eight-year period, Kevorkian participated in more than one hundred thirty assisted suicides. On five occasions, prosecutors tried him for the death of a seriously ill person; three trials ended in acquittals and a fourth in a mistrial, before he was finally convicted in 1999.

Derek told me that he and Jack "never hit it off," despite the fact that they were "fundamentally driving down the same track, seeking to allow all people who enjoyed a good life to then achieve a good death."

In his memoir, Derek wrote that Kevorkian "will go down in history as a major catalyst for reform by getting public attention via the media's morbid fascination."[7] As he told me: "There is only one person the American public associates with the right-to-die movement. It isn't Faye Girsh and it isn't me. It is Jack Kevorkian. His is the one name people know."

As I walked past Morganroth into the preview, large and colorful reproductions of Kevorkian's paintings were on display.

I had never seen his art before. The originals were estimated to fetch $100,000 to $150,000 apiece. They were startling. To call them crude and ghastly depictions of death is to minimize their horror. The subject matter included: dripping blood, giant rabbits, knives, Adolph Hitler, J. S. Bach, and a surfeit of skeletons. The paintings offered a window into the mind of a man clearly obsessed with mortality and destruction.

A painting entitled, *Fa La La La La, - La La, - La, - LA!*, for example, was meant to provide a visual commentary on the waste and commercialism of Christmas. Santa's foot was depicted as coming down a chimney about to crush a baby Jesus. A rotting corpse stood wrapped in Christmas garlands behind large boxes covered with wrapping paper and festive ribbons.

Against a far wall stood the exhibit's big-ticket item. Carrying an estimated value of $200,000 to $300,000—the Thanatron was one of the so-called suicide machines that Kevorkian jerry-rigged at home, with parts acquired at flea-markets and local hardware stores. The accompanying caption noted that anyone could use the device to "quickly and painlessly leave their daily suffering behind."

Kevorkian's patients self-administered lethal doses of medications or canisters of carbon monoxide with the devices. Reliance on the suicide machines repeatedly helped him to avoid criminal prosecution on a technicality—arguing that while he may have made the equipment, his patients were the ones who ended their lives.

Kevorkian would employ one of these instruments when he helped fifty-four-year-old Janet Adkins, an Alzheimer's sufferer. He could not find a suitable place for her to die and had to settle on the back of his rusty VW van.

Adkins was among the initial batch of people to reach out to Kevorkian for help, and her husband, Ron, and she were prepared to travel from their comfortable home in Portland, Oregon, to meet with him in Michigan. The couple had read and were impressed with a *Newsweek* story about him.

Adkins and her husband were both longtime members of the Hemlock Society, and their beliefs about accelerating death were clear and consistent. She was good-naturedly accompanied by Ron to four separate sessions with Kevorkian, during which her medical situation and motivation for dying were reviewed (three of the meetings were recorded). When Kevorkian recommended that she consider participating in an experimental dementia research protocol at the University of Washington, she immediately acquiesced and underwent what proved to be an unsuccessful six-month course of investigative treatment.

After her death, the Alzheimer's Association would subsequently publish a letter from Ron in the national newsletter, *Advances*:[8]

> My wife, Janet Adkins was excited by life. She was a woman of many ideas and interests. She was a talented musician and an avid reader. She liked pushing the limit and trying new things, such as trekking to Nepal.
>
> When she was diagnosed with Alzheimer's disease at age 53, she was devastated. She weighed the options of letting the disease take her mind and body or exiting early with the assistance of a doctor while her intellect was still intact. We had openly discussed end-of-life issues, and her choice was not to let the disease progress.
>
> We made an informed decision and a personal choice, one that was right for Janet. Most importantly, we opened end-of-life issues together as a family. I encourage others to do the same.

To the present day, people remain divided in their opinion of Kevorkian. My good friend, Dr. Carl Kjellstrand—always a contrarian—is representative of the admirers and wrote a fulsome opinion piece.[9] Much like the right-to-die advocate Faye Girsh, Kjellstrand is convinced that the man was a hero, in accordance with the classic Greek definition, and in the face of danger and adversity displayed unflagging courage and willingness to sacrifice himself for some greater good to humanity.

However, there are three things that one regularly hears from those who were outraged by Kevorkian and his right-to-die campaign. The first was the man's insatiable hunger for the spotlight. His public relations pranks included appearing at an interview while restrained in an old village wooden stock, and his arrival at a court hearing dressed in Colonial-era garb to symbolically demonstrate how the laws and criminal statutes concerning the care of the dying were antiquated.

Medical professionals disliked that Kevorkian was a pathologist—someone trained to examine cadavers and arrive at diagnoses from tissue biopsies—who posed as a clinician. Pathologists are generally the final word in diagnosis, and they are accustomed to exposing medical failures. Kevorkian embraced that aspect of the role, but he pursued it with living, breathing, miserable people who underscored modern medicine's limitations. Many of the patients who sought out his assistance had suffered from treatment complications and were deeply disappointed with the care they had received.

Others continue to fault Kevorkian for disproportionately assisting in the deaths of women and those who were not actively dying.[10] But more than anything else, doctors asked, why did Kevorkian select for his first patient someone who was suffering with an illness that destroys cognitive abilities and can potentially influence the delicate balance necessary to make sound life-and-death decisions? Why pick a disease that kills in slow increments over the span of decades, rather than a terminal illness like pancreatic cancer, metastatic carcinoma, or acute leukemia that ends life within a span of months? Why start with a medical disorder that is so fraught with ethical complexities? Why dementia?

I believe that the answer is one that even today, most physicians don't want to hear or accept: that the deterioration from dementia is a fate worse than death. I suspect Kevorkian felt the same way, and he was always supremely confident that everyone would eventually see things *his* way.

As I wandered through the gallery exhibiting Kevorkian's grotesque paintings and personal effects, I had an opportunity to spend a few minutes talking with Morganroth. He was a Michigan attorney who represented Kevorkian in several of the legal cases and developed a warm friendship with him. Morganroth explained that Kevorkian made a serious error in judgment in his final trial in 1999 by believing he could represent himself.

"Although an attorney was appointed," Morganroth recounted, "he was a disaster, and Jack turned to me for advice." But by that time it was too late. Kevorkian was found guilty of second-degree murder for his role in the death of Thomas Youk, and he received a sentence of ten to twenty-five years in prison. If the jury had found him guilty of first-degree murder, it would have carried a life sentence. But, in the end, the length of the sentence made little difference to the elderly physician.

Kevorkian was always ready to go to prison if it could raise awareness about what he considered to be America's tyrannical euthanasia laws; however, in previous cases, his cause had been well represented by the moving testimony of bereaved next of kin on his behalf. Such family members were frequently Kevorkian's most steadfast defenders. Their words touched the hearts of the jury when they declared that the slender man sitting before them was a saint. The families passionately argued that, when all other physicians failed to help their loved one, Kevorkian alone stood up and responded courageously and compassionately.

Because of Kevorkian's hubris, however, his maladroit efforts to represent himself in the last trial led the presiding judge to rule that Youk's widow and brother could not testify. When Kevorkian went out to dinner with the family that evening, they expressed their bitter disappointment at being denied the opportunity to describe to the jury the suffering of their loved one, his emphatic wish to die, and their overwhelming gratitude to the man who had responded to his final request.

The verdict might very well have been different if they had testified, but then again, this case differed in several ways from previous trials. It was not an assisted suicide but an instance of voluntary euthanasia. Youk, a fifty-two-year-old Detroit native, suffered from Lou Gehrig's Disease and had lost voluntary muscle control over most of his body. Accordingly, Kevorkian did not employ a suicide machine but instead injected the medicine himself directly into Youk's vein.

Jack Lessenberry is a journalist from the *Detroit Metro Times* who covered all of Kevorkian's trials and probably got to know him better than any other reporter. After originally euthanizing Thomas Youk, Kevorkian went to the reporter for advice about how to reach a national audience and ratchet up the debate to a new level. Lessenberry knew Mike Wallace, and he suggested that Kevorkian approach him for an appearance on *60 Minutes*. The columnist would later characterize himself as having inadvertently become "a minor instrument of the good doctor's own demise."[11]

To his credit, Kevorkian routinely videotaped patient sessions and thereby left a record showing how he actively tried to discourage people from hastening death without first exploring other treatment options. To the best of my knowledge, these tapes have largely been kept confidential (I stumbled upon one television documentary that featured excerpts from four them),[12] but when Kevorkian was invited to appear on *60 Minutes*, he broke with his usual practice and provided the Youk recording for broadcast to a national audience.[13]

Not surprisingly, the most damning and incontrovertible evidence at the subsequent trial was the segment of the videotape in which Kevorkian could be seen administering the fatal injection.

"Are you sure you want to go ahead now?" Kevorkian asked.

Youk nodded.

"We're ready to inject. We're going to inject in your right arm."

Kevorkian could be seen administering the barbiturate, Seconal, followed by a muscle relaxant and potassium chloride; the latter short-circuits the electrical system of the heart.

He then looked at the electrocardiogram tracing and turned to the camera, announcing, "Now there's a straight line. His heart has stopped."

Following Kevorkian's instructions, when Mrs. Youk and her brother later returned to the house they called the hospice. They asked that someone be sent over to certify the death. It was the hospice staff member who spotted Kevorkian's name on a Federal Express receipt, became suspicious, called the police, and initiated the formal investigation.

Three days after the broadcast, Kevorkian was charged with first-degree murder and delivering a controlled substance without a medical license (his had been suspended some time earlier).

Before delivering the sentence, Judge Jessica Cooper stated, "You were not licensed to practice medicine when you committed this offense. . . . And you had the audacity to go on national television, show the world what you did and dare the legal system to stop you. Well, sir, consider yourself stopped."[14]

Although momentarily disappointed with the outcome, Kevorkian was still optimistic that he could turn it to his advantage. The journalist Lessenberry was in the court and observed, "What he thought was once he was convicted, people would surround the prison and demand his release and the world would be safe for euthanasia. . . . [But] the prosecutor looked at me and said, 'Prisoners don't usually get to hold press conferences.'"[15]

Later, reflecting on the case, Lessenberry would write:

> Jack Kevorkian, faults and all, was a major force for good in this society. He forced us to pay attention to one of the biggest elephants in society's living room: the fact that today vast numbers of people are alive who would rather be dead; who have lives not worth living.
>
> Yet legally they are helpless to do anything about it. A young woman may legally destroy a healthy young embryo growing in her body. Yet if she has a terrible and incurable disease—bone cancer, say—that dooms her to death and tortures her with pain, she legally can do nothing to end her suffering.
>
> That's why people paid attention to Jack Kevorkian.[16]

HEMLOCK

When *Jean's Way* was first published in America, it was not particularly successful. However, all the television networks eagerly sought out Derek Humphry to relate the story. He was a guest on *Good Morning America*, the *Donahue Show*, and other trendy programs, where his honest approach and British accent drew wide appeal. The public began to write to him with their questions: What drugs did Jean use? How can you kill yourself rapidly and painlessly? How should families talk about this subject?

Mike Wallace interviewed him on *60 Minutes*, the most popular TV show in the United States at the time, and asked, "What are you going to do now?" Not having consciously thought about the topic, Derek says he was practically as astonished as the television audience when he heard himself saying, "I'm going to form an organization and fight to change the law." Perhaps thinking that Derek was kidding, Wallace laughed uproariously at the remark.

Derek wrote a series of articles on death and dying in the *Los Angeles Times* and his final one addressed euthanasia. He got to know a lot of people, particularly on the West Coast, who were interested in making choices about dying. California had just passed the world's first living will law in 1976. It went into effect in 1978, just as he arrived. As he told me, "The subject was hot in California."

Furthermore, three weeks after Jean's death, a twenty-one-year-old woman named Karen Ann Quinlan lapsed into a permanent vegetative state after ingesting alcohol and Valium at a party.[1] Her parents, staunch Roman Catholics, knew their daughter would not want to be kept alive by extraordinary means, and they fought for the right to make legally binding treatment decisions on her behalf. They were aided in this battle by the support of Monsignor Trapasso, then pastor of Our Lady of the Lake Roman Catholic Church in Mount Arlington, New Jersey. He cited church teachings and a 1957 declaration by Pope Pius XII that held there was no moral obligation to continue aggressive medical care to sustain life in the absence of realistic hope of recovery.[2] In 1976, the New Jersey Supreme Court allowed the withdrawal of Quinlan's mechanical ventilation, thereby permitting her to die.

But, to everyone's surprise, she didn't.

The artificial feeding was continued, and it wouldn't be until *nine* years later, in 1985, that she eventually succumbed to pneumonia. At the time of her death, Karen Ann Quinlan was thirty-one years old, weighed sixty-five pounds, and had been comatose for a decade.

In 1983, another case caught the media's attention. Nancy Cruzan, then twenty-five years old, lost control of her car and was found lying face down in a ditch with no heartbeat or respiration.[3] Cruzan sustained permanent brain damage from lack of oxygen, but her life was maintained by use of a feeding tube that provided nutrition and hydration. After several years, a court determined that, like Quinlan, she was in a persistent vegetative state. Although her breathing and circulation continued unaided, she was largely oblivious to her surroundings, had no cognitive or reflexive ability to swallow food or water, and had developed a spastic quadriplegia causing her limbs to atrophy. In 1990, the United States Supreme Court determined there was no hope for recovery, and they found sufficient evidence to establish that she would not have wanted her life sustained. The justices ordered the feeding tube removed.

There is a sad and lesser-known postscript to Cruzan's case, however, that led her attorney, William H. Colby, to use the plural in the title of his book, *Long Goodbye: The Deaths of Nancy Cruzan*.[4] Colby wrote about how Cruzan's father, Joe Cruzan, later hanged himself in the carport of the family home, leaving behind a suicide note. He was exhausted by the legal fight and had been a target of intense criticism by right-to-life proponents. For example, the Rev. Joseph Foreman, told reporters after Cruzan died: "I sympathize with the hardship of caring for a helpless woman, but I have no sympathy for a family who solves their problems by starving their daughter to death when there were hundreds of bona fide offers to care for her regardless of her condition. Even a dog in Missouri cannot be legally starved to death."[5]

The family would respond with a statement that Joe Cruzan was "proud he carried out his daughter's wish and helped others in the same situation, but knowledge and pride could not fend off the depression of her accident and the loss of a daughter."

Cruzan's and Quinlan's cases—highlighting the difficult choices involved in handling situations when brain-damaged people were placed on life-support systems—woke up the world to the extent to which medicine had changed. The public had not previously appreciated the dilemmas that the new medical advances and modern intensive care were creating. Most people had barely heard of breathing machines, kidney dialysis, cardiac stimulants, and artificial feeding, while media attention was almost exclusively focused on the life-saving potential of these devices and treatment protocols.

Now people were confronted by the fact that the modern medical miracles were just as likely to draw out and prolong the process of dying. Even if people survived, they might no longer be able to interact with loved ones, resume activities that were important to them, or physically function the same. The ethics and morality of starting, withholding, and withdrawing treatments seemed like a quagmire. The cost in human and financial terms hadn't been sufficiently considered. Only after a period of unrealistic optimism was the public given an opportunity to reflect on the drawbacks of temporarily and incompletely salvaging lives that would otherwise have ended.

In 1978, a play by Brian Carter premiered in London that addressed these issues directly. Derek was invited to the Mermaid Theatre's opening night of *Whose Life Is It Anyway?*[6] The play's lead character is a sculptor who becomes paralyzed from the neck down following a car accident. He demands to be allowed to die, but neither the doctors nor the hospital administrators are willing to accept his ultimatum. The play's successful reception led to a Broadway production that won Tom Conti the 1979 Tony Award for best actor, and in a gender reversal, Mary Tyler Moore won a special Tony Award for her performance the following year. A popular Hollywood film with the same title was released in 1981 starring Richard Dreyfuss.[7]

When my son Jake and I visited Derek, he told us how timing was crucial for Brian Carter and for himself. Originally written six years earlier as a screenplay that was broadcast on television, *Whose Life Is It Anyway?* had received barely any attention from the public. Carter then rewrote it for the stage, but it took years for him to find someone willing to produce the play on Broadway. "And then just like that," Derek loudly snapped his fingers, "he got it at the Mermaid, and it turned out it was the same month that *Jean's Way* came out. So, between Cruzan, Quinlan, *Whose Life Is It Anyway?*, and *Jean's Way*, the oyster was opening up! The oyster was pretty much opening up to intelligent, thoughtful people across the English-speaking world. It was a case of a set of ideas occurring at the right place at the right time."

Immediately following the *60 Minutes* broadcast, where Derek had blurted out his intention to form a right-to-die organization, he came to a decision. He arranged for fourteen like-minded friends to meet at a home in Brentwood. It was 1980, and all of those assembled agreed there was a need for a group to promote lawful assisted suicide. Derek joked that they already had the *Good Housekeeping* seal of approval, because the magazine had just begun serializing *Jean's Way*. "All the earlier efforts in the United States to promote euthanasia, dating back to the 1920s," he explained, "had been nascent and scattered." But now a unique opportunity seemed to present itself.

There was consensus that a new organization should be formed, but when the ebullient Englishman asked who would join in this endeavor, not one person stepped forward. He repeated his call for action, and a single individual, Gerald Larue, now a professor emeritus of religion at the University of Southern California, spoke up in favor of the plan and plaintively asked the assembled, "How can you say you want it, but not support Derek?"

Some of the group abashedly answered that their children attended Catholic schools and might suffer consequences. Others worried that clients would abandon their businesses if they were identified with this cause. Still others said they feared their houses could be bombed, because there were a lot of abortion clinics being attacked at the time. The meeting ended uncomfortably.

After the room had cleared out, Derek turned to Larue and announced, "You're the president, I am the CEO, and my wife is the treasurer."

"Why me?" asked Larue

"Who else?" said the bushy-eyebrowed man.

They decided to name the organization the "Hemlock Society" to evoke the careful consideration Socrates gave before swallowing a drink infused with the poisonous plant. A press conference was called on August 12, 1980. One reporter asked whether the Hemlock Society was going to be in the Yellow Pages, and although the organizers hadn't thought of it until that very second, they enthusiastically declared that it would be. Earlier in the day, a friend of Larue's had joined the organization. Accordingly, when the reporters inquired, "How strong are you?" the reply was, "We are growing every day." Derek was anxious about whether the reporter would have a follow-up question as to how many people were in the Hemlock Society, but fortunately he did not.

Before long, though, their numbers did expand. In short order, a thousand American men and women had joined the group and, not long after that, the number of dues-paying members doubled. People were attracted to the Hemlock Society's dual mission of providing information to dying persons who thought about accelerating their deaths, and passing legislation permitting carefully regulated physician-assisted suicide. According to Richard Côté, at its peak the Hemlock Society had fifty-seven thousand paid members spread across eighty-six chapters throughout the United States. Coté wrote, "The self-deliverance genie had been forever freed from its bottle and had taken on a robust, self-sustaining life of its own."[8]

While previous organizations had campaigned for greater use of living wills, Hemlock's members were less interested in that issue. Derek put it succinctly, "Bugger living wills! How do I kill myself?"

Derek decided to write a book on how to take one's own life, and he sought legal advice about it. The attorney told him that if the book was absolutely true and based on people's lives then the law could not touch him. Derek promptly sent a letter to all the Hemlock Society members inquiring whether they had a story to tell about having helped someone to die. He received a string of replies, and he followed up by flying all over the country to conduct interviews. In 1982, Derek published, *Let Me Die Before I Wake*.[9]

He then began researching *Final Exit: The Practicalities of Self-Deliverance and Assisted Suicide for the Dying*.[10] The book is now widely recognized as being a suicide manual, and it has sections on death-accelerating practices, advance care planning, and the legal ramifications.[11]

Hemlock and the writing project became Derek's passions, and he left the *Los Angeles Times*. The manuscript began to take shape, but as with *Jean's Way*, he found publishers were wary. He decided to self-publish in 1991.

A reporter from the *Wall Street Journal* called him and asked, "Who is going to *hate* this book?" Derek promptly provided a list of names of people he thought would despise *Final Exit*. Between the *Journal*'s provocative article and the Hemlock's new membership, the original printing of forty thousand copies quickly sold out. The following week, they printed another hundred thousand books and these, too, were immediately purchased. The pattern kept repeating, swelling Hemlock's and Derek's bank accounts.

Final Exit was translated into twelve languages. The strongest foreign sales have ironically been in the Catholic countries of Italy and Spain.

Derek has never been formally investigated by law enforcement other than in the aftermath of Jean's death. He has directly assisted very few people to die, and they were relatives or dear friends. He told Jake and me: "You never really know what will happen when you're helping a stranger to die. Even if you know them a bit, you can't be sure to whom they left their money, or whether they are in the middle of a quarrel with someone, or who is going to be mad when they find out about the death. With your own intimate family and friends, you know the circumstances."

He then proceeded to tell us about two cases, and first emphasized that in most instances of assisted dying, and especially those that follow the legal state protocols, things go smoothly and without a hitch. But this is not guaranteed. Proponents are hesitant to acknowledge these unfortunate circumstances because they rightfully believe that opposition spokespersons will seize hold of them to make the case that the practice is unsafe and unwise. To Derek's credit, he prefers to be open about such matters, but for the sake of prudence I have slightly altered the identities of the participants from his account.

"I've taken part in only one Oregon death with dignity, and it didn't go very well," Derek exclaimed.

> She was a forty-eight-year-old woman who got brain cancer. I knew the parents much better than her. She had come home to die—you are allowed to do that even if you don't live in Oregon. You can come home to your parents, to your family. They called me, and I witnessed her death request. I signed for it.
>
> But her parents then called me and said, "We want you to be here."
>
> "But she doesn't need me," I said. "You've got it all properly organized."

They said, "We'd like you to be here, Derek." So, I agreed and went down to their farmhouse outside of Medford.

She decided to die at 11 o'clock in the morning. Along with family and a couple of friends, I sat with her. She picked up the drink, drank it, and said, "Oooh, that's awful." She then passed out.

But hours later, she was still alive and her parents were going bonkers. I went out in the garden to occupy myself with a book. . . . I tried to keep out of the way but not run away. Her mother was going around, literally tearing her hair out, saying, "What is going to happen?" and, "She was supposed to be dead!" and, "What can we do?"

I tried to calm her, and said, "She's bound to die. She has taken a huge dose. Perhaps it won't be until the early hours of the morning." I went in to look, and the breathing was very shallow.

The family phoned the doctor who had written the lawful prescription, and he said, "Perhaps she'll wake up, and we'll have to administer it all again." That sent them over the edge. They were mad, angry, and frustrated.

In the garden, the mother said to me, "What can I do?"

I said, "If you put a plastic bag over her head, given that the breathing is so shallow, she will die very quickly." But I also made it explicit and told her, "It is your decision, because in any case she will die during the night." Nothing further was stated, and we all went to dinner.

Around the farmhouse table, the father, brothers, and sisters sat. They were a lovely family. They all knew what was happening in the next room. Suddenly, the mother came in and began eating her dinner. She looked up from the food and announced, "Fran is dead."

The mother told me later that she had put a piece of plastic over her daughter's face. She wanted to stop that narrow, shallow breathing. It was all very moving. The family was very sensitive and caring. But that was my only lawful experience, and it didn't go too well.

Derek stared at Jake and me. He said: "Now, if I was in that position again, I would've told the daughter to first have a couple of scotches or a vodka to accelerate the medication. She would've died in half an hour. I would also never watch a friend just use ten grams of Seconal. The Swiss are now using twelve grams. The daughter was a young woman, and she was strong from having always worked on farms."

Before our visit to Oregon, I had read about Derek's disastrous second marriage and therefore had distinctly mixed feelings when he brought up the subject. Ann Wickett was described to me by Derek as having "a severe borderline personality disorder." She was being treated for breast cancer at the time she filed for divorce; the marriage had completely self-destructed. However, Wickett proceeded to publicly accuse Derek of abandoning her. Although Wickett's cancer was in remission and she was not terminally ill, she nevertheless became convinced that she was going to die from the disease.[12] Based on her situation, Wickett decided there were subtle pressures being brought to bear on vulnerable people like herself, which contributed to any decision on their part to embrace euthanasia and assisted dying. Wickett gave interviews to multiple newspaper reporters condemning Derek and the Hemlock Society. She appeared on the *Sally Jesse Raphael* and *Larry King* shows, and tried unsuccessfully to obtain a book contract. Derek countered with a four-page statement, entitled, "Why My Marriage to Ann Wickett Failed."

In October of 1990, several months after the divorce was finalized, Wickett filed a $6 million lawsuit against Derek and the Hemlock Society. In it she asserted that he had committed libel and interfered with her cancer recovery. She also expressed regrets and added details—whether true or false remains unclear—as to the circumstances around her parents' deaths. That was the second case (or third if you include Jean) that Derek told me about in which he actively played a role in helping someone to die.

Derek has publicly mentioned but never written about his involvement in the deaths of Ann Wickett's parents. Once again, I have chosen to slightly alter some of the details.

In 1986, Robert Kooman was ninety-two years old and slowly dying of congestive heart failure, while Cynthia was seventy-eight years old and had undergone a series of crippling strokes.[13] The couple were members of the Hemlock Society and lived in Boston, where Robert was a retired banker. One day, they called up Derek and their daughter, and announced, "We want to die. And not only do we want to die, but we want to die together. Will you help us?"

Derek and Wickett flew to Massachusetts and moved into a spare bedroom. It was evident that Wickett's parents were firm in their resolve. Although her activities of daily life had been impaired by the strokes, Cynthia was not terminally ill. Derek took his mother-in-law to a nearby park in her wheelchair. It was quiet and peaceful amid the verdant hedges and bright beds of flowers; they sat together on a bench in the dappled sunlight. He said, "Cynthia, you don't have to die. We will take you back to California. There is a nursing home near us by Santa Monica beach. You will always be close to us."

"No, Derek," she said. "I want to go with Robert, I'm not staying."

Derek was concerned about how the Kooman's niece might react to their deaths, as there had been conflicts among family members. He told the elderly couple, "We can't help you unless we find out how your niece feels about this. Please arrange for her to come for breakfast so that we can all talk."

The next morning the niece arrived, and Derek said, "Tonight your aunt and uncle are going to take their lives. It's their decision, and we're supporting them. But what will you do?"

The niece replied, "I give you my word that I will say nothing and do nothing. I just don't want anything to do with them."

"That's good enough for me," said Derek.

Derek spent the balance of the day with Wickett and her parents. Then the elderly couple had a light snack for dinner, and the Seconal was mixed up in a blender with ice cream for Robert and yogurt for Cynthia. They had slept in separate bedrooms for many years that were down the hall from each other. Derek went and sat in Robert's room, while Wickett accompanied her mother.

Robert said, "I'm ready to go now." He spooned down his ice cream and began to get drowsy. He murmured, "Goodbye, Derek. Thank you very much." Robert lost consciousness and was dead within fifteen minutes.

Derek understood that the same thing happened in Cynthia's room.

The couple had previously confided the exit plan to their general practitioner. After he was summoned to the house, he explained that he had given the situation considerable thought and that following a double suicide there was no choice but to notify the police. The chief of police arrived and the death certificate was signed without any repercussions.

A reporter from the *Boston Globe* called the following day, and Wickett spoke frankly about her parents' death. The obituary quoted the suicide note, which said they had had happy lives together—Derek's voice broke when he told me this—and because of many health problems they wished to end their lives.

"It was a good, honest obituary," Derek said, "that did not attempt to hide what happened."

Shortly afterward, Wickett threw herself into a writing project and published, *Double Exit*. The book went into considerable detail about the deaths.[14] She made it clear that her parents were "affronted and humiliated by the growing indignities of their deterioration" from aging, and this had directly led to a decision to end their lives. Wickett said that her conscience was clear, and she wrote, "They actually did it, and they did it right."[15]

However, she suffered afterward. According to friends, like Julie Horvath, Wickett was tortured by ambivalence.[16] "She felt guilty and remorseful," Horvath explained. "At the same time she'd rationalize, saying, 'I'm proud of what I did.' But then she'd start to cry, saying, 'All I wanted to do was help my parents.' She went back and forth. It ate away at her."[17]

Wickett would later make a videotape with a friend who had come for a visit, in which she detailed another version of the events. She maintained that her mother's suicide had been coerced. In the tape she said, "I knew my mother was not ready to die. I knew she felt pressure and that she couldn't survive without my father. I never forget that."[18]

Wickett also confessed that Cynthia's death had not gone smoothly. After ingesting the barbiturates, her mother began to choke. "I got really scared," Wickett exclaimed. "Derek had always said to me, 'Just use a plastic bag or a pillow.' And so there was a plastic laundry bag with her linen in it, and I took the bag and very gently held it over her mouth."[19] After a long pause on the recording, Wickett continued, "She died very peacefully. But I walked away from that house thinking we're both murderers."[20]

The day after making the videotape, Wickett learned that her lawsuit was unsuccessful. Hastily composing a few notes and a last enraged letter to her ex-husband, she hitched a horse trailer to her Chevrolet pickup and took off with Eben, her chestnut Arabian gelding. Wickett drove four hours into the mountains of Oregon. She parked and then rode the animal along a familiar trail to a secluded spot in the forest. Taking off his saddle so that he could safely return to the truck, she sat down by a tree and overdosed with barbiturates. Her body was found six days later.

Derek's experience with Wickett has undoubtedly influenced his present opposition to offering assisted dying to people with psychiatric disorders. His position, he told me, is that "mental illness is a minefield. I've been saying it at the Network for years that it is going to blow up in our face, partly because mentally ill people are liars. They will tell you anything to get their way and to get what they want. You can't believe what they say."

Derek explained to Jake and me that he has recently been bombarded by psychiatrically disordered people wanting help committing suicide. But he has repeatedly told them, "You're not going to get any assistance from us. I'm afraid it's morally wrong and it's legally dangerous. I don't think that the public is ready for assisted suicide of the mentally troubled, if they ever will be."

In 1990, Derek married an Oregonian, Gretchen Crocker. During the day that Jake and I spent with him, Gretchen quietly drifted in and out of the office and could not have been more accommodating or caring. I drove away from Derek's home, hoping that he had found a soulmate who would bring him some measure of peace in the years ahead.

15

❦

A WELL-WORN
SWEATER

I wrote a letter to Jack Kevorkian addressed to the Oaks Correctional Facility in Manistee, Michigan, inquiring whether we might conduct an interview. I never heard back from him, and later came to understand that this activity was discouraged at the state maximum security prison.

Being an ascetic, Kevorkian adjusted reasonably well to prison life, although he had miscalculated and originally thought he would be sent to a relatively cushy federal penitentiary. He also incorrectly believed that a series of appeals addressing the subjects of euthanasia and assisted suicide would work their way up through the judicial system to the Supreme Court. He was bitterly disappointed when the justices refused to adjudicate his case.

According to his biographers, upon visiting Kevorkian, they found him clad in the standard blue prison uniform with orange epaulets.[1] Like other inmates, he was kept in a cell twenty-three hours a day, excluding meal breaks. Kevorkian served his sentence at six different prisons, where he usually had the dubious distinctions of being the oldest and the best-known inmate.

When Kevorkian became eligible for parole, Morganroth applied to the Michigan governor to grant a pardon or to commute the sentence. The doctor was given an early release from prison in 2007 after serving eight years. As a condition of parole, he promised not to assist in any more suicides. Kevorkian was seventy-nine years old when released, and he suffered from advanced hepatitis C, hypertension, adrenal insufficiency, cardiac disease, emphysema, and arthritis.

During his television appearances, Kevorkian had always come across as belligerent and provocative. But he also offered a plethora of stimulating ideas about autonomy, the medical profession, and our society's reticence to respond to people's suffering. At the first press conference following his release, I was shocked by his appearance. Not unexpectedly the man standing in front of the microphone looked gaunt and angry. But he also seemed to me to be suffering from a cognitive impairment. Prison, the passage of time, and accumulated medical ills had combined to break him.

Who was this man of contradictions? He was a middle child and only son.[2] His parents survived the Armenian genocide that took the lives of 1.5 million people, and they witnessed unspeakable atrocities before immigrating to the United States. They settled amid the substantial Armenian community in Michigan, where there was work in the foundries and assembly lines of the automobile industry. Kevorkian's mother and father were strict, introspective, working-class people who believed that the suffering in Armenia required them to forego any desire for revenge but to instead live with dignity. As members of the Armenian Apostolic church, they fervently believed in the acceptance of God's will.

Kevorkian, according to Nicol and Wylie, rebelled against the philosophy of redemption through suffering and the passive acceptance of horror. He was resentful that his parents encouraged his sisters to develop their innate talents for art and music while insisting that he devote himself solely to academic pursuits. He passionately wanted to become an artist and immerse himself

in the beauty of music, but "the Kevorkian family expected greatness of him, and it was as if they all made an agreement to work
together to keep him from getting sucked into fantasies of a life in
sports or the arts. . . . He was the brilliant heir apparent."[3]

The expectations shaped his personality. From a young age,
Kevorkian sought to establish that he was the smartest person
in the room, the hardest working, best prepared, and the most
erudite. He cultivated a need to be the winner of every argument, every debate. Although gifted with a sense of humor that
was appreciated by classmates, he didn't hesitate to employ it to
shame and humiliate teachers.

His biographers describe the death of his dog, Wooly, in ado-
lescence as having been his first experience with the dying of a
beloved. They suggest that he was inconsolable, found the pain
unbearable, and this colored the nature of or absence of future
relationships. Perhaps.

Nicol and Wylie describe him as having embraced the role
of "eccentric bookworm," and said that he shunned romantic
attachments as unnecessary diversions from education. During
high school, the polymath taught himself to be fluent in Japanese and German—the languages of the enemy combatants in
World War II.

It was in college where Kevorkian first began wearing the
cardigan sweaters that made dressing simple and quick, and
it was there that he became consumed with staying physically
fit through a restrictive diet and exercise regimen. He became
bored with his first choice of engineering as a major, but then
discovered the possibility of a career in medicine.

Kevorkian was asked during his medical school admission
interview why he was likely to persevere with a medical career
having given up engineering, and he replied: "You might think
I'm cocky for saying this, but the reason seems obvious to me.
I'm one of the smartest guys you'll ever see walk through your
door, but I'm not doing this because of my ego. I'm doing this
because medicine needs me. You let me get into medical school,
and I'll prove it's the best decision you've ever made."[4]

Kevorkian was attracted to the specialty of pathology that
required its students to master the breadth of medicine and to

develop skills honed by countless hours in the laboratory and library. He was always comfortable conducting autopsies.

Internship was spent at the Henry Ford Hospital, where he encountered a woman dying of metastatic cancer. Kevorkian later wrote with characteristic impudence: "It seemed as if she was pleading for help and death at the same time. Out of sheer empathy alone I could have helped her to die with satisfaction. From that moment on, I was sure that doctor-assisted euthanasia and suicide are and always were ethical, no matter what anyone says or thinks."[5]

The Korean War was being waged and Kevorkian volunteered to serve in the military. He was ordered to Seoul; there he helped soldiers with battlefield injuries. In his spare time, he practiced playing on the flute songs by his favorite composer, Johann Sebastian Bach. He also taught himself Latin and Greek.

Returning home, Kevorkian began a pathology residency at the University of Michigan Medical Center. It was there that he embarked on the first of what became a series of bizarre research investigations about dying. The study entailed photographing the eyes of patients immediately following their demise, and it earned him his nickname, "Dr. Death." Although this work was correctly performed after first obtaining consents from the families and attending physicians, it was unquestionably macabre, and the results were unclear.

Other equally strange research projects would follow. Between these and his prickly sense of right and wrong, a short temper that frequently resulted in bitter arguments with colleagues, and a tendency to disdainfully express his boredom with others, Kevorkian worked as a staff pathologist in several different Michigan hospitals for distinctly short periods of time. He flitted from place to place and idea to idea until finally having a eureka moment when he discovered the social cause that would shape the rest of his life. And despite the early opposition by his parents, he simultaneously soothed himself with music and art, expressively playing his flute into the early morning hours and enthusiastically splashing paint on large canvasses.

In 2010, *You Don't Know Jack*, a glossy TV biopic about Kevorkian's life, directed by Barry Levinson and starring Al Pacino, was broadcast to considerable acclaim.[6] Pacino won an Emmy for Outstanding Lead Actor, while Adam Mazer received an Emmy for Outstanding Writing. Mazer looked down from the stage to an animated Kevorkian sitting in the audience and joked, "I'm grateful you're my friend. I'm even more grateful you're not my physician."

Dr. Jack Kevorkian was eighty-three when he died from "natural causes." In addition to the previously mentioned medical problems, he developed pneumonia and kidney failure. Morganroth told the Associated Press there were no artificial attempts to keep him alive and he did not suffer.[7] The nurses played recordings of Bach in his hospital room.

Geoffrey Fieger said that Kevorkian was too weak to hasten his own death. "If he had enough strength to do something about it," the attorney told a news conference, "he would have."[8]

The author Zoe Fitzgerald Carter observed "If that is true, there is something almost epically tragic about the fact that a man who fought so long and hard for patients' right to die on their own terms, wasn't able to take advantage of this option in the end. But then who is to say 'Dr. Death' didn't simply change his mind?"[9]

She makes the point that our personal beliefs may prove inconsequential when it comes to the actual circumstances in which we die. Even the staunchest pro-life, anti-assisted-suicide crusader may waver in resolve while in the throes of extreme agony or existential angst as the end approaches. Even committed aid-in-dying proponents, like Beth Weinstein and her loving family, may procrastinate and defer acting. My experience is that despite protestations to the contrary ("if that happens [dementia, ALS, cancer of the face, name your nightmare] then get a gun and shoot me!"), *everyone* would prefer to die naturally, and preferably in their sleep.

It is both glib and illusory to assume we can always maintain control. Carter recounts a wonderful anecdote about giving birth to her first child, in which, "somehow, between planning the perfect play list and specifying that I didn't want an episiotomy, I forgot to factor in throwing up, forgetting to breathe, and the uncontrollable urge to yell obscenities at the nurse." She concludes, "So much for my beautiful birthing experience."[10]

This is not to say that we shouldn't define and regularly express our desires, as well as complete both legal and semi-official forms spelling out terminal care preferences and choice of health care proxies. Open communication between loved ones and the use of advance directives will give people the best chance for not prolonging dying and for planning one's death. Meanwhile, laws will continue to be crafted that implement safeguards preventing the abuse of vulnerable individuals.

Kevorkian was irascible, obdurate, incapable of cooperating with his fellow aid-in-dying activists, eccentric, and narcissistic. My friend and palliative medicine colleague Dr. Timothy Quill was critical of how Dr. Kevorkian "reinforces our society's penchant for seeking quick technological solutions to complex human problems."[11] The bioethicist Arthur Caplan summarized the man's impact, saying, "I think he's turned up the heat on this debate and, in some ways, will be remembered as the central figure who made America grapple with the question of assisted suicide and not allow them to turn away. At the same time, the tone and the tenor of the debate, the theater, the politics, the stridency, the militancy and, if you will, going out on the fringe and dealing with individuals who very few people would want to have the right to die—I think we can blame him for that, too."[12]

But if you look behind the man's public persona into his family's history and personal dynamics, then perhaps his behavior is more understandable. I think of Kevorkian as being the prodigal son of two Armenian genocide survivors. Like my friend Dr. William Breitbart, whose parents survived the Holocaust by joining the partisans, such adult children are left with a charge and a debt to pay. Bill, who is the chief of psychiatry at Memorial-Sloan Kettering and an adamant opponent of assisted dying, recently wrote, "My legacy was not merely one of loss, death and suffering. My legacy was to be revealed to me . . . as much more; a legacy of transcending suffering and loss through care and love and the value of 'Compassion.'"[13] I suspect that these words apply equally to Kevorkian, even though his interpretation of all these attributes would radically differ from that of Breitbart.

Kevorkian was remembered by his friends as a martyr. The epitaph they chose for the tombstone reads, "He sacrificed himself for everyone's rights."

Jack Kevorkian willed his possessions to his niece and sole heir, Ava Janus. She and Morganroth decided to dispose of the estate in an auction, and they hired a fine arts and celebrity memorabilia appraiser who estimated the value of Kevorkian's paintings alone at $2.5 million to $3.5 million. There were seventeen Kevorkian works of art at the Armenian Library and Museum of America in Watertown, Massachusetts. He had left them for safekeeping when it appeared that the Youk case would lead to imprisonment. Whether this was a loan or a donation became the crux of the legal dispute that Morganroth alluded to in our first conversation.

Among the other items that I saw at the preview was Kevorkian's iconic blue cardigan sweater. The description noted the presence of small paint dots near the arm cuffs and stated, "So in addition to him wearing this for public events he also wore this while painting his remarkable art." The cardigan was noted to have small repairs on the right shoulder (presumably by Kevorkian's hand) and carried an estimated value of $2,000 to $3,000.

The doctor's black plastic hair comb was estimated at $800 to $1,200. Also on display were his driver's license, medal for winning a spelling bee, license plate, and prescription bottles. His beloved silver flute was available for bidding, as was a bulletproof vest worn during court appearances after receiving death threats.

I was not present for the actual auction on the following day, but it must have been a tremendous disappointment to Morganroth and anyone who hoped the sale might rival those of Elizabeth Taylor, Jacqueline Kennedy, and other celebrities whose most mundane personal effects garnered stratospheric bids.

None of the paintings sold. Neither did Kevorkian's comb, spelling bee medal, and most of the other memorabilia. According to the auction firm, the highest bid for the Thanatron was

$65,000. The bulletproof vest brought $5,000, and the well-worn sweater went for a relatively modest $500.

Almost one year after the auction, the *Detroit News* reported that the dispute between Dr. Jack Kevorkian's estate and the Armenian Library and Museum of America over the ownership of the seventeen original paintings was settled.[14]

Morganroth explained that under the agreement the museum would keep four paintings, and thirteen were to be returned to the estate.

"Of course, we are happy it's resolved," the attorney told a reporter. "The settlement recognizes the need for his art to be preserved . . . while returning artwork to his heir." He went on to note that the paintings were expected to be offered for sale at private galleries.[15]

"We had opening bids of $100,000 for some," Morganroth said. "But when we told interested persons we couldn't guarantee delivery because of the pending litigation, the bids dropped off."

In 2015, Jack Kevorkian's niece, Ava Janus, donated his papers, medical records, video and audio recordings, photographs, and musical compositions to the University of Michigan Bentley Historical Library.[16]

As for me, the auction fulfilled my premonition. The sight of the man's modest possessions greatly saddened me, his Thanatron left me chilled, and the paintings were pure torture.

The more I have heard and read, the greater is my ambivalence about Kevorkian. He was undoubtedly a brilliant individual who was justifiably venerated by the patients and families whom he helped. But he was also obsessed with death and unable to cooperate even with those political activists who shared his beliefs. As a psychiatrist, I have a substantial tolerance for psychopathology, but I don't regret having missed the opportunity to meet him.

However, in my capacity as a writer, I must admit to having more than a twinge of regret at not interviewing Kevorkian. Andrew Solomon has called him the Malcolm X of the right-to-die movement, and wrote that "he should not have gone to prison, but civil disobedience comes at a cost, and he paid it."[17]

My favorite recollection of Kevorkian involves the last few seconds of an interview that took place on *60 Minutes*—not the infamous broadcast that led to his guilty verdict, but an earlier conversation with the avuncular host, Andy Rooney.[18] During the interview, Kevorkian ranted, raved, polemicized, but also managed to display a lighthearted charm. Rooney's final question was: "What do you do for fun, Dr. Kevorkian?"[19]

Without the slightest hesitation, he replied, "Irritate people!" And the broadcast ended with everyone in the television studio—the other guests, Rooney, and his entire camera crew— all heartily laughing.

16

BRING OUT YER DEAD

In the 1975 motion picture *Monty Python and the Holy Grail*, the delightfully surreal British comedy troupe depicted an imaginary scene set in medieval Europe where the victims of the Black Plague are being tossed into a cart to be hauled away for burial.[1] Eric Idle, the cart's driver, slowly ambles through town while loudly intoning, "Bring out yer dead."[2] He then argues with John Cleese over whether the last body tossed in the wagon is actually deceased. The so-called corpse, clearly an elderly relative, maintains that he is quite alive and definitely "not dead." Cleese, meanwhile, has already handed over the ninepence disposal fee and is eager to move along. The hilarious scene—yes, it's ghoulish, but it is also very, very funny, particularly with English accents—was turned into a song and reappeared thirty years later in the Tony Award-winning musical *Spamalot*. It concludes with Idle banging the Dead Man Who Claims He Isn't on the head with a mallet, followed by the profuse thanks of the grateful Cleese.

In 1996, a group of disability rights activists incensed at Jack Kevorkian's euthanasia campaign adopted Not Dead Yet as the name of their organization.[3] For the past ten years, I have scrupulously followed their regular online postings. The group's

4

spokespersons are incredibly eloquent in condemning society's misrepresentation of the lived experience of disabled people and in articulating their position that attempts to legislate assisted dying are manifestations of the devaluation, oppression, and abuse of the chronically ill and elderly. They view Kevorkian as having gotten off far too lightly when he was sent to prison.

I have long wanted to meet and interview members of Not Dead Yet. They are understandably sensitive to being exploited and misquoted. Bizarrely, my chance to hear from a few of them arrived when I attended the biennial meeting of their arch-enemies, the World Federation of Right to Die Societies.

The protestors milled about on the street in front of the somewhat seedy Embassy Suites Chicago hotel where the conference was being held. They consisted of roughly forty people, most clad in neon pink T-shirts with the logo "Not Dead Yet" boldly printed on the front. A racially diverse group, many of the individuals were in their twenties and thirties. By contrast, Not Dead Yet's board members, who delivered speeches during the next couple of days, were mainly white men and women in their fifties and sixties, and most were attorneys.

One of the protestors explained to me that the board members assembled in Chicago from New York, Boston, Montreal, and other cities to attend this all-important protest vigil. They expected to be joined later by members of ADAPT (Americans Disabled for Attendant Programs Today), part of the militant wing of the disability rights movement. The activists from this latter organization regularly engage in nonviolent direct actions of civil disobedience with the goal being "to ensure the civil rights, liberty and freedom of disabled people of all ages to live in our own homes in the community, rather than in nursing facilities or institutions."[4] They had recently shut down a Senate Finance Committee hearing that was debating a bill to repeal Obamacare, and numerous activists were arrested during a protest over another bill, HR 620, that would make it more difficult to file lawsuits under the Americans with Disabilities Act.

Not Dead Yet president Diane Coleman, who has a neuro-muscular disease called congenital myopathy, announced in

Chicago, "We are here to contradict the message . . . that it's better to be dead than disabled." Coleman has required a wheel-chair since age eleven, and for the past couple of years she has used mechanical breathing support most of the day as well as at night. She is an attorney who directed several nonprofit disability-related organizations before heading up Not Dead Yet.[5] At a similar protest, she condemned the right-to-die movement as, "a wolf in sheep's clothing: the trappings of compassion, but the reality of corporate greed and social contempt for ill and disabled people who are seen as expendable."[6]

A few children and adolescents clad in the hot pink shirts were sprinkled among the protestors, and they enthusiastically marched back and forth on the sidewalk carrying hand-written placards that read, "Killing Is Killing," "Disabled and Proud," and "Death Does Not Cure Anything!" Every so often, the group would chant slogans, such as, "We don't need your suicide; Not Dead Yet keeps us alive!"

A few protestors obviously had major mental illnesses while others appeared to be developmentally delayed. Several were dressed in Halloween costumes and masks: ghosts and goblins were in evidence, the Grim Reaper strode alongside a Big Bad Wolf, and a faux doctor clad in green scrubs with a surgical mask was fiddling with his toy stethoscope. But there was nothing make-believe about the people zipping around the sidewalk in electric wheelchairs. The drivers were adept from years of maneuvering their chairs, and they were clearly enjoying themselves. The mood at the gathering for this deadly serious cause was a strange mélange that kept shifting between merriment and defiance.

Not Dead Yet board members were taking turns delivering formal speeches in front of a large banner, but frustratingly, the portable sound system was defective and their words were muffled. From her wheelchair decorated with a bright blue sign that had a picture of an old-fashioned bell and the caption, "Give Me Liberty—Don't Give Me Death," Coleman tried to articulate the purpose of the demonstration, but the loudspeakers crackled and faded in and out. As Coleman finally wheeled away from the microphone, it was unclear whether she knew that her speech had gone largely unheard. I suspected that she is convinced people rarely pay sufficient attention to her message. Coleman was a study in contrasts, looking simultaneously exhausted and invigorated, sick and resilient. Her formal remarks had been typed and copied, and they were included in a packet that Gary Arnold handed to me.

Frankly, I had never had a conversation before with a "little person," and I didn't know whether to bend my creaky six-foot-one frame down or to drop on one knee in front of Gary. I chose the latter and continued to genuflect each time that I spoke with the other protestors who were in wheelchairs. While it felt a bit like bowing before royalty or bishops, it also seemed like the polite thing to do. As a physician, when I go to patient bedsides, I never stand and look down upon them; if they are reclining, I usually request that they put up the head of the bed while I'll pull up a chair so that we can approximate being eye-to-eye with each other. My impression is that we are more likely to have a meaningful conversation if it begins with a respectful physical arrangement.

Gary was wearing a blue hoody sweatshirt on top of his pink shirt and had a satchel of press releases slung over a shoulder. He lives in Chicago and works at an organization called Access Living that provides resources for people with disabilities to live independently.[7] He is the Access Living public relations coordinator, and his organization opposes efforts to legalize assisted suicide and related life-ending practices.

Back in 2005, Gary was present when Not Dead Yet staged another demonstration in Chicago objecting to the removal of Terri Schiavo's feeding tube. Schiavo was in a persistent vegetative state, and Gary told me, "If we don't know what a person wants or doesn't want, then we should do everything possible." For the current protest, Access Living asked him to provide media outreach.

Gary is forty-four years old and describes himself as being a "person with dwarfism, a person with short stature." Born in Madison, Wisconsin, he left to attend college, and after graduation moved to Chicago. He originally worked for the Association of Community Organizations for Reform Now (better known as ACORN), sometime after Barack Obama had ceased his role as one of its leadership trainers. During the period in which Obama was running for the presidency, Gary was a community organizer driving into neighborhoods, ringing doorbells, and speaking with people about how to address urban poverty and improve the quality of their lives.

I asked Gary about dwarfism and its impact on his life. He told me, "My professional path and disability rights stuff would never have happened if I did not have a disability."

In addition to his job at Access Living, he is the president of the board of directors of Little People of America.[8] This is a national organization that mainly serves to provide social support. "Dwarfism is a relatively rare disability," he explained. "If you are person with dwarfism you are going to grow up to likely be the only person in your school or community with that condition. People will treat you differently, and especially when you are young that can be alienating. The most important role of Little People of America is to give people some space to share their common bond. You can be different in every other way—politically, economically, religiously—but you also have this shared experience." He described attending national meetings, which bring together two thousand or more members, a grant program to financially assist with the cost of higher education, and a program to help people adopt children of small stature. The organization also sponsors educational outreach to schools and other settings.

I asked Gary about the demographic diversity evident in today's protest rally. He commented wryly, "Disability does not discriminate. Anyone can join the community at any moment." He said, "It is a natural part of life and is going to impact everybody. If you yourself are not going to acquire a disability then the chances are that a family member or someone you are close to will. That is why it is so important to integrate disability issues into almost all broader issues: health care, housing, education, and employment. There is a disability component to each one of those."

I asked what accommodations he requires because of the dwarfism, and these turned out to be in his words, "pretty minor." They included having a chair at work with a support for his feet (that would otherwise not reach the ground) and pedal extenders in his car. He considers himself fortunate that both are simple and inexpensive to install.

The action in front of the hotel continued in fits and starts, and a folksinger wearing a broad-billed leather hat drove her bumper sticker–covered wheelchair up to the microphone. The audio equipment was still malfunctioning, and most of what she sang was inaudible. But her songs were well known to the protestors, who happily joined in the choruses.

John Kelly rolled up in a wheelchair to the microphone and gave an impassioned speech based on a recent editorial he had written and the arguments he used in his campaign two years earlier that contributed to the defeat of the Massachusetts death-with-dignity ballot referendum. Opponents, such as John, insist on consistently labeling the practice "assisted suicide," in contrast to the host of less pejorative but verbally vague euphemisms employed by proponents. John and his organization, Second Thoughts Massachusetts, were part of the well-funded victorious coalition, and I respected his efforts, even if I didn't agree with many of the assertions in his speech and our subsequent interview.

"In reality," John told me, "two-thirds of the people Dr. Death, Jack Kevorkian helped to die were non-terminal, disabled people. Assisted suicide is the ultimate denial of choices."

While acknowledging that the current death-with-dignity statutes in America all require people to have a disease likely to end their lives within six months, John contended that physicians are hopeless at making accurate prognoses, stating, "Ted Kennedy was given two to four months to live and he lived fifteen months!" I thought to myself, *This is true to an extent, but it was obvious from the start he had an incurable malignant brain cancer that would inexorably kill him.*

If anything, Kennedy's doctors tried to put a positive spin on his condition, announcing that the surgery for his malignant brain tumor was a success and he should experience no permanent neurological effects. But the medical team originally had said the focus of treatment would be radiation and chemotherapy, and they acknowledged afterward that the brain cancer had been "debulked"—doctor-speak for acknowledging they could only remove a portion of the cancer.⁹ Kennedy appears to have wanted to put a brave face on his situation, and a spokesperson quoted the senator as good-humoredly telling his wife, "I feel like a million bucks. I think I'll do that again tomorrow."

Having researched and developed a prognostic instrument for people receiving dialysis, I agree that doctors are not soothsayers. Nevertheless, we can identify with a fair degree of certitude the subgroups and often the individuals who are facing death within a short time period.

John continued his arguments and cited Oregon Health Department statistics that indicate 90 percent of the patients who make use of the state's death-with-dignity law do so because of a "loss of autonomy," and 40 percent endorse "feelings of being a burden." He maintained that neither of these factors should *ever* be acceptable reasons for someone to choose to die. In his opinion, disabled people and seniors are buffeted by poverty, the lack of available independent home care, and the horror of institutionalization in nursing homes. These factors combine to coerce them into accelerating their deaths. Again, I thought, *It is shameful but true what he's saying about the disabled and elderly, but why shouldn't losing one's autonomy or becoming a burden be an acceptable rationale for assisted dying? And isn't the word, coercion, a bit strong?*

John agreed with the comment of his colleague, Bob Kafka, a national leader of ADAPT, who had said, "The last thing we need is for those in power to make a public policy choice, during this time of vast budget cuts in Medicaid health and long-term care, that an early death is the cost-saving answer to these very real human needs."¹⁰

John did not cite but would also have agreed with Daniel Sulmasy, who wrote:

> [When] people living with disabilities are so fearful of legalized assisted suicide and other forms of medically assisted killing . . . it is not so much that they anticipate being lined up in wheelchairs and forcibly injected (at least not in the

near term). It is the assault to their dignity that comes with social sanction of the idea that lives characterized by incontinence, cognitive incapacity, and dependence on others are unworthy of life and so can be ended by direct killing.[11]

These sentiments make a certain degree of sense to me, and I worry that our government could unjustly balance the budget in the future by removing rules and practices that enable our most vulnerable citizens to survive. I appreciate that medical aid in dying has the potential to become "a seductively inexpensive alternative" to comprehensive palliative care.[12] But where I differ, again, is that I fail to see why people—even if elderly or disabled— should *not* be permitted to truncate the process of dying. Why shouldn't they have that choice if *they* feel like an undue burden on loved ones or if *they* believe their autonomy has been irreparably compromised. Again, I don't think that John, or Kafka, and Sulmasy are entirely wrong—we differ on the emphasis.

When he was twenty-five years old, John sustained a spinal cord injury that left him paralyzed below the shoulders. During his introduction on Not Dead Yet's website as its regional director, he wrote, "I have the same amount of physical function as the suicidal characters in the movies '*Act of Love*,' '*Whose Life Is It Anyway?*' and the Spanish movie '*The Sea Inside*.'"[13] John went on to write, "The *only* time I get to see someone like me on the screen is when they want to die or raise money for the cure."

Admitting that he and his family were vulnerable to the commonly held belief "better dead than disabled,"[14] John blogged that at the time of the accident his father thought it would have been preferable if he had died.

In 2000, John was a graduate student at Brandeis University. His attitude radically changed during a protest held in Boston where one of the flyers being handed out read, "We don't need to die to have dignity." It resonated powerfully, and he described himself as having since become one of "the trouble-making disabled people, not the peaceful death-loving disabled people that everyone likes to have around."[15]

During my interview with John outside of the Embassy Suites Chicago hotel, we talked about how society misunderstands the disabled. He disputed that there is anything wrong about requiring or accepting accommodations and support. "The other half of human experience," he told me, "is to be cared for! To adapt is a wonderful feature of being a human being."

"When I became disabled," he explained, "I could no longer feed myself, and my worries were, 'Will people stare?' But you know the food tastes the same! It tastes exactly the same. It tastes really, really delicious!"

In newspaper pieces, he reminded me, one often sees joyous wedding photographs in which the bride is feeding the groom, or there is a shot of the groom messily popping a piece of cake into the bride's mouth. "But," by contrast John said, "if they want to show someone who deserves to die, they illustrate this with an old person being fed pabulum,"

With a snort he continued, "Well I don't eat pabulum!"

Our conversation shifted to motorized wheelchairs and the frequency that they electrically short-out in the rain. "Unless you cover the control with a plastic bag," he said, "one dare not go outside." He mentioned how numerous supporters of his organization, Second Thoughts Massachusetts, who opposed the Commonwealth's ballot question couldn't attend a scheduled hearing of the Joint Committee on Public Health when a storm made streets impassable for them and they risked becoming snowbound. Despite the obstacles, he managed to get to the State House, where he testified: "Being stuck inside for days on end without relief is another way that disabled and older people get the message that we are not as valuable as other people. If we were as valued, the sidewalks would either be clear or [this] hearing would be postponed."

My reaction to his words was visceral, and I remarked, "It hardly makes sense to me that we have unmanned rovers zipping along the Martian surface for months at a time but engineers haven't mastered a means to provide you and your peers with dependable mobility in inclement weather here on Earth."

While agreeing with my sentiment, a week later, John posted the following nuanced but acerbic account of our sidewalk meeting:

> Afterwards, a tall affable white man dressed in the jacket
> and slacks of the academic elite came over and asked me

for a copy of my speech. "I liked what I could hear of it'" he said. He told me that his name was Lewis Cohen and he was writing an article for the *Atlantic Monthly*, and working on a book about assisted suicide. He told me he was a Massachusetts palliative care doctor who pushed for the assisted suicide referendum question in 2012, and congratulated us for our victory.[16]

I found a clip of Cohen from 2012, in which he said of the Massachusetts assisted suicide bill, "This is something that gives people confidence." Against the evidence and disabled people's own experience, Cohen said that doctors are able to predict someone's death. He did agree with me—and even started his tape recorder, when I talked about the class makeup of the early and current death proponents: white, wealthy, well-educated, secular, and relatively fit. These people, I said, approach life as a buffet table of choices, in which they are in control and can predict outcomes. For the rest of us, life is immediate and chaotic, with daily struggles to get our needs met uppermost in our minds. I suspect that Cohen is one of the disturbingly large group which understands and accepts many of our criticisms, but supports assisted suicide anyway as a boon to himself and his class. I would think being a public advocate for legalized assisted suicide would put your qualifications for easing people's pain into question.[17]

John's critique was accurate and insightful. I am now admittedly a sixty-nine-year-old, highly educated, secular, reasonably healthy, white, married, heterosexual male. Until becoming quadriplegic, John and I shared many of these same physical and socioeconomic characteristics. However, that was then. Presently, John and I can't help but look at the world from different perspectives—literally. Before the accident he, too, stood six feet tall, but now describes himself as being four-foot-six (in his chair).

John's observation was also correct that his fellow disability activists on the street looked nothing like the right-to-die activists I would encounter upstairs in the hotel conference

rooms, but frankly, they also did not resemble the anti-euthanasia opponents I previously met while writing my first book
on this subject. The latter had included Terri Schiavo's brother,
Robert Schindler, and others, whose opinions on the issue were
shaped by their religious faiths or conservative social values.
Those other opponents of assisted dying share many of the same
demographics and differ from the proponents upstairs only in
superficialities: a profusion of crucifixes around their necks, and
eye-catching, anti-abortion pins and political buttons condemning same-sex-marriage.

I am grateful to John for highlighting the importance of
economics, and especially poverty, in shaping the meaning of
"choice" for different people. According to 2016 Census Bureau
data, the employment rate of working-age people (ages twenty-
one to sixty-four) with disabilities in the United States was 36.2
percent, which is to say that nearly two in three are unemployed;
the median annual income of households with working-age
people with disabilities was $43,300; and the poverty rate of
working-age people with disabilities was 26.6 percent.[18] While it
is an overstatement to suggest that proponents of assisted dying
are uniformly prosperous, it is true that people who live on the
edge and lack a safety net will experience their lives and the end
of life quite differently from those who are economically stable.
While both rich and poor desire the best possible quality of life—
including its last phase—the beliefs and available options can
differ according to socioeconomic circumstances.

Since my interviews with the activists on the sidewalk,
I have had the opportunity to listen repeatedly to the recordings and muse over their words. Three things strike me. Gary
made the point that he would never have become an activist if
he had not had the fortune or misfortune to be disabled. As will
be apparent in my descriptions of his counterparts among the
right-to-die spokespersons, they, too, would never have become
compelled to participate except for having been fortunately or
unfortunately immersed in the experiences of dying loved ones.
No one abstractly chooses to be an activist on either side of this
issue; our encounters with illness and death dictate whether this
will become a personally meaningful cause.

After reviewing my conversation with John, I was also impressed with the importance of family and community. He did not elaborate on the statement that his father thought he'd be better off dead than having to accommodate to a high spinal cord injury, but I can only imagine the impact of this opinion on him. When any of us suddenly becomes ill and relatively helpless it is natural to turn to family—but what happens if we can no longer depend on them? What happens if they hold different views and pull away from us? What occurs if they are simply unavailable?

In 2016, there were seven potential family caregivers for every person over eighty, and one-quarter of these were millennials, one-third simultaneously were holding down a full-time job, and one-quarter were working part time.[19] However, by 2030 the ratio of potential family caregivers is estimated to decrease from 7 to 1 down to 4 to 1. What will happen then?

In my work with dialysis patients—who can be in their twenties but on average are seventy—I am always shocked at how many individuals go through treatment on their own without anyone except the clinic staff lending a hand. They often live alone and they fly solo. This is not only dispiriting but must often feel like an impossible Sisyphean ordeal.

The third issue that was raised for me by my interactions with the Not Dead Yet activists has to do with the paramount importance our society accords intellectual and cognitive function. This was evident in the Not Dead Yet protests held around Teri Schiavo's hospice care and more recently in an active case involving Jahi McMath. The latter instance of brain damage is less known.

In 2013, McMath was a thirteen-year-old African American girl who ostensibly had complications at an Oakland, California, hospital from a surgery, in which doctors removed her tonsils, adenoids, and soft palate to treat sleep apnea—a condition that had been causing her to be chronically fatigued and unable to concentrate at school.[20] During the surgery, she sustained an "anoxic brain injury" presumably from severe blood loss. McMath was determined by the medical team to have brain death, but her family began questioning whether her brain was dead, and they also argued whether this should be equated with the death of a person. They refused to allow medical staff to remove the ventilator and insisted that she receive artificial nutrition and hydration.

McMath—dead or alive depending on your definition—was transferred with her ventilator to another hospital located in New Jersey, which along with New York, are the only two states where families can reject the concept of brain death if it violates their religious beliefs. The laws in both states were originally written to accommodate Orthodox Jews, some of whom maintain that the presence of breath signifies life. In a similar manner, the notion of brain death has been rejected by some Native Americans, Muslims, and evangelical Protestants.

Further complicating matters was the family's perception that racism was a factor in her treatment, and according to McMath's mother, "No one was listening to us. . . . I can't prove it, but I really feel in my heart: if Jahi was a little white girl, I feel we would have gotten a little more help and attention."[21] The family was sufficiently concerned that following the surgery, McMath's uncle slept in a chair at his niece's bedside to make sure that no one at the hospital would, in his words, "kill her off."[22]

In a *New Yorker* magazine piece, Rachel Aviv quoted Alan J. Weisbard, emeritus professor of law, bioethics, Jewish studies and religious studies at the University of Wisconsin Law School, as saying, "I think that the people who have done the deep and conceptual thinking about brain death are people with high I.Q.s, who tremendously value their cognitive abilities—people who believe that the ability to think, to plan, and to act in the world are what make for meaningful lives. But there is a different tradition that looks much more to the body."[23] Weisbard is especially troubled by circumstances where "minority communities should be forced into a definition of death that violates their belief structures and practices and their primary senses."

Aviv also cited Robert Truog, the director of the Center for Bioethics at Harvard Medical School, who has made the point that even in situations involving irreversible coma, African Americans are twice as likely as whites to ask that their lives be prolonged as much as possible. Furthermore, research has suggested that black patients are less likely to receive appropriate medications and surgeries than white patients, and they are more likely to undergo unwanted medical interventions, like amputations. Truog said about the McMath case, "When a doctor is saying your loved one is dead, and your loved one doesn't look dead, I understand that it might feel that, once again, you are not getting the right care because of the color of your skin."[24]

Given these issues, I can grasp why a disabled, chronically ill, nonwhite, religious, ethnic minority, or elderly person might fear the existence of any socially sanctioned means for people to hasten death—be it withdrawing or withholding treatment or the legalization of aid-in-dying practices. I can appreciate why they might distrust medical staff or even their own families to always support their decisions. I can understand how they might be overly sensitive to the possibility of coercion—and maybe that is the correct word—because coercion comes in different forms and is not always obvious.

On the second day of the protests, a contingent of activists from ADAPT arrived. Their tradition of civil disobedience extends back nearly four decades. Taking a page out of Rosa Parks and Martin Luther King's playbook, ADAPT has in the past demonstrated on behalf of wheelchair accessible public transportation by blocking buses and staying in the streets all night. In the "Capital Crawl," dozens of activists left their wheelchairs and walkers at the bottom steps of the Capitol building and crawled their way to the top before filing into the rotunda. Their actions contributed to passage of the landmark Americans with Disabilities Act, which was signed on July 26, 1990 by President Bush.[25]

With the arrival of ADAPT in Chicago, the protestors launched two civil actions. On Friday evening, they blocked the hotel doors. John later blogged how he weighs 550 pounds—if you total up his body and electric wheelchair—and how he parked himself in front of an exit door. John remained there, immovable, until the police eventually convinced him and the others to depart.[26]

I was in the hotel the following morning when the second action took place. Several Not Dead Yet and ADAPT members snuck into the hotel. As the conference delegates were about to descend for breakfast and their first scheduled meeting, the protestors simultaneously shut down all four elevators. John joined Diane Coleman in the atrium to watch, chants began to echo in the hotel lobby, and a Not Dead Yet banner was briefly suspended from an upper floor.

According to John:

> No elevator moved for almost an hour—we shut down the hotel! (We were told that we were a fire hazard, but promised to get out of the way if there was an actual fire.) I eased over to the stairs, and watched conference attendees sputtering and muttering out of the stairwell, some complaining that "It's not fair."
>
> A hotel official came over and told Diane that she would have to leave the hotel because she was not a guest. Diane calmly said that she was invited by one of the hotel's guests . . . explained to him that many different people and disability groups were participating, and offered to call up the leadership team to discuss how to resolve [the] immediate situation. That was not satisfactory. She also agreed to leave, but only as the last person out. When the police did get the elevators going again, escorting protesters out one by one, the chanting started up [again]. . . . We rejoined the ongoing vigil, and the civil disobedience concluded with our message [having been] delivered.[27]

Naturally, the proceedings were filmed and promptly posted on YouTube. The video depicted the main group on the sidewalk joyously greeting the appearance of each activist, who was accompanied by several police officers. Coleman brought up the rear and her exit was met with jubilance.

No arrests were made, and both the street demonstration and the conference itself continue unabated. However, Gary Arnold and the others were deeply disappointed that despite their efforts at seeking publicity, the media largely ignored these occurrences.

17

THE FEDERATION

pstairs in the cavernous conference center of the Embassy Suites Chicago hotel,
people milled about, scanned the room
for familiar faces, and greeted each other warmly. Faye Girsh
stood proudly at the podium, looking out at those who were
gathered for the twentieth biennial conference of the World
Federation of Right to Die Societies.[1] The organization, mainly
known as the Federation, was officially founded in 1980 and
is comprised of fifty-two right-to-die groups from around the
world. It was a beautiful fall day in 2014. Approximately three
hundred people from twenty-four countries had assembled in
Chicago and were being hosted by America's most radical aid-
in-dying volunteer organization, the Final Exit Network (FEN),
and Derek Humphry's Euthanasia Research and Guidance
Organization, better known as ERGO.

As Faye gazed around the room there were a lot of lined
faces and gray heads to be seen, but there were also a fair number of younger, healthy, new people in attendance, and they
represented the future of the global aid-in-dying movement. She
felt excited and optimistic while calling the meeting to order.

171

I felt comparatively youthful while observing the crowd: the slowly moving couples holding each other's hands, the aluminum walkers squealing, and the occasional wheelchairs silently rolling along. People were eagerly anticipating several days of lively talks and discussions. Sport coats, slacks, and conservative clothing predominated, and although there was diversity in evidence, the assembled appeared to be predominantly white and middle-class. A few Asians and African Americans in attendance were engaged in friendly conversations that swirled around the antechamber of the conference rooms. English was predominant, but here and there French, German, Swedish, Japanese, and other languages could be heard.

The only person clad in an obvious costume was a deathly pale, thirty-four-year-old woman with long blond hair, who was drifting around, propelled by the Brownian motion of the crowd. "I am Lady Liberty," she told me and anyone else that asked. "Give me liberty at my death." Her homemade gown and the foam rubber crown on her head, obviously purchased in New York where the tour boats embark for the Statue of Liberty, attested to her claim. She acknowledged having a lifelong history of mental illness and was running away from a strictly observant Catholic family. A lengthy bus trip had brought her here because she wanted to applaud the courage of those who gathered to celebrate their right to choose when and how to live and die. Lady Liberty had read about this self-determination movement, and she enthusiastically—but also somewhat pathetically—wanted to be a part of it.

I'm not sure if Jim Kinhan from New Hampshire was present, but he was the sort of individual that Lady Liberty would have especially admired and hoped to meet. During a town hall meeting, eighty-one-year-old Kinhan, terminally ill with colon cancer, would later question presidential candidate Hillary Clinton about her views on Oregon and other states that had passed death with dignity laws.[2]

"If worse came to worse, I can always move," Kinhan would tell a reporter after receiving an ambiguous answer from Clinton. "But I don't wanna move to some other fucking state. I wanna do it here in my home. I wanna die laughing." To this he added: "I want to go out smiling, blessing my children and grandchildren, and go to whatever comes after."

"The worldwide death with dignity movement is rapidly growing because increasing numbers of people believe that being able to control your own death is the ultimate human right," said Ed Gogol, president of Final Options Illinois.[3] He eagerly explained, "Mentally competent adults who are suffering intolerably have a basic human right at the end of life to choose a peaceful, dignified, and pain-free death." Rejecting the concerns of the opponents protesting outside that people would be coerced or encouraged to hasten dying, Gogol's emphasis on freely made choices was echoed by others throughout the conference.

The Chicago meeting focused mainly on the different laws being enacted in various countries along with the questions that confront end-of-life complexities: Should assisted dying be restricted to terminally ill people? What about those people who likely will live for years and not just six months with unendurable suffering? How about the mentally ill or the demented? And should aid in dying be extended to include children?

In a taped video that welcomed Federation attendees, the eighty-two-year-old archbishop emeritus of Cape Town, Desmond Tutu, affirmed his support of assisted dying.[4] He wanted it to be available as an option should he ever find himself terminally ill or in a situation of unbearable suffering. A couple of months before, in the lead-up to a fiery debate about the legalization of physician-assisted dying that took place in Britain's House of Lords, the retired Anglican prelate wrote that laws preventing people from being helped to end their lives are an affront to both them and their families.[5] He arrived at this position following the "self-delivery" (suicide) of a young, desperately ill South African man, Craig Schonegevel. Tutu also took the opportunity to condemn as "disgraceful" the treatment accorded to his friend, Nelson Mandela, who was kept alive through numerous painful hospitalizations and propped up for a photo shoot with visiting politicians shortly before his death at age ninety-five.

Archbishop Tutu said, "You could see Madiba [a nickname for Mandela] was not fully there. He did not speak. He was not connecting. My friend was no longer himself. It was an affront to Madiba's dignity."[6] Tutu concluded, "I have been fortunate to spend my life working for dignity for the living. Now I wish to apply my mind to the issue of dignity for the dying. I revere the sanctity of life—but not at any cost."

One of the keynote speakers in Chicago was Veronique Hivon, the minister of the National Assembly in Québec, who introduced the Act Respecting End of Life Care. The Act had passed by a resounding 94–22 vote that June, making Québec the first province of Canada to pass such legislation, and thereby affirm a right to compassionate care at the end of life, including continuous palliative sedation and medical aid in dying. I was in the audience when Hivon said, "There was such a strong public will to see improvements in end-of-life care in Québec. . . . The whole society was behind it, which gave incredible strength to the movement."[7] In June 2016, the Québec decision proved to be a bellwether for the entire nation of Canada as the Canadian Supreme Court ruled that medically assisted dying and clinician-administered medical assistance in dying (voluntary euthanasia) were legal.

Laura Belli of the National Council of Scientific and Technical Research in Argentina presented the changes taking place in her country, where legislature had passed two years earlier permitting patients who have intolerable pain from a terminal illness or incurable conditions to refuse treatment. In cases where patients are unable to speak for themselves, the law allowed relatives or legal proxies to help make decisions. While refusing life-prolonging measures is hardly the same as active assisted dying, the Catholic Church had strongly rejected the legislation. The law's passage by a vote of 55–0 marked a radical change in a country that is 76 percent Catholic.[8]

Between sessions, I briefly joined Derek Humphry, who sat behind a bridge table situated in the antechamber. A handsome bronze medal that he had been awarded for his five decades of commitment to the cause was perched in front of him. It wasn't clear to me just why Derek was pensively sitting at the table with his back to the wall, but people kept spotting him and approaching for a few minutes to chat. When I walked over, the author,

Richard Côté, was seated by Derek's side, happily snapping photographs.

I interviewed Richard a couple of years ago after his book chronicling the right-to-die movement was published.[9] He was a jovial South Carolinian, who published historical prose as if it were a bodice-ripping yarn. Derek remarked to me with evident amusement, "In his book, Richard portrayed me as something of a sex maniac."

Dr. Lawrence Deems Egbert Jr. and his wife, Ellen Barfield, were trying to locate the room where he was supposed to speak. Ellen is a Mother Earth–like figure, and she was clad in a brightly colored peasant dress. Her husband mainly looked exhausted and befuddled after an arduous train trip from their home in Baltimore. This mode of transportation takes between nineteen and twenty-one hours, but the couple is both by necessity and inclination always frugal. Larry is in his eighties, but his body has been honed by daily bike riding (neither he nor his wife own a car). At the meeting, however, he looked frail and uncomfortable having had a recent bicycle mishap in which he fractured his pelvis. It was uncertain whether he could resume cycling.

Larry had told me during one of our frequent interviews how proud he felt at being invited to address the meeting. However, the invitation was prompted by a legal ordeal; he and his organization, the FEN, were hit with three separate indictments for assisting in suicides, and as a result, he was facing the possibility of incarceration and the loss of his medical license. He had been forced to step back from his work at the FEN.

Faye would later introduce him as being the most embattled aid-in-dying activist in the nation. Like Jack Kevorkian, the original Dr. Death, to whom he has been compared, Larry was physically and mentally worn down by the legal melee.[10] Rather than giving an optimistic and feisty report, as Faye would have preferred, Larry told me that he intended to announce during his speech he was "personally feeling depressed and drinking more than usual." Faye tried to dissuade him, but Larry has always followed his own compass and that is exactly what he did.

Following Larry's speech, I approached Robert Rivas, the general counsel for the FEN, who was sitting in the antechamber.

Rob was intimately involved in all the legal cases, and he sat in an overstuffed chair, reviewing notes and strategy on a laptop. He observed to me, "That was just Larry being Larry."

Shortly afterward, I would have a chance to greet Dr. Richard (Dick) MacDonald, whom I also knew from interviews. Dick was at that point the FEN's senior medical director, and his words to me echoed Derek's belief that "even when the law allows certain people to die, a physician-assisted death in a medical facility is not what patients want. They want to die at home, with family and loved ones surrounding them."

During the next several days, I listened to a series of emotionally moving and intellectually stimulating talks. However, some presentations were surreal. I fled, for example, from the opportunity to see videotapes showing people ingesting barbiturates or ending their lives with helium gas.

There were plenty of controversies and recent developments on the minds of participants. In an address to the Association of Italian Catholic Doctors in November, Pope Francis had weighed in on the death-with-dignity movement, saying it offers a "false sense of compassion," and he labeled euthanasia as being a "sin against God the Creator."[11] In addition, during the summer the beloved comedian and Oscar winner, Robin Williams, had hanged himself, which his wife attributed to anguish related to the progression of Lewy body dementia.[12] At the time, the American media largely focused on whether Williams had psychiatric problems and if his death could have been prevented, rather than concentrating on the suffering associated with this particularly virulent, debilitating, and irreversible neurodegenerative disease.

At the Federation meeting, Tone Stockenström, a journalist from the *Humanist* magazine, interviewed attendees. She would assert that humanists "are likely to support many aspects of the issue. But what about when it concerns children? What about the mentally ill? What about the people directly affected by another's death?"[13]

She concluded that "These and other questions present a complex set of ethical issues on which humanists will have a range of opinions."

Dr. Faye Girsh, the president of the Federation, is a forensic psychologist who back in 1983 had been volunteering with the American Civil Liberties Union when she was asked to conduct a psychological evaluation of Elizabeth Bouvia. It would be Faye's introduction to the right-to-die movement.

Bouvia was a patient at California's Riverside General Hospital. According to a story in the *Disability Rag* by Mary Johnson, there is nothing straightforward about Bouvia's saga.[14]

"I'm trapped in a useless body," Bouvia had told the reporters she summoned to the hospital.[15] Twenty-six years old, mostly paralyzed by cerebral palsy, in considerable pain from severe degenerative arthritis, estranged from family, and considering suicide, Bouvia admitted herself to the psychiatric ward of Riverside General.

Bouvia decided that she wanted the hospital to keep her comfortable while she starved herself to death. Not surprisingly, the Riverside General had a different agenda and matters quickly got ugly. Staff force-fed her through a tube, which she resisted and tried to bite in half. They then inserted a nasogastric tube through her nose, and four attendants were required to hold her down while liquids were pumped into her stomach. All the while, she was hooked up to a morphine drip to ease the pain of the arthritis.

While some physicians considered this to be torture, others asserted that the hospital was correct to position itself squarely on the side of prolonging life. Bouvia telephoned not only journalists but also attorneys to come and hear her account and to fight on her behalf. She asserted that it was her right to die. The ACLU sent Faye Girsh as part of their team.

From the perspective of some disability activists, Bouvia was asking for the wrong thing. They point out that prior to the hospitalization, she had a miscarriage, her marriage to an ex-convict dissolved, and the state rehabilitation agency took back her accessible van and interfered with her plans to complete a master's degree program.[16] From their vantage point, what Bouvia needed was more attention to solving her personal and psychiatric problems, and like any disabled person she required basic accommodations to get back on her feet (figuratively). A disability rights picket was organized outside of the ACLU's Los Angeles office.

Her lawsuit and series of judicial appeals were accompanied by intense publicity. The matter was finally settled by an Appellate court ruling in Bouvia's favor that force-feeding constituted battery.

But after her victory in court, Bouvia promptly reversed course and declared that she no longer wished to starve herself to death.

She was interviewed on *60 Minutes* in 1986, and then ten years later she was featured in a second broadcast. In 1997, a new attorney managed to get disability payments placed into a trust fund that allowed her to live in her own apartment with twenty-four-hour-a-day in-home assistants. She required regular administration of morphine for pain and expressed ongoing ambivalence about remaining alive.

I have been unable to find any obituaries; Faye suspects that Elizabeth Bouvia is still probably among the living.

According to Faye, Bouvia had attended San Diego State University to seek a master's degree in social work, and she was "absolutely competent." Faye agreed with the plaintiff's stance that use of a feeding tube constituted a medical procedure. Faye believed that Bouvia ought to be able to refuse, and that decisions about voluntarily stopping eating and drinking—nowadays abbreviated as VSED—should likewise be left to individuals. For Faye, the case identified "an important civil liberties issue."

By contrast, what stands out for me as a psychiatrist is the tragic conundrum of an individual with a major physical disability that apparently had contributed to Bouvia's failed marriage, alienation from family, and difficulty securing employment, added to a medical system dedicated almost entirely to prolonging life, combined with a judiciary that had newly gotten around to decriminalizing suicide. All the above was filtered through a powerful personality that was hell-bent on engendering conflict and seeking maximum attention. Unlike Faye, if I had encountered this case it would probably have been the last time I ventured into the right-to-die arena.

But then again, unlike Faye, I didn't have the opportunity in 1986 to hear Derek Humphry present at a conference organized by the medical school of the University of San Diego. She was completely entranced by Derek's charm, eloquence, and radical ideas. Faye told me that she was convinced by his argument that the current law "allowed you to refuse unwanted medical treatments. But most of us don't have life-support treatments, and we should be allowed to die peacefully, too. We should not have to die violently with a weapon or in our cars or by jumping off tall buildings."

Derek's philosophy seemed touchingly humane to Faye, and she began a correspondence. "In 1987," she told me, "I opened a chapter of Hemlock in San Diego. In 1988, I tried to change the law in California with a ballot initiative. I was then invited to join the national board of Hemlock, which sponsored two close but unsuccessful legalization campaigns in Washington State and California."

According to Faye, "Things got more interesting in 1991, with the publication of Derek's book, *Final Exit*. It unexpectedly brought in a lot of money and Derek put $1 million into the Hemlock treasury. However, in 1992 he resigned following the whole rhubarb thing with his second wife."

"We all knew Ann," Faye said, "and none of us particularly liked her, but that is beside the point."

In 1996, Faye's husband died. She was still heading up the San Diego Hemlock Society chapter when she received an invitation to become the president of the national organization, which was now based in Denver. "I loved my job as a clinical and forensic psychologist in private practice," she explained, "but closed my office to move there and take the position."

"Practically all we offered at that time to people who called seeking help from Hemlock was that they read *Final Exit*. This was a barbaric thing to do to a suffering eighty-five-year-old person—the medications mentioned weren't [readily] available and all they really had was a plastic bag."

Faye proposed to the Hemlock board, "that we develop a team of volunteers who would go to [members'] homes and work with them—not directly to provide physical help or the means, but to tell them what to do and how to get the equipment that they needed. We'd be there when they died, if they chose that way. We called this program Caring Friends. I presented the tentative outline of Caring Friends at the Michigan meeting of Hemlock in 1997. In August 1998, was our first training, and twenty-eight volunteers assembled from all over the country."

"Shortly afterward," she continued during one of several interviews, "Derek started NuTech, a program to come up with alternatives to barbiturates, as these were increasingly difficult for people to obtain. In the second edition of *Final Exit* he had described using a plastic bag, but that was too uncertain. It was NuTech that came up with the helium method."

I would later ask Dick MacDonald and Larry Egbert to elaborate, but for now I listened while Faye talked about the second training of Caring Friends. In 1999, about twenty volunteers assembled to witness a demonstration of the helium method. "From then on," she explained, "that was the method we recommended to people. When the third edition of Derek's book came out in 2002, the helium method was highlighted."

While I am basically a "people person," interested in individual stories, from the very start of this project, I also realized that it would be important to grasp the social tsunami set in motion by Derek, Kevorkian, Faye, and their peers. I understood that it takes organizations to pass legislature or correct unjust laws or create protocols with explicit criteria. It takes an organized movement, be it the disability rights movement or the right-to-die movement, to create legislative acts that offer new options and freedom to millions of citizens. All of this begins with a small group of committed individuals working together, before society will incorporate novel ideas and expand the boundaries of acceptable behavior.

18

୨୦

CARING FRIENDS

As they were ushered into the living room of The Woman's elegant, prewar Manhattan apartment near Central Park, Dr. Richard (Dick) MacDonald and the volunteers from the Caring Friends program were jittery. The latter had taken part in the first training of the organization, but they didn't really know what to expect.

Like a classic diva, The Woman lay on an elegant settee looking impossibly sophisticated. She lived in an attractive residence that had high ceilings, thick walls, elegant plaster ornamentation, and generously proportioned rooms. She was a self-possessed, well-informed, highly educated, and cultured person in her early sixties, and the visitors were aware that she had been a successful executive in the fashion industry. But she immediately put her visitors at ease with a gracious smile and warm greeting.

The Woman knew exactly what she wanted. She wanted to die. But first, she wanted to celebrate. Whether you call it a party or a living wake, she wished to spend the next couple of days with her husband, best friends, and the small group of invited guests from Caring Friends. The latter provided her with confidence that she could effectively choreograph her death. Everyone present had come to support her "final exit."

When Dick told me this story, he simply called her "The Woman," so, I will, too. I asked if he wanted me to alter any of the details out of confidentiality concerns. Pausing to think about this, he replied in the negative. So, this account is taken almost verbatim from our interviews, and it offers a window as to the Caring Friends program in the 1990s. It is important to emphasize the service was provided solely to Hemlock members who often resided where there were no legal protocols for aid in dying. The state of New York, for example, has never passed a death-with-dignity law, and assisted suicide continues to be listed as a crime.

The Woman was married for many years and had no children. Her husband was considerably older than she and not in especially good health. It was apparent that after her death, he would almost certainly need to move to an assisted-living facility or make some other arrangements.

Five additional women arrived, who comfortably wandered in and out of the different rooms of the apartment. The six had been the closest of friends since college. They had spent nearly half a century intimately connected to each other in ways that only true female friends are able, and they had shared thrills, disappointments, tragedies, and the high and low points of careers, marriages, illnesses, and childrearing. The six women intended to use this opportunity to revel in the many years of memories that intertwined their lives.

All the assembled were prepared to respect the wishes of their dear host. The Woman had let it be known that she wanted to go out in style, and they were ready to share in a bountiful feast of the finest foods and alcohol.

This was the inaugural case for the newly formed Caring Friends program. Dick and the other volunteers were pleasantly surprised at their gracious reception. During the next several years, they would come to learn that patients and loved ones would almost invariably shower them with affection.

According to Dick, "People are appreciative that someone who doesn't really know them has arrived at this crucial moment to offer peace of mind . . . and the necessary information to prepare for when they choose to hasten their own deaths."

The Woman was a longtime member of the New York chapter of Hemlock. Her cancer began in the esophagus and despite treatment had widely metastasized. Having spread to her bones, she spent most of her days in the living room, dependent on opiates to control the pain. The cancer had reduced her to a state of emaciation, and her life was being prolonged with artificial nutrition and hydration provided through a feeding tube surgically implanted into her stomach.

The Woman had asked and received from her internist several prescriptions for an anti-nausea medication and nine grams of the barbiturate Seconal. This was the assisted dying regimen being used at the time in The Netherlands and Oregon.

Dick has acquired a vast experience with such matters, and he speaks softly and carefully. "Such a massive amount of barbiturate will overwhelm the brain," he told me. "It shuts down the centers controlling breathing and heart rate located in the brain stem. . . . One doesn't suffer with asphyxia (struggling to breathe) but dies from anoxia (the lack of oxygen). I always favor starting the antiemetic a day or two in advance . . . and in all the years that I used the medications, we never had a patient vomit up the barbiturate."

While it was often difficult for patients to obtain the necessary medicines from their physician, The Woman had a sensitive doctor who knew her intimately and was willing to acquiesce to her request. After filling the scripts at the pharmacy, her husband and a friend carefully took apart the ninety barbiturate capsules and dissolved the powder in juice. They could alternatively have used coffee or apple sauce with plenty of sugar added. Current protocols call for using the contents of one hundred barbiturate capsules (10 grams).

Dick has tasted a miniscule sample of dissolved barbiturates and says that it is an exceptionally bitter draught. He is impressed with the dogged determination required to swallow the necessary amount, even when buffered by a sweetener.

The strategy that Dick mentioned to people who wanted to obtain Seconal but couldn't confide the true purpose to their physician involved planning things well in advance and prevaricating. The individual would tell their doctor that they were going on a trip and needed a sleeping pill. They would explain that more common sedatives, like Ambien, Dalmane, Trazodone, and Valium, had proven to be ineffective; however, they had good success with Seconal.

When Andrew Solomon's mother did exactly this (as he described in a *New Yorker* article), her physician proceeded to write out a standard prescription for twenty pills.[1] Two months later she made the same request and he wrote another script. Meanwhile, she was simultaneously going through the same routine with a different doctor.

Dick explained the necessity for carrying out this charade multiple times to stockpile the required ninety or one hundred capsules. However, such an approach is no longer feasible, as most physicians won't offer this medication for insomnia under any circumstances.

Although he is far too modest to admit it, over the past twenty years Dick has been a brigadier general in the death-with-dignity movement. For a man approaching the ninth decade of life, he has a remarkable memory. I looked up several of the dates mentioned during our interviews and they were always spot-on.

Back in 1993, he noticed an advertisement in a medical journal stating that applicants were being sought for the position of medical director of the Hemlock Society. Dick had spent most of his life as an old-fashioned general practitioner, first in Canada, and later in Southern California. Hemlock decided it was imperative to hire someone to liaison with health care professionals at various levels. The organization realized it needed to enlist doctors and nurses to formulate and support a rational protocol if laws were ever going to be effectively changed. The Oregon ballot legalizing physician-assisted dying passed that year, but it was not allowed to go into effect because a right-to-life organization challenged it in the courts. It would not be until 1998 following the second Oregon ballot that the law was finally instituted. Dick was hired for a modest salary to work one day per week traveling around the country, speaking at medical conferences, and writing articles for newspapers, journals, and the organization's newsletter.

He secured the position after being interviewed by the Hemlock board and submitting essays, he told me, "about the early years of my practice—especially before the 1970s, when most people would not be hospitalized and chose to stay at home. During that period, I had helped a number of patients to die."

Dick graduated from medical school in 1952, and he went into a general practice where it was not unusual for him to treat terminally ill patients. In his quiet, easygoing way, Dick described how he and other physicians of his era readily accepted that it was rational for people to request assistance when suffering became unmanageable and their quality of life had drastically deteriorated.

"It was an open secret," he explained to me, "especially in general practice. Many of us felt that was part of what we owed to the patient. Back then, we were never criticized, either by our medical peers or by organized medicine or by church leaders for helping people. . . . Everyone understood that it was really comfort care."

Derek Humphry had just retired from his administrative role in the Hemlock Society. His book, *Final Exit*, had become so successful that he and Hemlock (the organization shared in the book's proceeds and received occasional bequests) were financially stable. According to Dick, Derek's preference had always been to advocate self-help rather than reliance on medical personnel. However, after he stepped down, the Hemlock board was persuaded by Faye to hire Dick and to shift the organization's emphasis to seek the aid of medical personnel and trained volunteers.

"I think Derek had a very pragmatic belief about physicians," Dick explained to me. "He knew some are supportive of their patients, as he had learned firsthand in England when he was able to get a physician to provide the barbiturates for his wife. But he also learned that organized medicine spoke out very strongly against . . . the Hemlock Society." Derek was open to involving physicians, but he had no expectation they would be helpful.

After Dick was hired, he began to approach other doctors, and the single most common explanation from colleagues who opposed assisted dying was that their religion prohibited this behavior. Dick grew accustomed to responding that he greatly respected their faith but hoped they would not impose their beliefs upon others. He asked them to respect patients who wanted to hasten death and to make referrals to physicians who were more likely to assist. As he traveled the lecture circuit, Dick quickly grew accustomed to medical staff and lay people coming up after his talks and saying, "I hope you are around when I am dying."

According to Dick, the creation of the Caring Friends program in 1998 was prompted by the suicide of a beloved member. When she became terminally ill, she was unable to obtain the assistance of others in helping her to die. She shot herself in the backyard and the body was found by a young woman going to work. The experience was traumatic to the Hemlock board, which felt that there was something awry if their own members were unable to access more dignified ways to end life. Waiting for the laws to change before acting or merely providing educational information in the form of books about which drugs would be effective suddenly seemed unacceptable.

Dick was asked to become the medical director of Caring Friends and to institute the first volunteer training course. It was conducted with the assistance of a retired hospice nurse, a social worker, and a Unitarian minister. The four senior instructors then assumed responsibility for determining when Caring Friends would offer "final exits." Two or three weeks later, in December of 1998, they heard from their first applicant—The Woman. By 2003, there were almost one hundred fifty Caring Friends volunteers.

When MacDonald started the group, he insisted that people for whom they would offer aid in dying had to be rational, able to provide documentation of an irreversible illness (even if it was not terminal and did not meet the six-month time period used by hospice), and afflicted by a medical condition that was accompanied by considerable suffering. If they had loved ones closely involved in their lives, those individuals had to be prepared to accept the death-hastening decision. It was essential for Dick that the means of accelerating dying be speedy and effective, which is why they initially recommended using barbiturates and only later switched to the helium method.

During the trainings, Dick taught the volunteers that they must feel the immensity of what was occurring and "make sure it goes very peacefully for the person." All the conversations during visits needed to focus on that individual—the person's life and final wishes. Everybody involved needed to understand the importance of the finite amount of remaining time. They were all likely to experience anticipatory grief, and the assisted dying represented a "sacred" opportunity for closure.

"No dying episode that I've attended is easy," said Dick. "I never get used to the idea the person we're visiting woke up that morning and said to him or herself, 'Well this is the last day of my life.' It's quite remarkable to me that they are so determined to complete life when they choose to. . . . It is absolutely what they want. There is usually such calm on the part of the loved ones who are present that you can tell that they, too, have already accepted the loss of their parent, partner, or child."

Dick is clear, "If we ever encountered an ambivalent person—and I can think of a couple of such situations—we have suggested that they not proceed." Caring Friends was built around the idea it would offer services to members of the Hemlock Society who had carefully formulated an end-of-life philosophy and now wanted to die. The group saw its role as providing information and support, and it was the responsibility of the individual (or their friends and family) to assemble the materials needed for any of the methods. Ultimately, it was up to the dying person to ingest the medications or to turn on the helium. The Caring Friends volunteers were prepared to be present in an advisory capacity. They came to share in the deaths out of compassion for their fellow human beings.

It was the second day of festivities at the Manhattan apartment of The Woman with esophageal cancer. Before agreeing to become medical director, Dick had supported (and he often uses this word as a synonym for *assisted*) numerous others to die. But while many of the deaths he attended through the years were bittersweet events, this first one for Caring Friends stands out in his memory because of the special closeness of the participants, the emotional honesty, the generosity in permitting him and the other volunteers to enter into The Woman's life, and the enthusiasm surrounding her leave-taking.

While doctors often have a well-deserved reputation for being emotionally distant and over-intellectualized, this was never the case for Dick. "Many of my patients became my friends, and many of my friends became my patients," he remarked. Serving in World War II helped shape his view that dying should not be prolonged. "Anyone who was in the military learned about the concept of triage," he explained. "You save the people you can, and make those that you can't save, comfortable."

The two days in the New York home had been spent with recordings of the hostess's favorite music playing in the background and poignant reminiscences proffered by the friends. While recounting stories from their common past, the women occasionally broke down, wept, and comforted each other. They railed against the cruel reality, and they frequently took refuge in humor. However, most of the time they simply accepted what was happening. Glasses were regularly lifted in toasts, and they ate with no attention accorded to the number of calories consumed. Their hostess was unable to eat normally, but she made do with her feeding tube.

The Woman had determined when and how the party would end. Turning to one of her friends, she asked for assistance to the bathroom so she could empty her bladder and bowels. According to Dick, "Most people are very thoughtful that way. They often will wear a diaper if they are afraid they are going to soil themselves. They do this even though we try to reassure them that with the peaceful manner they are choosing to die we don't see sphincter control loss. It just doesn't happen."

The Woman was accustomed to feeding herself meals of formulated liquid nutrients. The barbiturates had been dissolved into a liquid slurry and filled a large syringe. She was sitting up in a reclining chair, surrounded by everyone when she squeezed the mixture into the feeding tube.

"We make sure to have an opportunity before the exit time to talk with the family," Dick told me. "These women friends were 'family' to her. I explain how dying occurs according to the method the person chooses. We don't hide anything. We let them know it can be very difficult at times [to witness] very deep or stentorian breathing, [although] the person won't be having any distress because they are unconscious from the medication or the helium. He explained that family members choose whether to be with the loved one right to the end, to say farewell and be in another room, or to leave the premises entirely. "Amazingly," he said, "quite a few want to be there. We tell them that they will feel very proud of having supported the person. Often, we hear back from them that they were very glad to have been present. And it's not an easy thing."

The medicine had gone down the tube directly into The Woman's stomach, and within a couple of minutes she was deeply unconscious. Within half an hour her breathing stopped and death transpired. Dick believes that the short period of time between ingestion and death attested to how close she was to dying from the cancer, as more physically fit people might take two hours or more before respiration ceases.

Dick sat next to her and felt for a pulse. Such moments are in a sense "a let-down, but also a relief. One is relieved that it has been successful . . . that it has accomplished what they wanted most. And the person has had the dying process they wished." In her case, it was flawless.

"It is at this point that participants usually want to get busy and tidy up," Dick explained. "There is never a lot of wailing or gnashing of teeth. Instead there is quiet regret at the loss and a lot of hugging. If you have a planned death, most of the deep grieving has already taken place."

On this occasion, everyone sat for a while in the apartment and quietly chatted. They filled their glasses one more time and solemnly raised them in tribute. Dick observed, "I find that most of those who choose to be in control of their dying process have approached life optimistically. . . . It is common to hear them say, 'I've had a good life.' Accordingly, our toast is: 'To a good life and a good death!'"

Dick would then remind families to clean up and dispose of equipment, such as pill containers or the helium tanks and hoods, as most people wish their death to appear natural. Hoods were cut up so that if they were found by children they would not pose a health risk. The plastic was discarded in a dumpster along with the empty gas canisters.

Dick usually advised that if there was an arrangement made with a private physician or with hospice staff, then that individual should be called in a couple of hours. The doctor notifies the funeral director that they are available to sign the death certificate. If the family has made no arrangements, they are encouraged to phone the non-emergency line for the police and to say that their loved one was no longer breathing. They should explain that the person had been sick for a long time with a terminal illness and it was not an emergency. Despite that caution, unfortunately, sometimes emergency vehicles are dispatched because it is a death at home. Families are discouraged from making up an elaborate story and instead to simply say that they just discovered their loved one has died. Where hospice care is involved, the company should be notified to come and remove unused medications.

In two instances, Dick recalled, hospice directors and nurses had befriended the dying person and chose to witness the planned deaths. Throughout his many years of providing this service for Caring Friends and later for the Final Exit Network, none of Dick's cases resulted in a formal investigation or any legal problems.

Back in New York, the husband called his wife's internist and the funeral director. The following day, Dick and a couple of others met with the elderly spouse for a champagne brunch. The man would remain in touch with Dick for several years, and in his most recent letter the spouse wrote, "Looking back on it, I cannot imagine you having had a more perfect case."

19

THE METAMORPHOSIS
OF CARING FRIENDS

From 1998 to the summer of 2004, the Caring Friends program triaged thousands of calls, provided the number for suicide prevention hotlines to innumerable people with emotional and psychiatric problems, and maintained detailed records of 152 attended "exits." Dick MacDonald was personally present at more than two-thirds of these. In his capacity as medical director, he became accustomed to hopping on planes and traveling around the country to the bedsides of the dying. In a rare lapse from his usually exact accounts, he cannot recall for me whether the total of deaths he attended was 117 or 119.

The demographics of the people who chose to die this way are interesting. According to Dick, "Most of the exits did not have a strong religious affiliation." An exception was a Methodist minister who was attended at the end by her own minister. Dick also observed that among the membership of the death-with-dignity groups around the world there are very few non-Caucasians. He recalls presiding at the "exits" of one Latino, one Native American, and no African Americans.

According to Derek Humphry, "During his fourteen years in full-time service to the movement, Dr. MacDonald (Dick to everyone) did more in terms of actual help to the dying than anyone other than perhaps Dr. Kevorkian in the 1990s. But whereas Kevorkian trumpeted his actions, and confined them to Michigan, Dick quietly moved around America, and few—other than Caring Friends organizers—knew of his work. With great medical skill, careful regard for the law, and saintly empathy, Dick was at the bedside by request of many persons who were dying in distress."

When Dick stepped away from this work, he explained to me: "Being asked to be present with so many who proceeded to exercise their choice and control over that final important moment of life was both an honor and a privilege. I have learned much about dying and, perhaps more importantly, about living from many of those remarkable individuals." Later, he said, "We get a lot of [he cleared his throat] thanks. We get a lot of return from the appreciation of people. It is really remarkable."

Derek made the point that Dick always managed to remain under the radar. While the doctor agreed, he explained, "It's just that I guess [the authorities] don't have any complaints against me. Also, in my presentations to the public or medical people, I let them know that as a physician I don't feel like I am doing anything unethical. Indeed, I think it would be wrong to abandon patients at the end of life just because we can't do anything more for them."

It is difficult to find much about Dick's activities through online searches. Accordingly, I am especially grateful that he and I not only had the opportunity for several interviews, but that he was also willing to recount some self-revealing, autobiographical anecdotes.

Dick came from an English theatrical family that moved to Canada, where he was born. Following his medical training, he began working in California in 1965. He continues to maintain a close relationship with his five sons and a daughter, the youngest of whom was seven years old when Dick's wife suddenly dropped dead. This was in 1971, and she was forty-three years old when she collapsed in front of the family, could not be resuscitated, and likely succumbed to a cardiac arrhythmia. To better balance his professional life with the sudden increased responsibility for the children, he left his position as a medical director and took over another physician's general practice. He is pleased that his extended family pitched in and the children did a lot to take care of each other.

While the way his wife expired contributed to shaping his attitude about dying and his future role in Hemlock USA, Caring Friends, and the FEN, it was his mother's death four years earlier that was most consequential.

She had a huge lymphoma in her chest that had wrapped itself around the aorta and trachea and could not be surgically resected. During a hospitalization, a long, uncomfortable endotracheal tube was inserted down her nose and into her throat to keep the trachea from being compressed by the tumor. Dick came up from California, and he learned from his father and siblings that she had pulled the tube out by herself and did not wish to be resuscitated. The surgical staff had immediately reinserted it, and she was being kept isolated in the hospital. She would indicate to anyone who came into the room that she wanted the tube removed, but the staff had tied her hands and assigned a young nurse to sit by the bedside. When Dick arrived, his family were all perched uncomfortably in a nearby waiting room, and his mother was in a little cubicle.

According to Dick, "She was not heavily sedated when I walked in. She let me know with slight movements of her hands what she wanted and I took off the restraints. I told her some things about what kind of mother she had been, and how I was very fortunate and could never have picked better parents."

"What did you mean?" I asked.

"They were wonderful, loving people," he said, after a pause. "My mother was unfailingly cheerful and always optimistic. My parents never let us know how poor we were while growing up."

"What were you feeling when you saw her?"

"I was very upset when I saw how cruelly the staff was treating her. She had been abandoned by the chest specialist. They put the tube in, and I don't know what they were thinking. They had previously talked to my dad and said that there was nothing more to do. I was very angry. I then reached down and removed the tube. It was the right thing to do. I held her in my arms and she took her last breath. In a minute or two minutes, her eyes took on that startled expression that I've seen so often when there is an interruption of oxygen. She was gone and I kissed her goodbye."

"I was so focused on my mother," he said, "that I didn't appreciate there was the young nurse sitting at the foot of the bed. I suddenly realized there could be repercussions. But she turned to me and said very quietly, 'Thank you, doctor.'"

At this point in the interview, Dick began to cry.

Dick indicated that he had not previously considered how powerfully her death influenced his future attitudes. At the time, he remembers thinking, *That was no way to treat people at the end of life.*

Composing himself, he told me that after leaving the hospital room, he sat down with his family. All of them were indignant about what had been going on, and they knew that she would not live long after Dick arrived. They had said their goodbyes and everyone had kissed her. Now, each of his family members expressed gratitude for what he had done.

After I wrote this chapter, I listened again to the three times I interviewed Dick. Here was an octogenarian physician who had been a spokesman for Hemlock and an activist who traveled around the country, visiting sick and anguished people. He was an Angel of Mercy and an Angel of Death. He came into homes and offered the necessary information and confidence to die. The last time that we spoke, Dick was ninety-one years old, and he was still receiving cards from the families of people whom he had met through his activities. The Woman's husband invited him out for lunch each time he visited New York.

It seems amazing to me that throughout his years as Caring Friends' medical director, Dick never felt intimidated or fearful of being prosecuted for murder or manslaughter. But until he recounted this anecdote to me, Dick had been unaware that his experience in the small hospital room with his mother had clarified who he was and set in motion the future role that he would undertake. I now understand that his moral sense of righteousness nullified any apprehensions that other people might have experienced under those circumstances.

At the Federation meeting in Chicago and during subsequent interviews with Faye Girsh, I asked her for an account of what happened to Caring Friends.

"We had volunteers all over the country," she said. "We had a very well run and efficient program. Dick MacDonald . . . Saint Dick! I love him. Everybody loves him! He was a wonderful medical director. I hope he outlives me, so when I die he can be there. He's just wonderful!"

Faye then told me how her tenure as president of Hemlock came to an end. "In 2003," she said, "the board wanted a *real* administrator, and I'm not that! They asked me to become a senior vice president, but the board was obviously going in a more conservative direction. Paul Spiers—not my favorite person—became chairman."

I thought, *Paul Spiers? The guy who riffs on Hercules? How could he not be Faye's favorite person?* But on reflection, I realized that Paul and the other activists I met all had distinct personalities, and I was only in the position of interviewing them. I never needed to negotiate with Paul or the others over conflictual issues.

Faye continued, "Spiers decided he wouldn't be chairman of an organization that was named for a poison weed. A lot of money was spent on doing polls and focus groups and all kinds of foolishness. They dropped the name, Hemlock, and came up with End of Life Choices. That lasted for only a year because, of course, no one could remember the new name."

"What happened to Caring Friends?" I inquired.

"The handwriting was on the wall that it was going to be shrunk down to nothing. The plan called for End of Life Choices to merge with another right-to-die organization, Compassion & Dying, and the new name would be Compassion & Choices (C&C)."

Faye and some of the more radical activists were unhappy with these organizational changes and met to discuss other possibilities. Faye explained, "We decided not to replace Hemlock but to keep the Caring Friends program intact [but under another name]. Half of Hemlock had been dedicated to changing laws, and we decided to leave that to C&C. A new organization sprung up in 2005, the Final Exit Network (FEN), to directly help people. It didn't agree with the restrictions C&C had about helping people. . . . FEN was not limited to a medical model (with a doctor or nurse participating) and [it also] offered services to people with chronic illnesses [who were irremediably suffering]. In addition, we wanted to potentially be present when people died and to offer our emotional support. The FEN [membership] followed the same criteria as that of Caring Friends and differed only in that it was entirely a volunteer organization without [any] paid staff. Dick MacDonald was unavailable when it was created and Dr. Larry Egbert, one of his protégé's, became the medical director."

Dick knew Larry from Caring Friends, as Egbert had volunteered, trained, and accompanied him on quite a few cases. "I imagine he considers me to be a mentor," said Dick. "We are good friends. He accepted the experience I had, and he learned from me." Dick would later volunteer to help with FEN before eventually retiring.

Faye left Denver and traveled for ten months, reestablishing her home in California. She resumed work with Hemlock of San Diego—the former chapter continues to retain the Hemlock name. In 2006, Faye became a senior advisor and FEN guide. Derek had been instrumental in also forging a global organization, called the World Federation of Right to Die Societies. Faye would succeed him, and she was presiding as the Federation's president when I attended the Chicago meeting.

In an analysis of eighteen years of data about assisted dying in Oregon using the barbiturate Seconal, Dr. Charles Blanke reported that after ingestion, coma ensued within approximately four minutes and death within twenty-five minutes.[1] "The coma," he explained was "like being anesthetized. The blood pressure and pulse slow and the person doesn't react to discomfort, indicating they're not in pain."[2] Blanke's conclusions are based on a sample of 1,545 patients who legally obtained a lethal prescription between 1998 and 2015. On average, 64 percent took the drug while the others died from their underlying diseases. Thirty-three (3.3%) of the patients who ingested the medication had complications, including six who woke up. They would die later from cancer and their other illnesses.

Seconal was developed by Eli Lilly and Company as a sleeping aid, anesthetic, and anticonvulsant. It first became available in the United States in 1934. According to Catherine Offord, the medication's active ingredient, the barbiturate secobarbital, was widely prescribed in the 1950s and 1960s chiefly as a sleeping pill, but it fell out of fashion among physicians due to problems with accidental overdoses, the abuse potential, and the emergence of benzodiazepines (another class of drugs) as safer alternatives.[3] In 2009, Seconal retailed for around $2 per capsule; the price then gradually spiraled up to around $15. However, when the rights to produce it were sold in 2015 to Canada-based Valeant Pharmaceuticals, the company promptly doubled the price to $30.

According to Offord: "Just one month prior to Seconal's price hike, California had proposed legislation that would make it the fifth state to allow medical-aid-in-dying, in which terminally ill patients given less than six months to live could choose to end their own lives with a physician's prescription for a lethal quantity of a drug—Seconal being the drug of choice. . . . But some healthcare practitioners called the move exploitative, whether or not the timing was deliberate." Spokespersons from Valeant denied the existence of ulterior motives for the cost increase, stating that the company did not promote it, sold only about a thousand prescriptions in 2015, and expected to earn less than $3 million in sales in 2016.

The alleged price gouging resulted in further attention being paid to Valeant, which was already being investigated after steeply hiking the prices of two cardiac drugs. Either way, the retail cost of 100 capsules of Seconal required for a death with dignity now carried a whopping price tag of $3,000 or more, with a recent podcast suggesting the cost in California is between $5,000 and $6,000.[4] While California Medicaid and several private insurance companies cover the cost, for some unfortunate people, such as those dependent on Washington Medicaid, the drug is unaffordable even if they are qualified to use it under their state's law.

George Eighmey, president of the board of directors of the nonprofit organization Death with Dignity National Center and a former state representative who helped pass Oregon's legislation, remarked that Seconal has become "prohibitively expensive," and as a direct result, doctors began to actively seek alternatives.[5]

Dick MacDonald was equally familiar with another barbiturate, pentobarbital, first developed more than eighty years ago and distributed under the brand name Nembutal. It, too, was marketed for insomnia. Physicians like Dick understood that ten grams of either the liquid or powder forms of Nembutal would cause a progressively deep sleep followed by a peaceful death.

The drug was widely employed as an anesthetic for veterinary surgery, and as people who sought to use it for hastening death ran into difficulty getting physicians to write barbiturate prescriptions, an underground network of smugglers began bringing Nembutal up from Mexico. Dick explained to me that, "People would go below the border and purchase quite a few vials. The couriers did not charge exorbitant amounts for this service. . . . A prescription was not even necessary. The couriers would merely say that they had a large animal and wanted to do a little surgery. . . . The main supply used to come from Tijuana. . . . But that has pretty much dried up lately."

According to Derek, the July 2018 newsletter of the Exit International organization lists forty-three websites that claim to sell Nembutal. They are scams, and potential buyers lose between $500 and $700 when they attempt to purchase barbiturates over the Internet.

Nelson and Offort have pointed out that as Seconal became exorbitantly priced and Nembutal less available, different combinations of drugs were then investigated that could be manufactured by compounding pharmacies.[6] These businesses mix drugs into products on a prescription-by-prescription basis and are not regulated by the US Food and Drug Administration.

Doctors with the End of Life Washington advocacy group proposed combining chloral hydrate (a sedative), morphine sulfate (an opiate analgesic), and phenobarbital (the barbiturate frequently used to treat epilepsy).[7] The cost came to a more reasonable $500.

Unfortunately, chloral hydrate turned out to be very acidic and when swallowed it is irritating to the mouth and throat. Although this problem with the so-called Washington compound became widely known, it was still selected by more than a third of patients from that state who were offered the option in 2015 presumably because of price considerations.

The following year, another combination was tried that did not contain chloral hydrate, and consisted instead of diazepam, digoxin, morphine, and propranol (it was dubbed DDMP).[8] But this mixture turned out to be slow-acting, and the group of physicians from Washington proposed yet a new compound that increased the dosage of three of these drugs. The compounded drug formula is known as DDMP2, retails for $700, and is now being extensively used in California.[9] According to the Washington group, death ensues within two hours.

Canada, the Netherlands, Belgium, and Luxembourg have each passed laws permitting medically assisted dying with oral medications, but they have also legalized voluntary euthanasia, or what Canada calls clinician-administered medical assistance in dying, whereby a physician can administer a lethal drug dose by injection (usually intravenously). According to Nelson, this second option allows for greater flexibility, lower costs, and fewer medication-associated complications.[10] She reports that less than 1 percent of patients in Ontario choose to end their lives through oral self-administration of pills, and almost all the Canadian patients are choosing to rely on clinician-administered medical assistance in dying.

According to Dr. Madeline Li from the Department of Supportive Care at the University Health Network–Princess Margaret Cancer Center, when Canadian patients opt for lethal injections, a series of drugs are administered in sequence. This begins with midazolam (for sedation), lidocaine (a local anesthetic), propofol (to induce coma, myocardial depression, respiratory depression, and to lower vascular resistance), and rocuronium (to cause respiratory muscle paralysis).[11]

In 1998, the complications and scarcity of effective oral medications for hastening death led to the formation of an organization called NuTech (New Technologies in Self-Deliverance).[12] Derek Humphry was its founder, and he was specifically interested in the development and promotion of nonmedical methods to hasten death. Derek prefers life-ending practices that require minimal involvement of health care professionals, and accordingly, he has discouraged the use of intravenous substances or other practices that need physicians, nurses, or medical technicians to be in attendance. According to its website, "NuTech's philosophy has been to acknowledge the importance of technology and technical development in the creation of better, more effective and peaceful ways for a person—in the context of old age or illness—to end their life."[13] The Holy Grail the organization has sought would be a lethal chemical or combination of agents that will be humane, effective, well-tolerated, inexpensive, readily available, simple to administer, and fast acting.

NuTech is uninterested in drawing attention to its activities or membership.[14] Search online for the name and one will encounter links to computer software, reservoir life cycle, regenerative medical products, seeds, cleaning supplies, security services, and fishing lures—anything but methods to hasten death.

NuTech's research is conducted by a small international group of scientists, physicians, aid-in-dying activists, and a few deep-sea divers. The latter were recruited because they had first-hand experience using helium in their tanks to prevent oxygen levels from getting too high and causing the bends. They were the ones who came up with another, more deadly, use for the gas, and to employ it at home to cause planned deaths.

NuTech's members initially began experimenting with helium during meetings. One volunteer said that after a couple of breaths he felt dizzy, as if he had had a couple of drinks, while most of the group reported having had no unpleasant symptoms whatsoever. Those who continued inhaling the gas became unconscious in about half a minute. Naturally, after they passed out, their colleagues then quickly shut off the canister, removed the bag that had been used to administer the gas, and the individuals awoke to full consciousness a minute later. They consistently denied feeling any distress throughout the test.

Helium is widely available in the form of small containers sold at party stores to inflate balloons. The apparatus necessary to administer the gas is simple to construct and requires widely available plastic tubing and a plastic bag that is slipped over the person's head. A resourceful activist from Florida made it even easier by manufacturing and selling inexpensive mail-order kits before her business was abruptly shut down by authorities.[15]

Dick was initially wary of the helium method. He was repulsed by the idea of using a plastic bag to administer gas. In the early days of the Hemlock Society, he had witnessed people following the recommendations outlined in the first edition of Derek's book, *Final Exit*, to ensure death following an overdose by covering one's head with a plastic bag. Individuals like David and Reba Raff secured the bag with rubber bands or by tying pantyhose around the neck and would thereby decrease the concentration of oxygen they were inhaling. Unfortunately, this technique resulted in the buildup of carbon dioxide, which triggered "air-hunger" and a panicky feeling of suffocation. Dick had watched people's faces through the bags, and he felt that some of them were dying uncomfortably from asphyxiation.

However, the helium gas technique radically changed matters. It resulted in anoxic deaths, not deaths by asphyxiation. Carbon dioxide did not increase. Instead the helium replaced oxygen in the person's body; their brain and other organs then rapidly ceased functioning. Beginning with his first case using helium, Dick was surprised at how acceptable it was to patients, their loved ones, and the volunteers—perhaps because people had become accustomed to anesthesiologists administering gas in operating rooms or dentists using nitrous oxide gas in their offices. As Nembutal and Seconal became less available, the helium method was increasingly recommended by Caring Friends. It would later become FEN's chief means to accelerate dying.

But before one rushes out to purchase a few tanks as an aid-in-dying insurance plan, it is important to know that over the past couple of years, manufacturers have been diluting the helium in balloon-inflation tanks with ordinary air. This is because of the rising cost of the inert gas, but it has inadvertently made helium from these tanks unsuitable for hastening death.

A modest annual award is now offered by Derek through ERGO to incentivize other innovative approaches.[16] I am of two minds about these efforts. I had a viscerally disturbing telephone interview with a member of NuTech, a physician living on the New York–Canadian border, who described testing out his ideas with farm animals. My head was flooded with horrific images of the Third Reich's obsessive attempts to find more effective techniques to kill Jews, homosexuals, and others "undesirables" in the concentration camps, and I couldn't get off the phone soon enough. I had a similar reaction to reading about experimental protocols, including a four-drug cocktail with the powerful opioid fentanyl, that are being tried in different states to execute convicted murderers.[17] On the other hand, I would like a reliable method to accelerate dying for people seeking medical assistance who have grievous and irremediable conditions, and I realize that these won't materialize merely by wishing.

Protocols involving inhalation of nitrogen are now being explored as a method by different states to carry out the death penalty.[18] Nitrogen is a widely available inert gas that should work in the same manner as helium through rapid replacement of oxygen in the body. Oklahoma's attorney general, Mike Hunter, has been quoted as saying that use of nitrogen to execute people is "the safest, the best and the most effective method available."[19]

Gas chambers had been constructed in United States prisons for this purpose since the 1920s, although they originally relied on hydrogen cyanide. This method proved to be unsatisfactory because it can cause visible suffering for ten minutes or longer. It was last employed in 1999.[20]

The current president of FEN, Janis Landis, believes the "science behind inert gases is quite well settled," and her organization considers nitrogen inhalation to be a reasonable method.[21]

FEN presently directs people to information about how to acquire and use it.

In 2017, Dr. Philip Nitschke came up with a unique way to administer the gas when he announced his invention of a euthanasia machine—the "Sarco capsule."[22] The Sarco can be 3D printed from plastic and has been described as resembling a luxurious one-person spaceship. When a person lies in the capsule, he or she can activate the mechanism with a code, at which point liquid nitrogen rapidly lowers the oxygen level and death occurs in a few minutes. According to Nitschke, an Australian activist, the capsule can then be detached from its base and used as a shiny coffin.

Nitschke has written, "Sarco does not use any restricted drugs, or require any special expertise such as the insertion of an intravenous needle. Anyone who can pass the [online psychological] entry test, can enter the machine and legally end their life."[23]

According to *Newsweek*, Nitschke has dubbed himself "the Elon Musk of assisted suicide" and considers the new machine to be his Tesla.[24] Inspired by Jack Kevorkian, Nitschke previously helped hundreds of people to have what he calls "rational suicides," although none have so far made use of the Sarco. The doctor fervently believes that anyone over the age of seventy who wants to die, for any reason, should be helped to achieve their desire.

He is not the only one who subscribes to this philosophical stance, but I am not among their number.

THE NEW DR. DEATH

The lawyer wore a conservative gray suit; the heavily tattooed and muscular prisoner was clad in a standard-issue orange jumpsuit. The two black men sat opposite each other across a table that was bolted to the floor in the overheated subterranean basement vestibule leading from the Baltimore City Jail to Courthouse East. They were engaged in a last-minute conversation about a plea bargain.

Two other men approached. One was a no-nonsense black correctional officer. By his side was a slender, elderly white man, Dr. Lawrence (Larry) Deems Egbert Jr., who usually moved with a gracefulness that belied his age. Larry's expressive eyes had a bemused look, but inside he was thinking, *I'm practically the only white person in this place.* Characteristically, the eighty-one-year-old, semi-retired anesthesiologist was fixated on the issue of institutional racism, even though he himself was clad in an orange jumpsuit. Larry would tell me later how he hobbled along, hands manacled, a chain around the waist, and leg irons secured to his ankles.

As he and the guard walked past the small conference table, the tattooed prisoner caught a glimpse of Larry's face and pointed. "That man right there? He's the real gangsta." The lawyer stared back at him with a puzzled expression.

"No bullshit. They say that for fifty bucks that man and his group will bump you off." He announced loudly, "For fifty bucks, they'll kill you dead."

Larry had never thought about things in quite those terms. But $50 was, in fact, the cost of membership in his organization, the Final Exit Network (FEN), which was the successor of Caring Friends. It had always seemed like such a small fee to lead to such immense consequences.

The previous morning, a bright and cheerful Wednesday, February 25, 2009, Larry had been working in his third-floor walkup office in an unassuming brick rowhouse in Baltimore, Maryland, when he heard fists banging on the door downstairs and a booming voice announced: "Open up! It's the police."

Thinking it was a prank, Larry cheerfully called down, "Cut the racket! The door is unlocked. Come on in!"

To his astonishment, four enormous homicide officers wearing helmets and body armor and brandishing guns ran up the stairs, yelling at the top of their lungs, "You are under arrest! Don't move a muscle! You are under arrest!" They seemed gargantuan and were trained to make a paralyzing first impression.

They succeeded.

Larry was terrified as the officers roughly grabbed his shoulders, swung him around, patted down his body and handcuffed his arms behind his back. They explained that he was charged by the state of Georgia for assisting in a suicide and they intended to wait in his office for the arrival of Georgia law enforcement representatives before bringing him to the Baltimore City Jail.

After establishing the octogenarian was not especially threatening and had no weapons, the police momentarily undid the handcuffs and allowed Larry to sit down. They permitted him to shift his arms to the front before reattaching the wrist restraints.

For two hours, the police and their prisoner awkwardly waited for the Georgia authorities. During that time, Larry's downstairs neighbors, who were fond of the old man with the slogan-festooned office ("We shall overcome Reagan" and

"Nuclear Free Zone"), debated what to do. They decided to call a local television station and the American Civil Liberties Union.

Consequently, plenty of curious bystanders were present when Larry was brought outside, and a television film crew chronicled his departure. The police officers rushed him past the small crowd, and the cavalcade quickly drove downtown to Baltimore's pretrial detention lockup. He then entered the formidable stone building—the oldest sections of which date from the 1850s—that overwhelmingly houses poor people of color awaiting trials for drug-related crimes. Larry was efficiently processed, fingerprinted, and given the orange jumpsuit. For his personal safety, he was locked in a cell normally reserved for psychotic inmates. While Larry had previously been arrested during civil protests, he had always been one of a crowd of activists and was never incarcerated. This time, Larry was to reside for nearly three days within a city jail that has roughly three thousand prisoners and has been described by the American Civil Liberties Union as being "a dank and dangerous place, where detainees are confined in dirty cells infested with vermin."[1] Like Jack Kevorkian, he would have the dubious distinction of being the facility's oldest inmate.

The physician was eventually brought upstairs to the historic federal courtroom to see the judge. Spotting his wife surrounded by supporters, including a Baltimore City Councilwoman and a Maryland State Representative, he grinned and waved his manacled hands, greatly upsetting the correctional officer. He was loudly instructed, "to put down your arms and behave properly." After the courtroom was called to order, Larry turned his attention to the judge who asked him if he understood his situation. Larry quickly relinquished all rights to an extradition hearing and agreed to pay bail.[2] He was instructed to travel to Atlanta to face criminal charges.

Larry didn't know it at the time, but his arrest followed an eight-state probe of the FEN in which the Georgia Bureau of Investigation concluded that, as its medical director, Larry had played an integral role in the death of fifty-eight-year-old John Celmer of Cumming, Georgia. Mr. Celmer had committed suicide in June. Larry and three other members of the Network were accused of not only assisting in his death and tampering with evidence, but also violating the RICO Act—the federal antiracketeering law that was enacted originally to prosecute the leaders of the Mafia and organized crime syndicates.

The FEN consists to this day of a largely underground group of volunteers, mainly in their seventies and eighties, who offer their services to the entire country. While the organization promotes the use of living wills, advance directives, do-not-resuscitate orders, and hospice services, it remains unusual in its willingness to not only help terminally ill patients but also people suffering from chronic illnesses. FEN volunteers are ready to aid people with dementias, Lou Gehrig's disease, multiple sclerosis, Parkinson's disease, muscular dystrophy, congestive heart failure, emphysema, and other slowly progressive and incurable disorders.

Larry and his associates are admirers of palliative medicine, the specialty that focuses on symptom management and brings attention to end-of-life issues. But while they agreed that its practitioners may relieve many patients of their physical complaints, they also correctly believed that suffering is a considerably more complicated social and emotional construct. Larry would expand the concept of suffering to encompass people who desperately did not wish to be confined to nursing homes, individuals who firmly resolved not to outlive their spouses, and those who adamantly had no intention of expending their remaining assets on futile medical therapies. If asked, he would have been willing to assist Chester Nimitz Jr. and his wife, Joan, along with David and Reba Raff, and Sigmund Freud.

As subsequent legal proceedings would reveal, the FEN did not exclude helping people whose families might take umbrage at assisted dying. The FEN also didn't require individuals to be physically able to swallow a lethal cocktail of medications—the only means of dying offered in states that have approved death-with-dignity protocols. In other words, the organization chose to follow broad—and many would say overly expansive—definitions for both suffering and ways to facilitate dying.

Larry's tenure as medical director began in 2004 when the group was founded. If distressed people applied to the FEN, he was the one primarily responsible for reviewing their letters and medical records. For nearly six years, Larry and a small committee were the final arbiters as to whether applicants were intolerably suffering and whether the FEN would help them to end their lives. Larry told me that he oversaw about three hundred deaths, roughly twice that of Kevorkian. He was personally present at the deathbeds of over one hundred people. When the police stormed into the office, at least twenty open files from new membership applicants sat on his desk awaiting attention; he was grateful that they didn't notice the pile of papers.

Larry left the Baltimore courtroom feeling relieved at the thought of soon being reunited with his wife and finally able to go home to shower, eat, and get a good night's sleep. He did not appreciate that he and his organization had been targeted by a law enforcement task force. He had no idea that authorities were actively gathering and preparing to provide evidence to local police and prosecutors around the country. He was unaware that, besides Georgia, two other states would issue criminal indictments against him. The cases represented a backlash against the successes and perceived dangers of his organization's role in the death-with-dignity movement. Larry could not have anticipated that *Newsweek* magazine would publish an article titled, "The New Dr. Death," that labeled him as being "assisted suicide's new face."[3] He certainly did not realize that a marathon ordeal was just beginning, or that at the same moment the police burst into his office they were also simultaneously rushing into eleven other addresses around the country, including that of his home.

Larry was detained by the police on a Wednesday afternoon and remained in jail on Thursday and most of Friday. During that time, his wife, Ellen Barfield, was in constant contact with family and friends, securing legal representation, coordinating the case with the American Civil Liberties Union, and staying in close communication with Derek and FEN board members. A deal was reached that her husband would be released on $60,000 bail to go to Georgia for the arraignment. Ellen needed to put up their house as collateral, and she had to first unearth the necessary documents to prove they owned the property. A lien was then placed and the money secured for the Friday afternoon hearing.

Ellen rode her bicycle to the courthouse. She sat on a wooden bench surrounded by friends and supporters. The proceedings concluded after only a few minutes, but she was sufficiently experienced to know that she should then return home while the bureaucratic wheels of justice slowly ground along.

Around midnight, Larry was finally taken out of his cell, given his clothes, and escorted to the room where his wife was waiting. She had come back with a friend who would drive them home.

As the couple walked out of the Baltimore jail rimmed with razor wire, it was early Saturday morning and the sun had not yet risen. In the harsh glow of spotlights, a sign suspended on the gate caught Larry's attention. He pointed it out to Ellen. It read, "Please Don't Come Back."

For Hemlock members approaching the terminus of their lives, the Caring Friends program was a valuable resource that quietly functioned in the shadows. So then how and why did Larry and his organization, the FEN, come under fire?

One answer is that a backlash was due. Derek Humphry and Jack Kevorkian had catalyzed a social movement in the United States, and there was inevitably going to be a societal reaction to maintain homeostasis.

But another answer is evident in the dissimilarities between the FEN and its predecessor, Caring Friends. It was these differences that were chiefly responsible for bringing unwanted attention and damage to the movement. During the 1970s and 1980s the Hemlock Society had expanded its membership rolls exponentially, as people were repelled by the idea of relinquishing control of the end of life to the medical establishment. In 1998, the leadership created Caring Friends to assist people who were irremediably suffering. Caring Friends limited its instructional and supportive activities through 2004 to existing members of Hemlock. They were individuals who likely had spent years communicating their end-of-life preferences to friends and loved ones.

By contrast, the FEN, which was formed in 2004–2005, decided to offer its services to anyone who met its basic criteria. By 2016, the FEN had more than three thousand members and about thirty exit guides.[4] While some of those who joined had long-standing beliefs in the right to die, the organization also attracted newcomers who were acutely or chronically distressed and had now discovered a means to end their misery. They frequently had family who were either unprepared or vehemently opposed to the idea of a planned death. This became especially problematic, as was evident in court cases, when people with nonterminal and other ethically more complex conditions sought and received the FEN's support.

Finally, there were activists in leadership positions at the FEN who mistakenly thought America was poised to embrace assisted dying and needed a final push that would be provided by advertising. Ted Goodwin had helped to set up the organization with Faye, and he gave interviews stating they would do everything in their power to adhere to the statutes and remain lawful. "But," Ted told me, "what we were doing was going to raise the ire of some law enforcement group that found we had run afoul of their legal code and [they would] then push the issue with their resources and power. . . . What I predicted over and over again was that arrests would be made. We didn't know when but were prepared as a group to take this risk because we thought this is something we need to do."

According to Ellen Barfield, "Sometime after he was brought to jail, Larry's eldest daughter asked, 'Why, Dad, have you been courting arrest?' But the answer is that he was not courting it. Larry and the other FEN people were willing to provide help, even though they knew there was a legal risk." She maintains that Larry never consciously wanted or sought such attention.

Nevertheless, his daughter's query is germane, and there is the matter of the Billboard Project.[5] During the summer of 2010, while Larry was awaiting trial in Georgia, the FEN board of directors launched a publicity campaign. Commuters from northern New Jersey (just outside of New York City) and San Francisco who were crawling along the crowded highways couldn't help but notice spanking new 14-by-48-foot billboards bearing the black and white message, "My life. My death. My choice. FinalExitNetwork.org." According to the FEN's newsletter, the explicit purpose of the billboards was "to provoke dialogue and create awareness of who we are." What the FEN's leaders didn't appreciate was that even if most of the country voiced support for the movement in opinion polls or at the dinner table, this still left millions of people who questioned or rejected its ideas.

The rollout of the FEN billboards continued the following year.[6] A new message went up in Chicago, Denver, Los Angeles, and South Florida: "Irreversible illness? Unbearable Pain? Die with Dignity. Join Final Exit Network."

Again, even if Larry had no desire to "court arrest," there were obviously people within the FEN who did not share his interest in maintaining a low profile. They saw an opportunity to get their message out and seized it.

However, throwing a media spotlight on the FEN was akin to resurrecting Jack Kevorkian. It mobilized hard-core opposition activists who claimed to law enforcement that FEN consisted of serial murderers who operated throughout the country. Opposition activists announced to the religious faithful that there was a radical group of individuals who were directly comparable to abortionists killing babies. They promulgated the ideas that those being killed were disabled, elderly, and vulnerable segments of the populace, and that all of the "slippery slope" arguments were justified.

The publicity campaign prompted the Archdiocese of Newark to issue a statement that the billboard's message "cannot be condoned. The Catholic Church teaches, and has always taught, that all human life has dignity and all human life is precious."[7]

The blogosphere lit up and critics labeled Larry and the FEN members as "suicide vigilantes." Stephen Drake, a Not Dead Yet research analyst, called FEN "the Tea Party of the right-to-die movement."[8] Attorney Wesley J. Smith, who relentlessly opposes aid-in-dying practices, warned that "beneath the loud assertions of [the billboards] lurks an ideology that would lead us toward for-profit suicide clinics—already proposed in Oregon—and a virtual death on demand social ethic. That is the ugly truth that simplistic billboard sloganeering just can't hide."[9]

In Georgia, the FEN's legal costs were anticipated to be enormous. Complicating matters, the state immediately froze the bank account and assets of the organization. It was Derek, the leading figure in the international death with dignity movement, who immediately responded by securing and hiring a legal team and raising funds to cover the expenses.

Derek explained to me that the FEN had about $400,000 in the bank when law enforcement swooped. Suddenly they were penniless. Even the World Federation of Right to Die Societies, which had nothing directly to do with the case but had an American account, found its assets frozen. After Derek was alerted, he rushed down to his bank, and by Monday had created and was running the Final Exit Liberty Fund. Although he made it very clear that contributions were not tax deductible, Derek was gratified by the public's generosity. The fund swelled to $150,000, and he rapidly began retaining attorneys and covering bail bonds. By then the FEN had unfrozen some of its money—some $200,000 that hadn't been properly seized. The organization went to court and argued that the Georgia authorities had acted illegally. All the assets were then restored by a judge.

On February 25, 2009, the Georgia Bureau of Investigation (GBI) had launched its investigation into the FEN. Review of documents later provided to Larry's attorneys include a PowerPoint presentation used to brief participants in an ambitious and carefully coordinated operation involving GBI and FBI agents, state troopers, and local police.

Law enforcement is not interest in subtleties. All the police want to do is uncover the truth as to whether a crime has been committed; they don't have a personal axe to grind. Regarding the FEN, the GBI's role was straightforward; it was not up to the agents to decide what laws they are going to enforce. Their job was to enforce all the laws. If aiding someone to die equated with killing them, then Larry and his codefendants from the FEN were not only potentially serial killers but mass murderers. And murder is the biggest crime—the ultimate crime.

However, from the police perspective the assisted-suicide laws are annoyingly complicated. The problem for law enforcement is the absence of a bright line delineating suicide from homicide, and police hate being placed in the middle of ambiguous situations. Police officers all too often receive contradictory and confusing orders. For example, when they are in training and go to the shooting range to qualify, the instructor invariably says, "We don't shoot to kill, we shoot to stop." But then the cop is applauded for firing off fifteen rounds from his or her 9 mm pistol and blowing a foot-wide hole through the heart of a paper target. The reality is that a cop learns to continue shooting until the danger is over. That means the targeted person has stopped moving, and it also likely means that he's dead. It is when things are fuzzy that police find themselves in big trouble with their superior officers, the politicians, and the public.

The GBI tried to keep things simple. It explained to the agents that the FEN was an organization dedicated to assisting people with non-terminal as well as terminal illnesses to commit suicide. The GBI's description was carefully worded and mainly accurate.[10] Assisted suicides, it stated, were generally accomplished by using helium tanks attached to a plastic bag or "exit hood" placed over the individual's head. In a document that I reviewed, the GBI omitted to say that patients were responsible for obtaining the gas, acquiring or building the bag, and ultimately pulling the hood over their own head. But the letter correctly explained that inhalation of pure helium resulted in the loss of consciousness and finally death. No mention was made in the GBI document as to how long it would take for death to occur or whether it involved any discomfort.

It was noted that an individual became a member of FEN after applying to receive the organization's services. During this process, the applicant's personal and medical information were sent to key members of FEN for review, and Dr. Larry Egbert was the final arbiter. If accepted, the individual was assigned two "exit guides" to assist the person with the preparation and completion of the suicide.

FEN first came to the attention of the GBI in June 2008 during an investigation into the death of a Georgia man, John Celmer.[11] Celmer was receiving treatment for cancer of the mouth and jaw. However, at the time of death, his disease was believed to have been in remission. According to a reporter, Charles Bethea, Celmer discovered an oral cancer that was likely caused by years of smoking (echoes of Sigmund Freud).[12] In September of 2006, he had his first operation, which involved cutting the skin along his throat from ear to ear and pulling up his face. The tumor was only partially resected, along with much of the floor of his mouth. Celmer then underwent radiation therapy, which unfortunately damaged his jaw and led to the loss of his teeth. By early 2007, a hole had formed in his lower jawbone below his chin.

Bethea wrote, "Everything he ate continued to fall through the hole in his jaw. He brushed his teeth and looked in the mirror and could see the sink through the hole." His speech was largely unintelligible, and working became too difficult to continue.

In 2008, Celmer underwent another disfiguring procedure, in which the surgeons attempted to reconstruct his chin and jaw using bone from his lower leg tissue and skin grafts from his chest.

Celmer had separated from his wife, Sue, several years before, but they lived in the same complex; she visited daily, and they remained close. The last surgery was considered to have been a "success," and he wasn't considered to be dying. Five days later, Sue Celmer was shocked to find his body.

Later when she went through his effects, she discovered a receipt for two helium tanks, computer messages pertaining to the FEN, several copies of the book *Final Exit*, and a handwritten note about buying a "hood." Sue Celmer was a deeply religious woman and was greatly offended that his life had ended this way. She also felt hurt that her ex-husband had not confided in her.

"We are not the Creator," Celmer would tell *Newsweek* magazine.[13] "We do not give life and don't have the option to take life." She would tell Bethea, "In God's eyes, John was murdered."[14]

Interestingly, Celmer's mother, Betty, would later say about the FEN: "If they helped John to die, that is what he wanted. I would never find them guilty for helping him."[15]

However, Sue Celmer was upset at her ex-husband's death, and she lodged a complaint with the police, asking them to investigate her suspicions about FEN involvement. The local law enforcement authorities then contacted the GBI.

At the request of the GBI, "controlled calls" were made by Celmer's stepson that encouraged the suspected exit guides, Ted Goodwin and seventy-six-year-old Claire Blehr, to talk about the circumstances of Celmer's death. A recording of calls between the stepson and the exit guides suggested that Celmer's hands were held and that the two exit guides later disposed of the helium tanks and exit hood.

The GBI set up a sting operation in which an undercover agent posed as a terminally ill man with pancreatic cancer who wanted to die.[16] He contacted the Network, provided false documentation of his illness and completed the application. The agent then had several conversations and preparatory meetings with Goodwin and Blehr.

According to John Bankhead, a GBI spokesman, the agent was instructed to buy two tanks of helium and an "exit bag," which resembled a plastic shower cap that he would pull over his head.

Excerpts from the agent's subsequent affidavit were posted online and played on National Public Radio.[17] They state that the junior exit guide, Blehr, described the procedure and how after taking two deep breaths the "lights would go out." Blehr explained that he would not be dead at this point, and that the helium tanks would continue to run for twenty minutes after they last felt his pulse.

Goodwin told the agent during a phone conversation that he and Blehr would remove the helium tanks and exit hood; the undercover agent's death would be attributed to heart failure. He explained that the first parts of the brain to irreparably cease functioning are those involved with consciousness, executive functioning, and speech. The brain stem, which controls breathing and the beating heart, continues to function even after other parts of the brain are irreparably damaged by the absence of oxygen.

In the undercover agent's affidavit, Goodwin said that he had been present for thirty-five deaths in the past four years. He and the agent agreed to talk once or twice a week until the exit event.

A rehearsal was arranged at the agent's house, but Blehr was delayed. Hidden cameras had been installed by the GBI. Film excerpts from the rehearsal were later broadcast during a *Frontline* documentary.[18]

When Blehr belatedly arrived at the house, Goodwin and she were arrested.[19] Over the next several hours, three teams of agents descended on different Georgia locations, while other officers executed search warrants in eight states, including Colorado, Florida, Ohio, Michigan, and Missouri. Three teams were assigned to Maryland, and they entered Larry's office, home, and the residence of a colleague. The FEN and four members of the group were charged with assisting in a suicide, racketeering, and tampering with evidence by removing equipment. Although Larry had never gone to Georgia or met Celmer, he was charged in his capacity as the medical director.

On April 1, 2010, the defendants in the Celmer case pleaded not guilty. Attorney Robert Rivas argued that the Georgia statute on assisting suicide was facially unconstitutional under the First Amendment. In 2011, the trial court judge entered an order denying the motion to dismiss the indictment and an order was made authorizing the defendants to appeal this decision before trial while suspending the prosecution until the appeals court's ruling.

On February 6, 2012, the Supreme Court of Georgia unanimously found the Georgia statute against assisting suicide to be unconstitutional. This led to all charges against the FEN and its members being dismissed. However, the GBI was not finished.

THE FINAL
TWO CASES

Following the conclusion of the Celmer case, I interviewed Ted Goodwin, and we spoke again in 2018. After witnessing several excruciating deaths involving his family, including that of his father from emphysema, Ted had originally become a dues-paying member of the Hemlock Society.[1] In the year 2000, he was elected president of the Atlanta chapter, and he was then brought on to Hemlock's national board. The organization was in the process of evolving, and he opposed the reconstituted board of Compassion & Choices. Ted argued against abandoning the Caring Friends program, and he resigned after his initiative failed.

Ted then arranged for ten activists to get together to discuss reconstituting Caring Friends with Larry as its medical director. He did not want to restrict the new program to members who were permanently ill or actively dying but believed "competent adults should have the right to determine where and when they are going to get off the train, if they are suffering more than they could bear." He said, "I wanted to advertise. I wanted to have a website and a speaker's bureau. I wanted to advance our society." The organization he had in mind, the FEN, would have oversight guided by proper medical considerations, but it was to be driven and supported by laypeople. "The endgame," he said, "was to catalyze a generational change."

A board of directors was formed, as well as an advisory board. The latter consists of people like Faye and Derek, who offered expertise from the sidelines. Derek loaned the organization $5,000, and later some of the board members contributed similar amounts.

Ted persuaded the board to also extend help to people who had major mental illnesses where there was evidence of long-term problems that were not solved by medications and other treatments. Several members departed over the issue, and it was at that point Ted became its president.

Ted described Larry to me as being "a man who works every day to advance social justice issues on a variety of fronts. He has done this for decades. He is generous. He is intelligent. However, he is the one who has been in the vise over the legal cases, in no small part because he is a physician. The authorities have decided to make an example of him. Larry is no spring chicken. It has to be hard on him and his wife."

"Why" I asked him, "despite the publicity does FEN function so secretly, so covertly?"

"Because," he replied, "it was born out of a desire by our members, those who were going to die by their own hands, to not have this known to others. . . . People who seek the assistance of the program almost always want the group to keep it confidential and not publicly reveal that this was a suicide. In practically all the cases, they think that suicide stigmatizes the memory they would leave with their family and friends."

During their investigation, the GBI learned that Arizona law enforcement was already in the process of pursuing another FEN case. It involved the death of Jana Van Voorhis, a fifty-eight-year-old Phoenix woman.

In 2007, Van Voorhis approached the FEN with a poignant story that she was suffering from cancer. I have heard two versions of what ensued: the first is that FEN naively accepted her account, while the other is that Larry and his screening committee understood that the claim was a delusional product of chronic and intractable mental illness. Either way, she was provisionally accepted by the organization, guides were assigned, and she ended her life.

Jaime Joyce, a friend of the Van Voorhis family, has written a thoughtful and gut-wrenching piece called, "Kill Me Now" that offers a detailed portrait of the circumstances.[2]

Joyce obtained access to the FEN telephone intake report. In it Van Voorhis claimed to have porphyria, an enlarged spleen, and lesions on her liver. She maintained that defective silicone breast implants had to be surgically removed. Van Voorhis reported having had multiple head injuries, overexposure to radiation, and a history of ingesting rat poison. She also claimed that she had breast cancer.

Van Voorhis may have been chronically psychotic, but she lived a privileged life supported by a trust fund. Her grandfather and great-uncle had been copublishers of Arizona's two largest daily newspapers, the *Arizona Republic* and the *Phoenix Gazette*. Because of her privileged social status, Van Voorhis's complaints were taken seriously, and her symptoms were thoroughly evaluated on multiple occasions by medical professionals and determined to be hypochondriacal and factitious.

Van Voorhis's emotional problems became manifest in childhood, and she was twenty-one when first psychiatrically hospitalized. As she got older, she was frequently admitted to the psychiatric units of different Phoenix hospitals. In May of 2006, her longtime psychiatrist, Michael J. Fermo, noted: "She reports having depressed mood swings, periods of irritability, difficulty shutting off her mind, especially at night, erratic sleep, low energy, nervous, socially isolative and an ongoing feeling that bugs are eating her. The patient has been increasingly becoming psychotic, claiming that roof rats have been overtaking her home, sneaking into her house, and attacking her."[3]

In July of that year, Van Voorhis's mother died.

Dr. Michael S. Roberts, a Phoenix oncologist, was accustomed to receiving regular telephone calls from Van Voorhis.

By his estimation she had been contacting the office ten times a week for the more than eleven years. Six months after her mother's death, Van Voorhis called Dr. Roberts, claiming to be bedridden and wanting to be moved to the hospice where her mother had last resided. She was convinced that recent "infections" were caused by Mexicans spreading pesticides across the border.

Because he followed the advice of his attorneys and never discussed specifics of legal cases with me, I don't know what Larry was thinking after he reviewed the medical records. Joyce has written that Larry decided Van Voorhis was a suitable candidate to receive help from FEN; however, on the bottom of her medical intake form he wrote in red ink and underlined the words "but stay alert."

Immediately after the death of Van Voorhis, the senior FEN exit guide called the woman's sister and claimed to be a concerned member of her church. The exit guide said she was worried about Van Voorhis's welfare and suggested the family check in on her. When the sister and brother-in-law went into the house and found the body, they initially assumed she had killed herself with an overdose, which made sense, given that it was less than nine months since the death of their mother. However, there was also cause for suspicion. According to Jared Thomas (the brother-in-law), "she was 58 years old, and she was in relatively good health. It was unusual to see someone that age dead in bed, especially when it was made to look so clean and sanitary, like she had died in her sleep."[4] As the family searched the home, they turned up FEN literature, a receipt for two helium tanks, and a suspicious message on the telephone answering machine.

For almost two months, they repeatedly called the Phoenix police, urging them to explore FEN's connection to the death. The police hesitated to get involved with an ordinary suicide, but as soon as they assigned two homicide detectives, evidence was discovered that exit guides had participated in the death.

Interestingly, a family member later told a reporter, "To be clear, we don't disagree with Final Exit Network's philosophy, but they need to be regulated or held responsible when they make errors like this."[5]

Larry was charged along with three other FEN members, and once again, he had been involved only to the extent of reviewing Van Voorhis's paperwork and deciding to offer the group's services.

Derek was enraged when he heard about Larry and the Arizona case. He told me, "I'm critical of him for signing off on that Phoenix thing without proper investigation. I've said so to his face. It was a massive blunder. . . . He didn't go within three thousand miles of the case, but he signed off [where a] woman had a clear-cut psychiatric illness and was not dying."

Derek is equally critical of the senior exit guide who flew down from Denver to ascertain the situation. According to him, she should have "asked the woman more about the family. If this family had known then what the woman was considering, they would have committed her once again to a hospital. The guide should've gotten back on the plane and flown home. It was bound to blow. . . . She was known in the area for saying outrageous things about the governor. She had been committed to a mental asylum. What a blunder on our part! I was furious, but there we are! People commit blunders."

Derek went on to explain, "I keep on saying to FEN, you must involve the immediate family. In both cases, the family was not involved. The family came and found the person had been helped to die. They loved the person, even the crazy woman. . . . They loved her and must have thought, *Why should she die?* We [the Network] must involve the family. . . . We work in a difficult field."

Two FEN defendants—both elderly and frail—pleaded guilty to a minor charge that ensured they would not be sentenced to a prison term.[6] The trial of the remaining two FEN staff began on April 4, 2011, and went on for two weeks. Larry was found not guilty by an eight-member jury; there was a split verdict for the remaining exit guide. The latter, an eighty-six-year-old retired college professor, then pled guilty to endangerment, which is a misdemeanor. He was placed on probation for a year and given a small fine.

Search warrants obtained by the GBI during their investigation of the Celmer case in Georgia resulted in acquisition of extensive

FEN paperwork, records, and computers. Upon review, the agents uncovered 523 names of individuals who had contacted FEN for aid in dying. Of these, perhaps 181 are surmised to have died with the group's help; this information was based on dates of death for the respective individuals. Thirty-six people contacted FEN but died without obtaining direct help. The records also revealed 306 additional individuals who were accepted as candidates for assistance; however, their status remained unknown to the GBI.

In a letter that was then mailed to law enforcement agencies around the country, the Georgia authorities provided listings of the names obtained from FEN records. A spreadsheet contained the individual's address, date of birth, and information regarding contact with the organization. In the letter, the GBI's Medical Examiner explained that helium is undetectable in routine autopsies. Due to the nature of the gas and the covert form of the assistance provided by FEN, local officials were warned that suicides might originally have been ruled as natural deaths. The letter explained that files were available from the GBI, and that local law enforcement was urged to determine matters of jurisdiction and whether to take further legal action.

For months following the letter, local police in different communities tried to track down leads and acquire evidence. They knocked on scores, if not hundreds, of people's doors, and discussed with prosecutors and district attorneys whether there were grounds for indictments. In only one state, Minnesota, was a decision made to pursue another criminal case against the FEN.

Doreen Dunn, fifty-seven, of Apple Valley, Minnesota, completed a Network application in 2007, stating that for a decade she had been living with unbearable pain following a botched medical procedure. In April, her husband came home and found her dead on the couch. She had not told anyone in the family that she planned to end her life.

Dunn was not terminally ill, but an autopsy concluded that she died of coronary artery disease. Her death was not listed as a suicide. Several years later, the case was reopened after the GBI sent the letter to Minnesota authorities and provided evidence that Dunn had applied to FEN.

Following an investigation, a seventeen-count indictment was issued against Larry and three other Network members. It charged the corporation separately, which would be brought to trial first.[7]

The initial trial took place in 2015, and Larry testified that he had flown to Minnesota on the day of Dunn's death. He and another guide went to her home where she died using the helium technique. They removed and disposed of the mask and tanks. The FEN's defense attorney, Robert Rivas, acknowledged that the guides were present with Dunn when she died. Rivas disputed whether the state had proof of assisted suicide.[8]

He challenged the Minnesota statute, which prohibited "advising, encouraging, or assisting [in a] suicide." The Minnesota Court of Appeals found the statute to be unconstitutional, but it still allowed the state to continue prosecution of the FEN on more restricted grounds.

At the trial, relatives said Dunn wasn't mentally competent. Her husband testified that he did not approve of assisted suicide.[9]

In May 2015, a jury found Final Exit Network, Inc. guilty of assisting Doreen Dunn's suicide and interfering with the death scene. This was the only time the national group was convicted of a felony for assisting a suicide. It was fined $30,000 and required to pay $3,000 to the Dunn family for funeral expenses.[10]

A decision was then made by Minnesota authorities to not conduct any further trials against Larry and his fellow defendants.

After the conviction, Attorney Rob Rivas differentiated between the FEN's Minnesota case and that of Michelle Carter, a teenager who was convicted in Massachusetts of involuntary manslaughter for causing the suicide of her depressed boyfriend through text messages and phone calls.[11] Carter had clearly encouraged the boyfriend to remain in a vehicle and to die from carbon monoxide poisoning. A Massachusetts court found that Carter could be convicted if her "conduct caused the victim's death."

"The requirement of 'causation' in the Massachusetts case makes all the difference in the world," Rob said. "FEN was not convicted of 'causing' Ms. Dunn's death."[12]

However, on October 2, 2017, The U.S. Supreme Court declined to hear the case, and the high court's decision signified that the 2015 conviction will stand against FEN.

Following Larry's criminal trials, he fought and lost a crucial battle with the Maryland Board of Registration of Medicine. His medical license was stripped. He was no longer permitted to conduct examinations and to testify in court on behalf of refugees who claimed to have left their countries of origin after being subjected to torture. This other social cause had given further meaning to his life when he could no longer volunteer on behalf of FEN. During our last interviews and at the Chicago meeting of the Federation of World Right to Die Societies, Larry was a broken man. Although he received medical care through the Veteran's Administration, it was insufficient. He died at home on June 9, 2016, of a heart attack.

Two months later, I sat on one of the simple wooden benches at Larry's memorial service at the Stony Run Friends Meeting in Baltimore. On the cover of the program was his photograph. In it he is casually clad in denim shorts, and happily sits beside a poster from the grass-roots antiwar advocacy group Another Mother for Peace, with its colorful sunflower illustration and logo, "War is not healthy for children and other living things." Listening to the eulogies, I thought of another physician-activist, Che Guevara, who had said, "The true revolutionary is guided by a great feeling of love. It is impossible to think of a genuine revolutionary lacking this quality."[13] I can attest there was a lot of love in that meeting room for a complicated man who had led a revolutionary life.

Larry told me once that he felt flattered to be compared with Kevorkian. But he also would have been the first to admit that beneath the surface gloss of every hero—and Kevorkian was no exception—is a flawed human being trying to do what seems right. Larry was always willing to acknowledge his own foibles during our interviews and to laugh about them. I don't know if he considered himself to ever be heroic—in fact, I tend to doubt that he did.

Perhaps what is most striking to me about the right-to-die activists that I've described— Larry, Derek, Kevorkian, Dick,

Ted, and Faye—are their commonalities. Such individuals spend their lives fighting for a social cause (or a succession of causes) with indefatigable dedication. They don't overthink the decision to live in this manner. They lack any sense of being extraordinary yet seem to be strangely oblivious to common worldly pleasures. They meld their self-identity together with a moral ideal and possess "an insane level of optimism, a certainty that history does change for the better and that achieving justice is only a matter of time."[14] They also perfectly mirror the deep confusion and ambivalence about our laws, policies, and norms about death and dying. On the one hand, they each show a ton of compassion—which seems to be an underlying motivation for just about all of them. But, in being overzealous or careless, they sometimes expose and lend fodder to opponents who worry about the cheapening of our society's reverence for life, and who fear that we have forgotten the terrible consequences of eugenics.

It was around the time of the Minnesota case that I noticed the medical-aid-in-dying movement had lost much of its momentum. It was worrisome. The colorful Jack Kevorkian remained the cause's best-known figure, but he had been effectively muzzled by being imprisoned, and then he had ignominiously died. The Hemlock Society peaked in popularity and evolved into C&C and other smaller organizations. Following the scandal surrounding his wife's accusations and suicide, Derek Humphry stepped away from the spotlight. While Derek continued to successfully provide financial support to Larry Egbert and other FEN criminal defendants, and he sponsored initiatives like ERGO and NuTech's small group of researchers who were trying to develop new ways for people to end their lives, there were no breakthrough accomplishments. To many, the FEN seemed to have become increasingly radical and misguided, and that organization struggled to survive its repeated assaults by law enforcement. All the while, the American Medical Association and much of the medical establishment remained adamantly opposed to assisted dying. While Oregon successfully passed the first death-with-dignity law in the nation, it had been challenged in court, and further efforts and a second ballot initiative were required before the act was finally implemented. Only a handful of sparsely populated northwestern states, including Washington and Montana, managed to legalize aid-in-dying practices, while multiple initiatives in different geographical regions failed judicial challenges or attempts to pass legislative bills and ballot referenda.

Most of the efforts to advance the right-to-die cause appeared to have been thwarted. The movement's leading activists had aged, and they were now mainly octogenarians and nonagenarians. If the inertia was to be overcome, then new, young, and inspirational leaders needed to appear.

Then they did.

PART III

$\mathbb{P}$aul Spiers and I were finishing lunch in Worcester, and he resumed his mythological tale:

When we left the siege of Troy and the suffering Philoctetes, a full decade had gone by. During that time, things had not gone well for the Achaean army. Battles were waged, much blood was shed, prisoners were taken, but each night the Trojans took refuge behind the walls of their noble city and the Greeks returned to their encampment. Both forces were frustrated by the stalemate.

It was at this point the Achaeans summoned a seer. The holy man prophesied that they would never conquer the city of Troy unless aided by the magic bow and arrows of Hercules. After much squabbling, the Greek kings and nobles arrived at a consensus and then commanded Odysseus to sail back to the sacred island and retrieve the precious weapon. If Philoctetes was alive, they wanted him recruited into the army.

According to Sophocles, Philoctetes was still among the living but in pretty rough shape.

Paul pulled out some notes that he had stashed in his back-pack and began to read:

> Chorus: Desolate, abandoned among the wild, rough-skinned, dappled beasts.
> Chorus: Truly worthy of pity!
> Chorus: He has to endure immense pain and hunger . . .
> Chorus: . . . incurable disease . . .
> Chorus: . . . and no one to help him with it.[1]

Paul continued:

> Following an otherwise uneventful voyage, Odysseus arrived at the island and found the pitiful man. Using all his wiles, Odysseus tried to convince Philoctetes to rejoin the crew. However, the wounded warrior adamantly refused his entreaties until Hercules suddenly materialized in front of them.
>
> The deity declared that if Philoctetes traveled to Troy with Odysseus not only would the festering snakebite be cured but he would fulfill his destiny and come to be hailed as a hero by all the Greeks.
>
> Not to belabor the point, Philoctetes agreed, and the prophecy was fulfilled. Cured by a gifted Greek physician and selected among the small group of warriors to hide inside the wooden Trojan Horse, he emerged to play a prominent role in sacking the city and ending the war. Plying Hercules's magic bow, Philoctetes was unstoppable. Among the many Trojans struck by his deadly arrows was Prince Paris, whose love-stricken behavior had originally precipitated the entire bloody conflict.

Paul sat back in his wheelchair with a satisfied smile on his face.

It was at this point in our interview that we could have discussed whether it is absurd to believe that myths from a group of people who lived nearly three millennia ago still contain relevant lessons. Or we might have discoursed on how philosophers have long been interested in Sophocles's play because it allows for an examination of the multidimensional nature of pain and the social stigma accompanying disability. We could have talked about our mutual fascination with the idea that even a demigod like Hercules preferred suicide to living with unremitting suffering. Likewise, we might have considered whether it is heroic to end one's life this way or to help someone hasten their death. But we didn't.

Instead, Paul said to me, "Pretty cool story, eh?"

"Yup," was my reply.

When we left the restaurant, I helped wheel Paul through the crowded, potholed streets in front of the courthouse. His van was parked in a nearby handicapped spot. I watched him trigger the remote control opening the doors. No further assistance was needed on my part as he operated the mechanical lift for his chair and swiveled into position behind the wheel. Paul honked his horn in a farewell flourish, gave a merry wave of the hand, and drove away.

I walked a couple of blocks to my car and then it was a straight cruise-controlled drive on the Mass Pike from Worcester to my home in Northampton. During the drive, I thought to myself, *Why don't most people know how Hercules died? Why can't we recall that part of the story? Does anyone remember Philoctetes?* I considered the words of Hercules and Hyllus, and whether those who participate in such deaths are murderers or healers. I couldn't stop thinking about the battle-hardened companions of Hercules and their reticence to fulfill his request. They must have been old-school warriors who didn't hesitate at murder, rape, and pillage—but they were taken aback at the thought of putting a suffering colleague out of his misery? And lastly, I wondered, *How do these things relate to our society's struggle over this taboo?*

I had enjoyed Paul's quirky mythological tale. The ancient allegory became part of my inspiration for embarking on this writing project. I was curious about proponents like Paul who sought to overturn the laws that made this a criminal act in most of our country. I wanted to learn about the backgrounds of those who worked to protocolize death with dignity as a medical option and who promoted other death-hastening practices. I wanted to collect and weave together these stories. Not just legends or parables but truthful accounts.

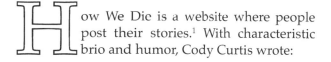

FOUR BOXES OF
CHOCOLATE

How We Die is a website where people post their stories.[1] With characteristic brio and humor, Cody Curtis wrote:

It's interesting how I was diagnosed—for my 52nd birthday I had gotten four, count them, four boxes of chocolate. And I ate them all. Afterwards I felt (deservedly) awful. I looked up my symptoms on the Internet and decided I was having a gall bladder attack like my father had earlier that year. It was a Saturday night so I didn't want to go to the emergency room. But I thought it was really weird, so a few weeks later I went in to see the doctor. She ordered an ultrasound.

When I went back to her office to get the results, she looked at me and burst into tears. She said, "Your gall bladder's fine, but you have a big mass in your liver."

The tumor was roughly the size of a grapefruit.

In December of 2007, Cody was diagnosed with cholangio-carcinoma. This is a deadly cancer of the bile duct, the tube that runs through the liver. Cholangiocarcinoma is an uncommon disease, occurring in only approximately two out of a hundred thousand Americans per year. Depending on the size of the tumor and whether it has already spread throughout the body, patients with this cancer are offered surgery, chemo, radiation, and sometimes a liver transplant. Even with aggressive treatment, however, this is usually a fatal diagnosis.

After Cody's general practitioner settled down, she discussed the implications of the finding and referred her to a local oncology (cancer) surgeon, Dr. Katherine (Kate) Morris.

Cody is a slender, silver-haired woman, whose face is distinguished by her high cheekbones and penetrating, thoughtful brown eyes. She communicates with considerable élan and her accounts are upbeat but realistic. In her posting, she wrote: "The good news was the location of the tumor made a resection of my liver possible. Your liver regenerates and within six weeks you have a new liver. I had the first surgery, which cut out about 60 percent of my liver. But there were complications and I ended up in the hospital for fifty days. I couldn't walk. I couldn't feed myself. My daughter lives in Washington D.C. She visited for a week and I didn't know she was there."

Cody knew going into the operating room that if the cancer persisted after resection of the tumor, chances of survival drop dramatically. "This is a pretty deadly disease," she explained, "the five-year survival rate for metastasized cancer is approximately zero. The three-year survival rate is about thirty percent. I didn't know it when I was first diagnosed, but the chances of the cancer coming back are about sixty percent. It was pretty awful in the hospital and recovery was tough."

When Cody and Kate met for the first time, the surgeon was thirty-nine years old. During the preceding three years, she had established a vibrant solo private practice based in Portland while also helping run the research and tumor banking program of a tertiary care center. She was happily married and was pleasingly satisfied with her professional and personal life.

In interviews, I routinely ask people to describe themselves, and Kate undoubtedly provided my favorite reply. Most physicians become flustered when asked. They are accustomed to formulaically portraying patients in medical records: "This is a fifty-eight-year-old, morbidly obese, widowed Hispanic man." But doctors are reticent to depict themselves in the same way, and although they are trained observers, most spend little time looking in a mirror or wryly considering their own appearance. Physicians are no more or less narcissistic than the general public, but in my experience, they are more likely to be surprised or even affronted by an author's description. Accordingly, in my interviews I almost always insert this question.

However, Kate gave me an immediate and simply delightful response: "I am hopeless at this, but will suggest, instead, a series of words to consider and words to avoid." Among her words to avoid were "stout, stumpy, Rubenesque, jolly, looks like Austin Powers minus the chest hair." Among those to consider were "a less anorexic Angelina Jolie, statuesque, willowy, serene, poised." Joking aside, she arrived at "I'm five feet four, have dark, shoulder-length hair, kinda hazel eyes, and teeth I should have had straightened as a kid, but refused to have braces." She followed this with the insightful observation, "I've a tendency to be willful!"

Kate grew up in a bucolic setting on the outskirts of Olympia, Washington. While not quite a ranch, her parents created a pastoral home that abounded with horses, cats, and dogs. One of her earliest lessons was that you don't allow animals to suffer. Raised as a Catholic and attending parochial school through eighth grade, Kate learned other lessons: people are responsible for themselves and their bodies, and autonomy is a cherished ethical principle that should always be respected. Her parents were professionally successful individuals: Kate's father, a computer specialist with an MBA, worked for the state of Washington; her mother was an attorney who in the latter part of her career became an administrative law judge. Kate moved to Oregon to attend medical school and complete a surgical residency. She then traveled to New York City and to the world-famous Memorial Sloan Kettering, where she did a surgical oncology fellowship focusing on cancers of the liver and pancreas. Portland, however, is not an easy city to leave behind, and she returned when offered an opportunity to establish a private practice and conduct clinical research. When Cody came to see her, she was one of a select group of surgeons specializing in the treatment of this disease.

Several years before Kate and her patient began to deal with the cholangiocarcinoma, Peter Richardson, a young Oregonian filmmaker, had gotten intrigued by his state's decision in 1994 to legalize physician-assisted dying. I would interview him in 2011, shortly after *How to Die in Oregon* was shown at the Sundance Film Festival. Peter's documentary vividly introduces the viewer to Cody, her devoted family, and her physician. By the film's conclusion, you know and care about each of them. I later learned that Kate had only grudgingly agreed to participate after Cody made a personal request. Even after her patient's direct appeal, the young surgeon was initially determined to silently remain in the background of the cinematic project.

However, Kate was transformed by her relationship with Cody. Kate has since become one of a small but growing number of medical professionals from around the country who have been enthused by the death-with-dignity movement. These people do not seek or welcome the role. Most are modest, highly intellectual, and intensely private professionals attracted to the field of medicine because it offers a challenge and an opportunity to help relieve misery. Most are workaholics who accept the drudgery and frequent frustrations of the profession because it is occasionally interrupted by the pleasure that comes with vanquishing an illness, ameliorating distress, or saving a life. Absolutely none of these individuals would ever have dreamed that their greatest accomplishment might entail helping patients to die. Not one would have imagined becoming a right-to-die activist.

Physicians like Kate do not fully understand why they are defying the deeply engrained taboo against death and why they have become combatants in this professional and cultural war. Previously, most have sought to live as inconspicuously as possible, but by taking this stance, they can't help but be noticed. They are not confrontational by nature, but this is a conflict in which most of the medical societies have lined up against them. Relatively few of their patients are likely to ever directly request assistance in dying, while many others will potentially be threatened or offended by their position in the societal debate. On the surface, their activism is not self-serving.

Because of their medical training, physicians like Kate are in an ideal position to offer compassionate terminal care and to assume leadership roles in the national and international aid-in-dying movement. However, this never began as a choice. It was their fate.

Cody and her husband, Stan, were born and grew up in Idaho. Stan, a mathematician, computer scientist, and entrepreneur has been responsible for several innovative start-up companies. He tends to downplay their mutual talents, and he told me that they came from "a small, little state and got a free pass as country hicks." This hardly explains his academic and professional accomplishments or Cody's MBA from Harvard—which she earned while becoming the first student of the program to intentionally get pregnant. In the early 1970s, the birth of their son was sufficiently noteworthy that she and Stan were featured in a documentary on dual-career couples. Stan proudly remarked that filmmakers and artists were always attracted to Cody because "she has a lot of style, is a good storyteller, and is quite beautiful."

Cody was hired as the financial officer at the Massachusetts Institute of Technology's artificial intelligence laboratory in Cambridge, where Stan also spun out his first start-up company. Their social circle included a variegated combination of medical researchers, academicians, clinicians, social activists, artists, and musicians. Cody was recruited from MIT to Oregon Health & Science University to work with the informatics group as their chief administrative officer.

Her fifty-second birthday took place on Halloween in 2007 and, as noted, was quickly followed by discovery of the tumor. Cody and her husband promptly sought advice from their extensive network of medical experts. They consulted with the leading authorities on liver cancer from Rochester and Sloan Kettering medical centers, and by Thanksgiving they were fully aware that the condition was both uncommon and life-threatening.

Accordingly, the couple was extraordinarily well informed when they arrived at Kate's office for the first meeting.

Kate, Stan, and Cody instantly liked and respected each other. The young surgeon was smart, articulate, and down to earth; she was also highly recommended by their medical friends. Her office suite was thoughtfully and tastefully designed, and it was apparent that her entire staff and she were fond of each other and worked together efficiently. The couple recognized that the surgeon was confident without being arrogant, and she was comfortable with the concept of a participatory or patient-led process. From the start, Kate informed them that their input and the opinions of outside experts were welcome, but she also conveyed a clear, understandable, and pragmatic roadmap as to the surgical approaches to the cancer and probable outcomes. During the ensuing years, and with her encouragement, the Curtis family received multiple opinions on everything from how to interpret individual tissue biopsies to advice on the advisability of proposed treatment alternatives.

Beginning with the first office visit, Kate was impressed by Cody's fierce determination to make the most out of whatever days and months of life remained. She was also struck by her patient's clearly articulated refusal to undergo chemotherapy and her reservations about having the recommended surgery. According to Kate, "She presented with a large right-sided liver cholangiocarcinoma and said, 'Doc, I'm not really sure I want this removed.' At the time, it was a potentially curable situation—it was resectable with no evidence of metastasis, no evidence of lymph node involvement."

There is an old joke that despite the high cost of living, life remains popular. In the end, Cody agreed to try the surgery that might cure her cancer. She was admitted to Oregon Health & Science University Hospital, and underwent a nine-hour procedure. The tumor could only be removed by first cutting through her liver and then reconnecting the severed halves. Afterward, Cody had a bumpy postoperative course, during which she was intermittently comatose and confused. Because of complications, a second operation became necessary, and this further extended her stay in the surgical ICU. It would take six solid months before she recovered. During that time, Stan took a family leave from his consulting job. Their son, Thomas, had just returned from the Peace Corps, and he maintained a daily vigil at his mother's hospital bedside. As Cody gradually improved, she and Thomas had lengthy conversations while slowly walking through the corridors. Their daughter, Jill, racked up frequent-flyer points traveling back and forth between the coasts.

The entire family and their attentive surgeon sighed with relief as the proverbial corner was turned and Cody finally began to believe that life could resume. Always upbeat, Stan describes the initial surgical procedure as "not having gone perfectly; there was a lot of intensive care. . . . Kate put a lot of effort into getting Cody out and restoring her positive attitude about life again."

During the ensuing months of recuperation, Cody and Stan decided the time had come for them to downsize and to fulfill some of their deferred life goals. Thomas and Jill moved out of the house to their own residences, and the family's home was quickly sold. The couple purchased a one-bedroom condominium in a historic building, the Alhambra, situated in Portland's fashionable Northwest neighborhood. They bought a building lot on the Deschutes River in the rain-shadow of the Cascade Mountains and began construction of shared cabins with their neighbors from the condominium.

The Curtis family is hardly utopian, but they have had a long-standing social commitment toward making the world sustainable and responsive to the aspirations of its inhabitants. They believe cities and neighborhoods must be reshaped and improved by establishing open standards between IBM, INTEL, and other high-tech innovators. They are advocates for fostering links between public and private community development. Previously, the couple had begun a start-up company in Palo Alto called People Power, designed to build a new generation of energy efficiency monitoring and control solutions for homes, buildings, appliances, and devices. The building project by the Deschutes River that was started with their neighbors similarly fulfilled a long-standing wish to create a harmonious rural outpost.

It was unfortunately at this juncture that a radiologist identified an abnormality on Cody's latest CAT scan, and Kate immediately recognized that the tumor had returned with metastases. The young surgeon was caught in the unhappy position of having to tell her patient that the cancer was back, had spread, and there were no longer any good curative treatment options.

During their very first office consultation, Cody had brought up the subject of physician-assisted dying and Oregon's death-with-dignity law. She and Stan had established with the surgeon that they wanted to keep this option in reserve. Having already gone down the path of a radical operation and a torturously difficult recovery, Cody returned to the office and emphatically made it clear that she didn't wish to go through that ever again. Holding her husband's hand, she looked Kate in the eye and quietly said, "You know what I want."

23

∾

ON HER OWN TERMS

D an Diaz greeted me at the door of his Bay Area home in California, accompanied by the loud barking of his beagle, Bella, and Great Dane, Charley. I was uncertain whether the dogs were merely excited by the arrival of a stranger or were being fiercely protective of their lonely master or both. In any case, I was relieved when they ceased howling as Dan ushered me into the living room and we plunked down on adjoining couches.

Bella took her accustomed position nestled into Dan's side, while Charley sprawled across my feet. Dan's wife, Brittany Maynard (pronounced Meh-NAHRD) didn't get around to changing her name when they got married. But she did have time to rescue the beagle from a Southern California shelter when it was around three years old. Charley, the Great Dane, was recognizable to me from an iconic photo that appeared in a series of stories from *People* magazine.[1] The first of these was titled, "Terminally Ill 29-Year-Old Woman: Why I'm Choosing to Die on My Own Terms." In the picture, the diminutive puppy can be seen nuzzling in the lap of a dazzlingly attractive woman. Brittany is a lithe brunette with an engaging smile. When I came to interview her widower, the dog was now a healthy 125 pounds of well-cared-for love incarnate.

Dan, forty-three years old, was also recognizable from the magazine photographs. He is a ruggedly handsome man who looks like a lifeguard—a job he relied upon to help support his attendance at the University of California, Berkeley. He bears a resemblance to the James Bond actor, Daniel Craig, and shares with him a habit of occasionally twisting his head around to give a quick grin. During a four-year period while assigned to a surprisingly treacherous deep-water lake, he rescued thirty-two drowning children and adults, including one pig-headed adolescent who managed to nearly kill himself twice in a single afternoon while showing off to friends. Dan marvels at how quickly the people whose lives he saved had gotten into trouble; one moment they were joyfully splashing around and the next they were sinking beneath the water's surface. He is obviously delighted to have been around to extricate them from trouble, but in recounting these exploits there is absolutely no conceit evident on his part. He also does not associate any of this to what happened to his wife, who had in an instant transformed from being a blissful newlywed to a terminally ill public figure.

During our first interview, it was evident that the preceding year's events had taken their toll on Dan. His facial features were deeply lined, and his eyes periodically reddened and overflowed with tears.

Dan lives in the home that Brittany and he purchased to begin their married lives together. It is an older, 1950s, one-story ranch built on a cul-de-sac with typical exotic California plantings and a small, drought-parched lawn. It looked elegant to the eyes of a small-town New Englander like myself, but one block away on Country Club Lane the houses are newer and larger, and adorned with intricate brickwork. Those mini-mansions sport vintage cars parked in circular driveways and have rolling green lawns, attesting to a desire by the homeowners to show off wealth. By contrast, the Maynard-Diaz house is a starter home for a middle-class couple, and now it has become a place of mourning and of single-minded devotion to furthering the right-to-die. Dan and I met on the day before he officially began his new job as a lobbyist for Compassion & Choices (C&C).

In the brief time they lived together, Dan oversaw the remodeling of the rooms, which are now open, spacious, and brightly illuminated, while Brittany was responsible for selecting the comfortable furnishings. The couple met at the University of California, where she earned a bachelor's degree in psychology followed by a master's degree at UC Irvine's School of Education. Brittany always wanted to see the world, and beginning as an adolescent she traveled widely. A talented amateur photographer, the walls of the house were hung with her framed pictures depicting those adventures. They competed for space with stunning wedding photos of the bride and groom that were familiar to me from the succession of *People* magazine and online articles.

Dan is by nature a neat and orderly man; everything—with one exception—was sparkling clean. He apologized to me when I noticed a shelf that was coated in dust and held his wife's ornamental rocks, crystals, and ammonite fossils.

"I try, but I can't do everything," he said.

"Who can?" I replied.

Casually attired in a polo shirt and shorts, he sat barefoot, a laptop in reach, occasionally bending over and checking facts as we spoke. Dan may appear to be California casual, but he is by nature a man who pays scrupulous attention to detail. He proceeded to recount Brittany and his story as if testifying in court. He is accurate, orderly, likeable, eloquent, and well suited to lobby legislators, and he is determined to preserve and further Brittany's legacy—as he told me several times.

The widower and I have since remained in contact, emailing and occasionally speaking on the phone. During the first visit, we eventually would leave his home to go to a local restaurant for lunch, and then take the dogs for a hike. I would meet him two years later at that same modest restaurant, where the owner clearly cared and fussed over him.

In one of his emails, he expressed his skepticism that anyone other than he could capture Brittany's "frame of mind, her personality, and soaring spirit." Dan wrote me that "no one would be able to convey that accurately." He is probably correct, and he intends to write his own account of the events.

We agreed that I would tell Brittany's story by using her words from the videotapes that she made, as well as offering the perspective of her best friend, Dr. Sarah Maufe, and relying on Dan's assistance in establishing the background. There are several recordings and opinion pieces available online from Brittany, including those produced with the help of friends and C&C,[2] CNN postings,[3] a tape aimed at legislators,[4] and yet another that was posted a year after her death.[5] All were made or written following the discovery of the cancer. Sarah's relationship with Brittany had begun well before those troubled times, and the young physician played an active role throughout the ordeal. I am exceedingly grateful to Dan for introducing me to Sarah, who had previously resisted being identified by the media and had refused to be interviewed by journalists.

The two young women shared a birthday, November 19. Sarah was two years older than Brittany when she moved into an apartment with her in Oakland the year that she finished college. Sarah had gotten a job as a behavioral therapist helping children with autism, while Brittany was a nanny for a pair of twins, one of whom, by coincidence, was autistic.

The two women became the "best of friends." They were instantly comfortable with each other and could be "silly together, dancing, and staying up all night talking over a glass of wine." They each had already begun traveling to remote places by themselves, savoring the strangeness, and experiencing the pleasures of different cultures. There was something about solitary wayfaring that brought each out of their comfort zone and made them accessible to a richer appreciation of life. The greatest joy of backpacking for a solo traveler is to meet and get to know random people on the road, and Brittany and Sarah were always eager for such encounters. Both women were unafraid to live simply and to hike in exotic locales, but Brittany pushed closer to the edge—going on arduous trekking and mountaineering expeditions, climbing rocky peaks in the ice and snow, and even joining a team that ascended Kilimanjaro. Wanderlust and the desire for an "adrenaline rush" were distinct elements of her character.

Brittany traveled to Laos, Vietnam, Cambodia, Thailand, Singapore, and Costa Rica. She practiced ice climbing on Cayambe and Cotopaxi in Ecuador, and she went scuba diving in the Cayman Islands, the Galapagos, and Zanzibar.[6]

Although they bonded instantly, what stood out for Sarah was her roommate's passion, "unmatched by anyone I have ever known." This was only enhanced by Brittany's tendency "to speak her mind." Sarah was in awe of how she would challenge "everything (!), which I loved and appreciated so much about her. She was unafraid to stand up for what she believed in."

At Brittany's "life celebration," Sarah would later tell the assembled about her friend's time in Nepal, where she volunteered to spend several months at an orphanage. This took place about three or four years after they first met. In preparation for the trip, Brittany collected donations of clothes, toys, pacifiers, and other things for children. Originally, she was assigned to work at a private orphanage, which turned out to have plenty of resources and was supported by a nongovernmental organization. But when she went to visit the city's public orphanage, Brittany discovered an entirely different situation: multiple babies sharing the same crib, overwhelmed staff who could not keep up with changing diapers, and everywhere the smells and sounds of wailing children who were rarely comforted. Brittany felt her time would be better spent in the public orphanage, and she immediately gave them the material brought from California.

However, after a week or two, she noticed that none of those things were being used.

According to Sarah, Brittany stormed into the front office and asked the staff person, "Where's the stuff I donated?"

The lady replied, "I don't know. Perhaps it is in storage."

"Where do you store things?" she demanded to know.

The staff member declined to answer, but Brittany refused to back down. Finally, the administrator conceded that various items were secured in a back room. Insisting the woman provide the keys, Brittany unlocked the door and proceeded to remove all the toys and items that she had given. She then walked through the halls, distributing gifts to the orphans. Brittany had instantly understood that this would never be accomplished if she didn't do it herself.

"She was like that," said Sarah. "She wasn't afraid to step over boundaries or to step on toes. Brittany did what she thought was right. If people didn't agree, she was still going to stand up for what she believed in her heart to be correct."

Following the nanny position, Brittany tutored children after school and taught English to immigrants. A pet lover, she volunteered at the town's animal shelters.

About her family background, Sarah said, "She had kind of a tangled upbringing. . . . I don't know a ton about her childhood, but her mother was a single mom who remarried after leaving her dad, then got divorced, and then met her current husband. So, Brittany had three different fathers through childhood."

Brittany didn't especially like high school, dropped out, and ultimately received a GED. Nevertheless, she worked hard and was accepted at the University of California, where she applied herself and did exceedingly well. Brittany trained to become a teacher and didn't care that such a career was never going to be lucrative. The work was fulfilling and that sufficed.

During that time, money was tight and scholarships and loans were needed to pay for her schooling. Only after marrying Dan could she afford to do more volunteer work; she was then able to tutor and help the needy because her income wasn't essential to cover the mortgage.

I tried explaining to Sarah that I appreciate dents and blemishes that lend character to antique furniture, and similarly, I didn't want to compose a polished hagiography of Brittany Maynard. Accordingly, I asked if she could offer me something other than the airbrushed images that the media and the right-to-die movement had cultivated—*People* magazine offered photograph after photograph of a flawless, picture-perfect wedding.[7]

Sarah tried her utmost to respond and said, "It's funny coming from the position of being best of friends. It is different from how the rest of the world is seeing her." Sarah struggled to articulate more.

"She was hilarious. She was so funny and really sarcastic," Sarah said. "She had a low tolerance for people who she felt were not good people. If they were racist or bad parents or would hurt others—those were the sorts she could not tolerate."

"We always just laughed," Sarah continued. "You just instantly loved her. My husband found her to be the favorite of all my friends because she was so willing to be herself, to be out there, to not hold anything back. If it got Brittany into trouble, she wouldn't care. There were no subtleties about her."

Frankly, Sarah's description of her own life sounds rather ideal, too. Sarah had wanted to be a doctor from the time she was nine years old. She said, "It is a cliché, I know, but I always had a desire to help people. I wanted to work with sick kids."

Sarah attended UC San Diego, did a year abroad in Sydney, Australia, and then took two years off and afterward went to St. Louis University Medical School. She tried to keep an open mind about her specialty, but fell in love with the pediatrics rotation.

In rapid fire succession, she took residency training at UCLA, met and married her husband, moved into a new house in Santa Cruz, had a baby daughter, and joined a pediatric practice. When I first spoke with her, Sarah's husband had left his job—that he hated—had gone back to school to pursue a career in music, and had become a stay-at-home dad. When I reconnected with her a couple years later, baby number two was keeping them fully occupied. She couldn't resist describing herself as "living a pretty amazing life."

Sarah and Brittany were always planning to travel together but could not settle on a date or a destination. Then the unexpected happened.

MY GOLDEN SUMMER

D r. Kate Morris never thought she would be directly involved with implementing Oregon's Death with Dignity Act (DWDA). She figured, "I'm a surgeon and usually it's medical oncology or cardiology or hospice or primary care doctors that deal with these requests. In retrospect, I can see I was in a little bit of denial, saying that I can support this intellectually, but I'm not actually going to have to face it. But then Cody came along."

When Kate realized that her patient wanted and intended to use the law, "It came crashing down on [me]. . . . Like, oh wow! Can I really do this? It's hard! It's not to say it isn't right. But as a physician it is difficult to wrap your head around it."

Momentarily paralyzed with indecision, Kate looked at the couple sitting across the way from her in the office. She said to them, "This is a really heavy thing. I need to think about it and talk to my family."

Cody replied, "No problem. I know it is a big thing and I know it is hard for you." Stan nodded in agreement.

After an otherwise typical, busy day, Kate went home. She absent-mindedly patted her cats, hugged her husband with real feeling, and continued to wrestle over the dilemma. She framed the problem as being "a sort of disconnect between what you know in your head versus what you feel when you're looking at your patient. The two of you have gone through a lot. You are very attached to her, and she's asking you to write a prescription that is going to end her life. I had a professor who used to say, 'There is the right thing and the wrong thing, and the easy thing and the hard thing— and you're lucky when the right thing is easy.' Well neither Cody nor I had been particularly lucky and none of this was easy."

Kate was supportive of the general concept of death with dignity. She had voted in favor of the first ballot initiative during medical school. While in residency training, she had the opportunity to vote for the second initiative. She was pleased and comforted when the bill passed both times, but everything remained more in the realm of theoretical until Cody—her cherished patient with whom she had just slogged through a year-long ordeal—requested assistance.

Over the course of the weekend, Kate talked endlessly with her husband, older sister, and mother. The first two are engineers; like any good obsessive-compulsive people, they were prepared to help her sit down at the desk and list the pros and cons. She literally got out a piece of paper and began writing, but she quickly found this approach to be fruitless. Her mother, "mainly worried about me getting hurt. After all, she is my mom."

Finally, it was her sister, a breast cancer survivor, "who cut through a lot of the crap by just saying, 'You know what? You're her doctor. You're going to have to help her!'"

With those words, her agony and indecisiveness ended and she committed herself to fulfilling the request. The following morning, she called up Cody and announced she was ready.

After her surgical residency, Kate had applied to a two-year fellowship in Surgical Oncology at Memorial Sloan Kettering in New York City where an interviewer remarked, "So you're from Oregon where you all smoke marijuana and kill your patients?" While at the time, she laughingly disputed the characterization, it was also her first realization that much of the medical community viewed the northwest as being a strange and quirky Twilight Zone.

What Kate soon came to appreciate while studying in New York is that each region of the country and every medical center has its own traditions and social mores. People specifically come to Memorial Sloan Kettering, a tertiary cancer institution, with the expectation that its staff will work miracles to not only preserve but save their lives. The celebrated author Susan Sontag sought treatment at Sloan for breast cancer, and she was not atypical of many of their patients in demanding absolutely everything possible be done. According to her son's memoir about the final months, Sontag could never accept that she was dying.[1] Although she wrote in her journal, "In the valley of sorrow, spread your wings," her son was unwilling to fictionalize or romanticize her illness, and to her lines he added, "This was not the way she died." Kate's fellowship training prepared her to medically manage death-denying people like Sontag and not necessarily individuals like Cody.

Kate sums up her own medical care philosophy as, "Personally, I would not be as aggressive as many of my patients have been. I'd probably be a more quality-of-life . . . go travel . . . go feel good as long as I can kind of gal. But everybody's different, and that's part of what makes being a physician so interesting."

Having had the opportunity to participate in many deaths, she observed, "It's one of the toughest and most enriching parts of my job, because you see people's real grace and beauty come shining out at the terminus of their lives. It's really an honor to be part of it."

Cody posted the following in How We Die:

Under Oregon's Death with Dignity law you make a face-to-face request to a prescribing doctor to get a lethal prescription (basically a massive dose of Seconal). Two weeks later you make a second request, which can be a verbal request. Another physician must attest that you are of sound mind and no one is coercing you and you do indeed have a condition that is irreversible. . . .

The outcome is clear in my case. If you're willing to look at what's likely to happen, it's fairly awful. People with this kind of cancer die of massive organ failure and it's not pretty. And I already did that to my family last year, bouncing in and out of the hospital. . . .

There are some experimental trials out there, and if I were younger and the children were younger I might be willing to close my eyes and hope, but there's no point in it now. I'm feeling pretty good and enjoying the sunshine. I have to pace myself, but I can still take care of myself. I can do the laundry. I can host book groups and talk to my brother on the phone. Food tastes wonderful again. I can hold hands with Stan and the kids and tell them I love them.

But I'll know when life's not worth living any more. It's really nice to have a way out, to die in comfort and with dignity. I don't want to die bed-ridden and weighing seventy pounds. I want the children to remember me as I am now, in peace and not in pain.[2]

Cody was pleased when she heard that Kate would comply with her request, and she immediately put her in touch with a C&C volunteer. This national organization has state branches, and in Oregon its members work with dying patients and their physicians around the DWDA. C&C volunteers are experienced sources of support who provide essential information. Kate promptly called up and spoke with a retired nurse who had been assigned to help. The young surgeon was determined to carefully follow the procedures as enumerated in the law.

The metastases were detected in February 2009, and after the necessary waiting period elapsed, Cody came to Kate's office for the Seconal prescription. During her career, Kate had written thousands of scripts. This time, however, she sat at her desk filling out the prescription form when she noticed that she had made an error. She tore it up and rewrote it. Shaking, she discovered another error, ripped up the next slip of paper and rewrote the prescription again. Kate did not want to hand over a prescription to her patient that had "cross-outs." It hardly requires a psychiatrist to understand why Kate kept making mistakes—she was obviously ambivalent about going ahead with this—but she persisted, finally succeeded, and gave Kate the properly filled-out prescription form.

But this also turned out inadvertently to be a mistake. The Oregon DWDA requires a physician to either bring the prescription to the pharmacist or to send it through the mail—and *not* to hand it over to the patient. The process is designed to prevent and circumvent any possible diversion of the barbiturates.

Cody explained, "[Even then] it's actually quite complicated to get the physical [medication]. Some pharmacies will not accept the prescription. Our insurance didn't cover it and it's expensive. . . . So now the drugs are in my bedside table."[3]

Although the DWDA of Oregon was passed in 1994, challenges delayed its enactment until 1997. The law requires all participating physicians to complete official forms that are sent to the Oregon Health Authority. The information is then compiled into an annual statistical report, which is available online.

While the numbers of dying people in Oregon who rely on this end-of-life option are incrementally increasing each year, they represent only a miniscule proportion of the state's total number of deaths.[4] In 2017, 218 people received prescriptions under the Oregon DWDA (compared to 204 in the previous year). As of January 19, 2018, there were 143 known deaths that had taken place in 2017 from ingesting the prescribed medications, including 14 who had received the prescriptions in prior years. Demographic characteristics of DWDA patients were like those from previous years. During 2017, no referrals were made to the Oregon Medical Board for failure to comply with DWDA requirements, and the estimated rate of DWDA deaths was 39.9 per 10,000 total deaths (0.4 percent).

Despite the claims and fears that are stoked by opposition spokespersons, legalization has not opened any floodgates. There are simply too many steps and safeguards built into the act. The process is arduous, and there are plenty of other ways that people can hasten dying, including withholding or withdrawing life-prolonging treatments and voluntary decisions to refrain from eating or drinking.

Since enactment of the law, a total of 1,967 people from Oregon have had prescriptions written and 1,275 died following ingestion of the prescribed medications.[5] Proponents are pleased to cite state reports from Oregon and Washington—the states that have the most data—that 16 percent and 26 percent, respectively, of patients who fill the prescriptions end up dying from their underlying disease and not the barbiturates.[6] The DWDA places patients in a position where they can end their lives at a time of their own choosing, but these findings suggest they aren't being pressured or coerced into killing themselves.

So, who makes use of this option according to the data sets? The annual report finds that the majority (80 percent) of deaths in 2017 involved people who were aged sixty-five years or older, and most of the sample had been diagnosed with cancer (80 percent).[7] They were white (94 percent), and well-educated (49 percent with at least a baccalaureate degree). The majority (90 percent) of individuals died at home, and (91 percent) were enrolled in hospice care either when the prescription was written or at the time of death. Everyone in the sample had health insurance.

The above data answer several concerns raised during the original Oregon initiative and in every subsequent attempt to establish death-with-dignity laws. In each of these campaigns, the opposition's main talking point has been that physician-assisted suicide disproportionately targets vulnerable segments of the population, and especially the elderly, disabled, uninsured, and those lacking in access to hospice and palliative care services. The statistical reports from Oregon and Washington document that most patients who make use of the law are older than the general population; however, this finding does not suggest ageism or elder abuse but instead reflects the reality that most people who contract cancer and other fatal illnesses are older. The data from the two states should serve to allay fears that eligible patients are financially disadvantaged, uneducated, or do not have access to either curative or palliative medical care. And if anything, the reports suggest that it is mainly privileged and accomplished individuals, like Cody, who are the ones making use of the law.

Admittedly, the data have limitations. Funds are unavailable from any of the states to conduct objective research, nor am

I aware of private foundations that actively support such efforts. The reporting forms offer the doctor's perspective, but the physician does not have to be present and is rarely around when a patient ingests the barbiturates. Consequently, much of the time we do not know what happens with a high degree of confidence, such as the occurrence of adverse outcomes and complications from the lethal medications. These would include a longer time to death than expected (possibly twenty-four hours or more), but may also involve awakening from unconsciousness, nausea, vomiting, and gasping.[8] When such problems are noted, essential details are lacking.[9]

There is also little or no follow-up to ascertain how families managed after the deaths or how they do in comparison to the bereaved following other forms of dying. Some deviations from the laws are acknowledged by the data, but the collection process is biased toward reporting everything as going without a hitch.

It was at this point that Cody, her family, and Kate were introduced to Peter Richardson, the independent documentary filmmaker. Peter had decided to make Oregon's DWDA the subject of his new cinematic project. Peter recognized he was tackling a polarizing issue that lent itself to considerable speculation and hearsay, and he decided there was a need to portray the reality of what people experience. The cinematographer wanted to challenge society's reluctance to accept the inevitability of death, and he wished to illustrate that these tragedies also contain the potential for triumph.

Peter had heard from C&C about Cody. The filmmaker quickly understood that she and her family had undergone an ordeal that began with the shocking discovery of cancer, the aggressive surgeries, and the probability that she was going to die during the complicated and lengthy initial hospitalization. "But then they got a do-over!" he observed to me. "They had tried the cure route. They looked at what medicine offered and decided, 'We're going to do it differently the next time.'"

In Peter's documentary, the silver-haired Cody appears to be consistently calm and composed. She exudes honesty and is incredibly candid. Her words are simple and unembellished. At one point, she looks directly into the camera and softly says:

"If I had an option, I would prefer not to die—thank you very much [and she chuckles ironically]. But given that I know I'm going to die, does an extra three months of fluid leaking through my pores sound that great?"

She answers herself, "Well, no! I'd rather go when I'm still feeling OK, and when I can still communicate with my family."

Peter does not see Cody as being exceptional. He believes that if given a chance, most people would want to confront death openly and to die surrounded by their loved ones. At the same time, he also believes that it is impossible to predict whether any particular individual who is terminally ill will choose physician-assisted dying.

Peter cites the case of Ray Camay, whom he also met and featured in *How to Die in Oregon*. Ray was someone who was very conservative politically, and he had been vehemently opposed to the Oregon law. However, once he received his own fatal diagnosis it completely changed his mind. He told Peter, "You never know until you're confronted with this choice and an uncertain end how you might feel."

Ray, a former opera singer who became a radio announcer, had throat cancer. The only treatment he could feasibly receive entailed having his voice box surgically removed. According to the filmmaker, "Of course, his voice was his identity, and so he chose not to have the surgery." Peter's camera follows Ray to a studio where he sits down in front of a microphone to record the eulogy he wants played following his death.

Cody saw the documentary as an opportunity to tell her story in a positive way and to deliver a personal message to a wide audience. According to her son, Thomas, she wanted to participate in the film because, "Taking her own life was a very difficult decision for her, but she felt strongly that others should have the same choice."[10]

Cody and Peter collaborated on the film over the last ten months, and she became its emotional centerpiece. When they first met, she was given less than six months to live. Cody was skeptical that she would survive even that long and set a date—Memorial Day—to take the medication. Then she outlived her prognosis.

Peter told me: "Basically, she kind of blew through the date, and she was doing really well. She had excellent palliative care through hospice, which is kind of one of these perverse realities I've learned about. Very often when people don't pursue a curative route, but rather a palliative care route, a lot of times not only is their quality of life better but they actually live longer. I think that was probably true with Cody, and if she'd continued with chemotherapy or radiation or other curative therapies she probably wouldn't have lived as long as she ultimately did. Certainly, her quality of life wouldn't have been as good by any objective measure."

Kate kept a close eye on Cody's symptoms, and she coordinated the efforts of the palliative medicine team and the staff from interventional radiology. Notwithstanding the presence of the metastatic disease, Cody began to feel physically well. Treatment with steroids improved her appetite, and she gained much-needed muscle mass. While she didn't especially appreciate the extra weight, it improved her strength and energy. Cody had a "reasonable" spring, and then began what she came to call, "my golden summer."

According to Kate, "Cody and Stan were both powerful, smart, go-getter people. They had lived fast. They worked a lot. They had raised their children who were now young adults, and as a couple they had lived incredibly busy and productive lives. They both knew that their time together would be limited, and this was to be a summer in which they could enjoy the pleasure of being with each other. Stan took more time out from his consulting work. Their son was nearby, and their daughter flew in from Washington, D.C., where she was living. It was beautiful. They are just a remarkable family."

Kate saw her patient every couple of weeks. Cody slowly, but joyously, hiked with female friends along her favorite Arboretum trails. She walked on majestic beaches with her family. The Oregon shore has a stark beauty—the shiny sand stretches unbroken; black rock formations jut out of the water, and the sun sparkles on small salty puddles. In a scene from the documentary, each member of the Curtis family is clad in brightly colored windbreakers that ripple in the wind, each takes a turn walking by her side, and they are obviously taking pleasure in each other's company. Cody looks ethereal, and one or another of the family is always lightly touching her, seemingly ready to grab hold if she stumbles.

During that summer, Stan took Cody for long drives exploring backcountry roads and collecting rocks for their garden. They dreamed about the cabin they were building, and they imagined an impressive basalt fireplace and imposing log stairway. Every dinner became an opportunity for trying out old favorite recipes and for storytelling. According to Stan, in the past, the Curtis family had given up or "forgotten" vacations so that they could host guests and visitors or help with their children's summer programs. This year was special—in his words, it was "self-indulgent."

Cody had often deferred her own pleasure for the sake of others, but now she was purely enjoying herself. She was self-confident, content with her accomplishments, and she didn't have a single unfinished task beyond talking, walking, and enjoying the sunshine. Her feelings were contagious, and the entire family could tell that she felt happy and loved. According to Stan, "It was the most romantic summer . . . one more day, one more chance . . . to kiss. Each day . . . each moment . . . was priceless!"

During this extraordinary period, Cody contemplated the existential meaning of her life. She constantly tried to make sense of two simple but profound questions: How do I want to live this day? And, do I want to be here tomorrow?

25

～○

DON'T SUGARCOAT IT

On New Year's Eve of 2014, Sarah and her husband went to a friend's house and spent the night. "Dan called us the next day, and he was crying," she told me. "He said they found a mass. They did a scan of her brain and found a mass. That was all he knew."

During the preceding few months, Brittany had been having headaches. They would occur especially at night, and she would take long showers trying to get rid of them. Sometimes she would begin vomiting or have visual changes. She saw a neurologist, who diagnosed migraines, and tried various treatments.

When Dan called on New Year's Day, 2014, Sarah and her husband immediately drove to the John Muir Medical Center. They found Brittany in the intensive care unit, where she was confused and disoriented—likely a medication side effect. By the following day, the medicine had been stopped and she was mentally clearer. Sarah and Dan arranged for her to be transferred to UCSF Medical Center, a teaching and research tertiary care center, where she would undergo further analysis of the tumor.

"In true Brittany fashion," Sarah said, "she was adamant about wanting to learn what was going on. She said: 'Give it to me straight and don't sugarcoat it. Am I going to die? What's the deal? If I'm going to die, I want to talk about my options.'"

By contrast, Debbie Ziegler, her mother, said, "At the beginning I hoped for everything. . . . First, I hoped they had the wrong x-rays . . . the wrong set of scans . . . it was all just a big clerical mishap. Your brain will do real strange things to you when you don't want to believe in something. You'll come up with fairy tales."[1]

Brittany accurately processed things right away and wanted to know, "So what are we going to do about this?"

Sarah spent time with her over the next couple of weeks in UCSF, where she ended up having a craniotomy (a surgical procedure in which the skull is opened) to remove part of the tumor. She then recovered remarkably well and demanded to get back to pursuing her passions and her ordinary routines. "Brittany wanted to resume the outdoorsy-life-to-the-fullest, because that was her way."

The exact diagnosis was uncertain, and her surgeons and oncologists went back and forth trying to grade the tumor. First, they thought it was a more benign grade 2, but after the surgery it was considered a grade 4 glioblastoma. Sarah tried to be helpful by diving into the medical stuff, researching treatment trials, and comparing notes with the UCLA physicians. When it became evident that this was a terminal condition, Sarah was the one to begin exploring the option of palliative care and the death-with-dignity route.

In Brittany's words:[2]

On New Year's Day, after months of suffering from debilitating headaches, I learned that I had brain cancer.

I was 29 years old. I'd been married for just over a year. My husband and I were trying for a family.

Our lives devolved into hospital stays, doctor consultations and medical research. Nine days after my initial diagnoses, I had a partial craniotomy and a partial resection of my temporal lobe. Both surgeries were an effort to stop the growth of my tumor.

In April, I learned that not only had my tumor come back, but it was more aggressive. Doctors gave me a prognosis of six months to live.

Because my tumor is so large, doctors prescribed full brain radiation. I read about the side effects: The hair on my scalp would have been singed off. My scalp would be left covered with first-degree burns. My quality of life, as I knew it, would be gone.

After months of research, my family and I reached a heartbreaking conclusion: There is no treatment that would save my life, and the recommended treatments would have destroyed the time I had left.

According to Sarah, immediately after the cancer was identified, Brittany was convinced that she was going to die. She had to be persuaded to undergo the surgery. After tests showed the cancer had continued to grow and spread, she set Sarah to investigating palliative medicine physicians in Washington State and Oregon, where death with dignity had been legalized.

Brittany explained:[3]

I considered passing away in hospice care at my San Francisco Bay Area home. But even with palliative medication, I could develop potentially morphine-resistant pain and suffer personality changes and verbal, cognitive and motor loss of virtually any kind.

Because the rest of my body is young and healthy, I am likely to physically hang on for a long time even though cancer is eating my mind. I probably would have suffered in hospice care for weeks or even months. And my family would have had to watch that.

I did not want this nightmare scenario for my family, so I started researching death with dignity. . . . I quickly decided that death with dignity was the best option for me and my family.

It was Sarah who found a skilled palliative care physician based in Oregon whom Brittany could relate to, and who was prepared to manage her symptoms and facilitate her fulfilling the state's requirements to apply under the act.

Brittany explained:[4]

> We had to uproot from California to Oregon, because Oregon is one of only five states where death with dignity is authorized.
>
> I met the criteria for death with dignity in Oregon, but establishing residency in the state to make use of the law required a monumental number of changes. I had to find new physicians, establish residency in Portland, search for a new home, obtain a new driver's license, change my voter registration and enlist people to take care of our animals. . . . My husband, Dan, had to take a leave of absence from his job. The vast majority of families do not have the flexibility, resources and time to make all these changes.

She went on to say, "I've had the medication for weeks. I am not suicidal. If I were, I would have consumed that medication long ago. I do not want to die. But I am dying. And I want to die on my own terms."

Brittany told Sarah that she did not want to go "quietly into the night," but wanted to follow Dylan Thomas's invocation to fight "against the dying of the light" by accomplishing some good during her remaining time. It was again Sarah who made contacts through her own friendship network that resulted in a reporter flying to Oregon from New York to conduct an interview for *People* magazine. According to Sarah, "Brittany was very open with her. . . . She is really an open book."

Sarah said, "I thought it would be a back-page story or opinion piece . . . and had no idea [that it would turn into] a media frenzy. . . . It skyrocketed out of control. Brittany would say, 'I can't believe how many people are calling me! She was inundated with people. . . . At no point did she ever realize it was going to get as big as it did. Overnight, she became a kind of superstar. . . . She did not go out looking for that. She had never sought publicity."

According to Sarah, Brittany was always a camera-shy person who preferred to take the pictures rather than be in them.

She had no experience with the spotlight. About the media attention, she remarked, "I think it is a good thing, but I'm so overwhelmed. I never intended for it to be such a big thing." She was extremely sensitive about the negative things that appeared in the press, and according to Dan, her feelings were easily hurt.

Brittany debated different courses of action with another friend, and they decided to approach C&C, the leading right-to-die organization in the nation, to assist in more effectively marshalling her efforts and making use of their public relations expertise.

When I interviewed Dr. Linda Ganzini, she clearly stated that she was not a death-with-dignity proponent or opponent. She was first and foremost a scientist. While conducting a series of research investigations, Linda conscientiously worked at maintaining a neutral position on this divisive subject. The two principal sources of information about the impact of the DWDA are the annual report from state's Health Division and Linda's articles that have been published in the most prestigious medical journals.

Linda was born in a small Oregon town and understands its people from the perspective of a native. She is a professor from Oregon Health & Science University, who is clinically trained in consultation psychiatry, geriatric psychiatry, and palliative medicine. There is a measured exactness in how she answered my questions during interviews. She speaks softly, seriously, and with considerable restraint. All the years that I've known her, she has worn her hair in an easy-to-care-for Prince Valiant style and dressed casually; her feet are clad in either sandals or hiking boots.

Over the past sixteen years in a book-strewn office with piles of articles stacked up around the walls amid photographs of her children, Linda has attempted to go beyond the simple demographics of the DWDA's annual report to ask such questions as: What are the psychological characteristics of patients who make use of this option? What has been the response of Oregon physicians to the act? Which ones are willing to directly assist in these deaths? How do hospice nurses, social workers, and chaplains view this end-of-life practice?

Linda explained that there is little evidence that vulnerable groups are being given prescriptions for lethal medication in lieu of palliative care. By the third year of the Oregon experience with the DWDA, physicians were granting only about one in six requests for a prescription, and one in ten requests resulted in deaths following ingestion.[5] She clarified that people often make requests for assisted dying too late during the course of their illness and are unable to survive the fifteen-day waiting period, or they are depressed and thereby disqualified. Other obstacles are being unable to find a willing pair of physicians or having a prognosis greater than six months. The law has been thoughtfully designed to be politically pragmatic and to not make it easy for people to obtain medically assisted dying. And even though the DWDA does not require loved ones to support the individual's request, family objections are realistically a factor that influence doctors to *not* provide their patients with lethal prescriptions.

When the act was first considered, among the many concerns raised by the opposition was that it would encourage a surge of non-Oregonians arriving to seek the lethal prescriptions—the way Europeans now travel to Switzerland to make use of the services of the Dignitas organization. Linda examined about one hundred forty cases and found only four patients had come from other states.[6] In three cases, the dying person moved to Oregon because that is where his or her family already resided. In her opinion, "suicide tourism" is unlikely to occur. Brittany Maynard was exceptional in many ways, including having sufficient time and the necessary assets to move her family to the state.

In a survey of thirty-five doctors who received requests for barbiturates, Linda reported that their patients were commonly described as "feisty" and "unwavering."[7] She found that the people who used the law were not so much depressed as they were determined. The greatest concern was not fear of pain but fear of losing autonomy, which was cited by 87 percent of the people who would take their lives with the drugs. Only 22 percent of the patients list fear of inadequate pain control as an end-of-life concern.

Linda's findings are mirrored by Oregon Health Authority statistics. In the 2018 report, the greatest concern of the DWDA sample was not fear of pain but worry over a decreasing ability to participate in activities that made life enjoyable (88 percent), the loss of autonomy (87 percent), and the loss of dignity (67 percent).[8]

During our interview, Linda concluded that compared to other dying patients, "If anything, this group of individuals seems less vulnerable." She pointed out that they often have substantial financial resources, have been successful in life, have not had difficulty making their needs known while interacting with medical staff, and had full access to end-of-life care because of excellent insurance. They almost always receive hospice and palliative care services because patients want them and their physicians would like to be confident that the requests for assisted dying are not prompted by untreated symptoms. In fact, she told me that "these people are 180° different" from what everyone was convinced they'd be when the law passed, "in terms of the vulnerability issues." They are certainly not passive victims. Rather, the most striking feature of their personalities is a lifelong need to be in control and hyper-independence.[9] It is hardly a coincidence that this description matches that of Cody and Brittany.

Linda has been especially interested in eliciting the attitudes of medical professionals about assisted dying. In one of her studies that took place two years after legalization, she sent questionnaires to approximately four thousand Oregon physicians (intentionally excluding pathologists, psychiatrists, and pediatricians, as they are ineligible to prescribe under the act) and received responses from 65 percent.[10] Her survey focused on the 144 respondents who reported that they had received a total of 221 requests for lethal prescriptions. The doctors, like the general population, are divided in support and opposition to assisted dying, and one-third of respondents were willing to write a lethal prescription under the law; 20 percent were uncertain, and 46 percent were unwilling.[11] The DWDA's regulations anticipated this and explicitly stated that a physician can decline participation for any reason whatsoever, and that he or she is not obligated to find another doctor to prescribe lethal medications for their patients. Some doctors agreed in principle with the act but balked at the thought of writing the lethal prescription for their patient; others were contractually prevented from prescribing because they worked for a religious institution or a medical system that objected to the practice.

Among patients who approached their doctor for aid in dying, family members knew about the request in 80 percent of 143 cases, and the physician spoke to a family member in 73 percent.[12] Thirteen patients did not confide their intentions to their family, seven patients had no family to inform, and nine patients did not inform the responding physician whether the family was aware of the request.

Linda examined how other health care professionals from Oregon view the act. In her surveys, she found that about 56 percent of psychiatrists endorsed support of assisted dying, as did about 70 percent of the psychologists.[13] Approximately 40 percent of hospice chaplains reported that they were in favor, while hospice nurses polled about the same as physicians with roughly an even split, though hospice social workers were comparable to psychologists in having a noticeable majority in favor.[14]

Not surprisingly given her training, Linda focused attention on the psychological aspects of the DWDA. She would prefer that the law required formal rather than informal screening of depression by having physicians administer standardized questionnaires. Linda has acquired some data suggesting that there are people with major depressions who go undetected during the process of requesting death with dignity.[15]

I have some concerns about the value of using standardized psychometric questionnaires and similar instruments for assisted dying. These are frequently relied upon in psychiatric research and for quick screening of clinical populations to ascertain the likely presence of depression or suicidal thoughts. But I think that in the context of life-limiting diseases, clinicians should be more cautious about labeling someone as having depression. Clinicians need to understand that a wish to die does not directly correlate with depression, and that it is not the same thing as suicidal ideation. It also doesn't mean that a person lacks the capability to participate in decisions. The social circumstances and the underlying disease's symptoms may each contribute to the incorrect impression that these people have a psychiatric disorder, but false positive psychiatric diagnoses are especially likely when questionnaires are used. I am disinclined to take away someone's right to assisted dying because of an overblown concern based on them having scored as depressed on a quick checklist.

On the other hand, I am more comfortable arriving at such a diagnosis from an interview that establishes that the person has had a family history of an affective disorder, has suffered from clinical depression in the past requiring treatment, or has made suicide attempts when physically healthy.[16]

I am admittedly an outlier among my peers in believing that in the context of a terminal illness, depression or other psychiatric disorders should only be exclusionary factors when they are of psychotic proportions and interfere with a person's capacity to meaningfully participate in medical decisions.

I don't think that psychiatrists are necessary to make these determinations or that they should function as gate keepers. Ordinary physicians—primary care practitioners or surgeons—routinely determine whether their patients retain the capacity to make vital decisions and whether they have major psychiatric problems. I don't think that it should be any different for death with dignity, and psychologists and psychiatrists can always be tapped as consultants for ambiguous situations.

Linda also focused her research attention on the families of people who died having used the DWDA.[17] Reassuringly, she found no elevated rates of abnormal grief or depression among survivors. If anything, family members appeared to believe that the death was a good experience for them and their loved one.

ENOUGH IS ENOUGH

D r. Kate Morris continued to see Cody in her Portland office each week to make sure she was medically stable. In the fall of 2009, the surgeon had been planning to embark with her husband on a long-awaited trip to Africa to celebrate a fortieth birthday. Hesitant about leaving, she was persuaded by her patient that the backup arrangements were more than adequate; Cody insisted that she depart as scheduled. The exotic vacation proved to be enchanting to the animal-loving physician, but upon returning from Zambia three weeks later, she found Cody was rapidly failing.

Over the course of a year, Cody had begun to have generalized body pains. The disease affected her breathing and left her completely exhausted. Her skin turned yellow, and food lost its taste. For a time, she looked model-thin, and things then progressed to the point that she appeared emaciated. Because of liver failure, her abdomen once again became swollen. Upon meeting her, a stranger might think Cody was three months pregnant, a couple of days later she would appear to be six months pregnant, and shortly afterward she'd look on the verge of going into labor. When the fluids were removed from her belly with a catheter, the cycle would quickly repeat itself. She began to have infections and require multiple courses of antibiotics. Throughout this ordeal, Cody remained mentally clear. She quipped and gave fashion tips on the Cholangiocarcinoma Foundation's online discussion board.

Cody posted, "I'm pretty thin now but still can't wear most of my old clothes because my stomach sticks out, yuck. There's an Adidas exercise pant with a stretchy waistband I wear almost every day. Wish I could find another pair. Or yoga pants, if they are low-slung, work. Since I have a huge surgical hernia (which I would have had fixed if the tumors hadn't recurred) wearing a back belt helps. That sort of disguises the whole waist problem too! I wear longer jackets that cover things up (easier now that the weather is cooler)."[1]

Concerning her wish to be able to continue exercising, she wrote on the same site, "I was a swimmer and walker and not heavy to begin with. . . . Isn't it awful—when you get to 50 and the wheels just start falling off, cancer or no cancer!"[2]

Her advice was, "Anyway, taking care of yourself means looking as much like your old self as possible, in my humble estimation. I try to wear make-up every day. And I've got a great haircutter, who cut my hair (what there was left of it) and made it look good when it was growing back in. And that made a huge difference too."

However, humor and optimism did not blind her from the conclusion that she was not going to survive until Christmas, and Cody decided she wanted a combined holiday celebration and leave-taking. She needed to say goodbye. It surprised nobody when she told her doctor, "Kate, this is not really what I signed up for."

The C&C volunteer contacted the surgeon and awkwardly reported, "Cody has decided to 'hasten' on this coming Monday." This was followed shortly afterward by a call from Cody, who said, "I understand I kind of shocked you with my decision." She then inquired if Kate would come and be present at her bedside.

Kate's reaction? She told me, "It wasn't even a question. I wanted to be there to support her and her family." Kate suspects that a Monday was chosen to allow Cody and her husband to have a final weekend together.

According to Stan, the fluid buildup and multiple infections from her poorly functioning liver were getting terrible. He called up their daughter and said, "Jill, your mother is not going to make it to Christmas. It could be a fever and I won't know until it is right on top of us. Get ready!"

"Cody had her friends over and they kind of shopped her closet," Kate said with a rueful giggle. She had previously given away the jewelry to her daughter. However, during a subsequent good period she felt "compelled" to purchase a few more items. One friend asked, "Are you sure you want to give this away?" To which Cody good-naturedly replied, "Well what am I going to do with it?" Kate repeatedly witnessed how extraordinarily smooth and generous her patient was at putting everyone at ease during this trying period.

Over the previous months, Cody and Kate found much to converse about besides health matters. They deliberated on the meaning of life, the impact of having children, and the importance of maintaining moral values, but they also chatted merrily about pets (Kate has two cats), style, and fashion. Cody always maintained a strikingly attractive appearance with her carefully cut salt-and-pepper hair, and a thin black line tattooed on each eyelid to offset her pale lashes. Because of the tattoo, she looked like she had just applied eyeliner even during her worst moments when she was in the surgical intensive care unit. Both women enjoyed talking about shoes and earrings, while one of the first things Cody noticed in Kate's office was the surgeon's use of comfortable microfiber patient gowns; Cody purchased one of her own to bring along for the hospitalization. Cody appreciated that most physicians create hierarchical offices; however, Kate was responsive to such matters and had empowered her staff. Gender equality was meaningful to Cody, and she admired Kate's persistence and fortitude in carving out a career within a traditionally male medical specialty.

Two days before she planned on dying, Peter and Cody met to carefully negotiate the filming. Cody made it clear that she would be uncomfortable with a cameraman in her bedroom, and she didn't want to be filmed ingesting the Seconal or taking her last breath. She desired to have some privacy with her family, physician, and the C&C counselor, without any outsiders intruding. However, she was agreeable to having a small microphone in the room that could be used for audiotaping. She wanted the public to experience the immediacy of her death and hoped that this would dispel many of the fears and misconceptions surrounding assisted dying. Cody suggested that a camera might be focused from outside the apartment on the lace curtain of her window, fluttering in the breeze. The viewer might be able to see the fluctuating silhouettes of those who were inside. The result is certainly the most tasteful, delicate, and purely artistic visual scene in the entire documentary, and it accomplished Peter and Cody's mutual goal of portraying a highly dramatic event with respect and restraint.

Cody was dedicated to the cinematic project and wanted it to accurately convey her personality, beliefs, and experience. This was not a simple task, or even necessarily possible, because Cody was a complex person who combined seemingly incompatible traits. While she grew up on a ranch in rural Idaho, she also had a father who was a respected professor of economics. Cody was an accomplished intellectual who excelled at Harvard, but she was always far more invested in caring for her husband, family, and community. She and Stan led very mindful lives, and both desired to be in control of their destinies to whatever extent possible.

Given her training in economics, it is perhaps no surprise that when Cody became ill, she was particularly sensitive to financial considerations. According to Peter, "That was certainly an aspect of her social consciousness. She was aware of the cost of care, and that was part of the calculus for her making this decision [to use the death with dignity procedure]. It was not, 'Oh, we can't afford this or that treatment,' but rather, 'why would I undergo a treatment if it can only get me so little time and cost the medical establishment money?'"

The filmmaker observed, "She had spent the last eighteen years of her career working at Oregon Health & Science University and was always trying to calculate when is enough enough? What is the rate of return? Where is that inflection point?"

Cody was a "numbers person" but also a highly emotional woman, and there was something about her situation that kindled an irresistible desire to tell the story, to explain how she had come to this point. She was intensely aware of crossing an unimaginable threshold by choosing to decide on the manner and timing of her death.

Having decided that December 7 would be the date when she would take the Seconal, Cody Curtis nailed it down with the announcement, "My surgeon has a full day of clinic and she'll be done at six. So, six o'clock it will be!"

Naturally, on the appointed day, Dr. Kate Morris was busy right up to the last minute. When she did leave the office, the first available parking spot seemed like it was eight miles away from Cody's condominium. The anxious surgeon rushed along the slippery Portland sidewalk while thinking, *You can't be late for something like this!*

Finally arriving at her destination, she rang the doorbell and stepped into a warm and brightly lit hallway that was festively adorned with green and red popcorn balls. Arms reached out to embrace her, and she was greeted by Stan, Thomas, Jill, Cody's parents, the C&C volunteer, and assorted other family members and friends. Kate had been prepared for wailing and despair. Instead, she found a group of people united by friendship, joy, and love.

Walking into Cody's bedroom, her patient looked up at her from the bed, smiled broadly, and handed over a final parting gift to the self-proclaimed "crazy cat-lady" surgeon. Beneath exquisite wrapping was a garish, leopard-spotted pair of women's pajamas. "So, it's the cat's pajamas," Kate remarked, prompting laughter. This continued until Cody gently but firmly said, "Well, I'm ready."

The Curtis family planned the last evening to also be a Christmas party. Their holiday tradition called for a lengthy sing-along. Before Kate arrived, Jill had provided sweet harmonies while the participants loudly sang Christmas carols. Sing-alongs have special meaning to this family, which cherishes them as being an unsophisticated, country thing, linked to their farmstead roots. Familiar songs would be sung each year, including Cody's favorite, which coincidentally had to do with flying away and dying.

Throughout the sing-along, Stan kept his composure until the line in You Are My Sunshine that goes, "please don't take my sunshine away." He remained shutdown throughout the next stanza:

"The other night, dear, / As I lay sleeping / I dreamed I held you in my arms. / When I awoke, dear, / I was mistaken / And I hung my head and cried."

Cody had immediately noticed his silence, and she quickly suggested they all join in a happier song. The assembled broke into a raucous chorus of Jingle Bells. When all were sung out, she thanked her mother for joining them in this bittersweet event, and the older woman recounted with pride and joy the circumstances surrounding the day when Cody was born. Everyone looked at each other and declared the moment to be "practically perfect."

"Cody's parents were not in on the story until the very end, but they figured it out. They got it," said Stan. "It is one of the amazing parts about her death." Cody's mother is a nurse, and she and Cody's father had struggled over their daughter's decision to end her life this way.

After Cody announced her readiness to take the medicine, Thomas and Jill hugged and kissed her, and then they and the filmmakers left the room. According to Kate, "That was difficult to watch because they were crying, and Cody was crying, and everyone else was crying."

The volunteer mixed the medicine into a drink. Kate asked if Cody wanted her to remain, and the patient answered in the affirmative, which was what Kate had been hoping would be her response. The surgeon felt responsible to support her throughout the entire experience. Everyone gave each other hugs, including Cody's elderly parents. She then drank down the medication cocktail. Smiling and wiping her mouth, Cody turned to them, laughed aloud, and explained, "The room is spinning. In the past, that has not generally been a good sign." Her last words were, "This is so easy. I just want people to know this is so easy."

"She finally drifted off after about half an hour," Kate explained. "She started to snore. The C&C volunteer and I took turns holding her chin up, a gentle maneuver that is called a "jaw thrust," which relieves the temporary respiratory obstruction. She wouldn't have wanted to be seen or heard snoring."

Afterward, the sounds of the Curtis children crying in the next room became noticeable; their grandparents left the bedroom to comfort them. About forty-five minutes later when Cody was fast asleep, Stan said that he was alright and wanted some private time with her. The volunteer and Kate found it difficult to leave, but they also wanted to respect Stan's wishes.

When Kate returned home, her husband was away on business, and there was no one to talk to. She put away the pajamas, hugged her cats, and began crying. Stan telephoned her apartment around 9:30 that night to say Cody had died, and Kate called the funeral home where arrangements had been made in advance to pick up the body on the following morning. In these situations, the doctor does not need to perform an examination for the formal declaration. The funeral home completes the official certificate and the explanation for death is listed as being "natural causes." The form was later mailed to Kate's office for her signature.

WHAT SHE WANTED

arbara Coombs Lee began our interview by saying: "Having choices at the end of life enables people to subdue the fears about how they might die so that they can allow mortality to come into their consciousness and be more present in their lives in compassionate ways. That is all the better for humankind. It is about improving the way we humans live our lives, because we understand how precious, how very, very, precious every moment is."

I thought to myself, *Who talks like that?* The answer was: an eloquent woman and veteran activist for whom choice is essential.

Barbara started out as an English literature student at Vassar College but chose to leave after a year for Cornell University's School of Nursing, where she prepared to follow in her mother's footsteps. Upon hearing that she wanted to go to nursing school, her college advisor had disparagingly remarked to the stunningly beautiful woman, "If it doesn't work out, you can always become a stewardess."

But nursing was only one of many career changes that Barbara would make, as she also completed training and practiced as a physician assistant and then as an attorney. Despite graduating second in her class at law school, as a woman, she had difficulty finding employment. The silver lining was that in 1991 she ended up as a committee member on the Oregon Senate Healthcare and Bioethics Committee. In addition to her grounding in law, Barbara brought to the position nearly twenty-five years of experience working in medicine.

It was a remarkable year for Oregon, as the committee chair, Bob Shoemaker, introduced an advance directive bill, and Senator Frank L. Roberts proposed one of the first aid-in-dying laws in the nation. Roberts was a revered statesman, widely known as the "Conscience of the Oregon Senate." At the time, he had advanced prostate cancer. As a complication of the radiation therapy, he had sustained a spinal cord injury and used to scoot around the capital in a wheelchair. Senator Roberts was married to the governor, and he knew that the prostate cancer was going to kill him. Barbara said to me, "One might think that all these elements would have allowed him to get his bill through the legislature? But quite the opposite. It didn't even get a serious hearing. It received what is called a courtesy hearing, which is when witnesses testify on the bill, but a vote is not held."

Barbara understood. The politics of the day called for Shoemaker's advance directive bill to take precedence, and for the public to not have to simultaneously consider an assisted-dying bill. But at the Roberts hearing, she felt it was a travesty that there was no one representing patients, let alone dying patients. She said, "Just about everyone who attended wore a clergy collar and had come to the capital building to testify against the bill, preaching that it would be the downfall of Western civilization. Then the bill died. And then about a year and a half later, Roberts died in the governor's mansion with his wife by his side." The senator, unfortunately, had exactly the kind of death that he had hoped to avoid, drifting in and out of consciousness for several weeks.

Barbara ended up becoming a Unitarian, because the one minister who testified in favor of Roberts's bill was from that denomination. It was two years later in a church bulletin that she learned that people were gathering to draft an initiative to place on a state ballot. Barbara had been working at the Senate for four years and knew about composing bills, and she volunteered to help.

Barbara spent the next ten months laboring on it. She suspects that she was the only person in the core group of five or six people who was not already a member of the Hemlock Society. They met weekly to struggle over the bill, and they tirelessly changed and refined it. One of her proudest moments came when Judge Reinhardt wrote his opinion and took special note of the bill's meticulousness. She was pleased they had drafted a sensible outline for a feasible medical practice.

"I must have missed the meeting," she said, "where the group decided I was going to be the chief spokesperson among the three petitioners." Either way, that year she campaigned on behalf of the initiative throughout the state of Oregon.

The law was constructed so that depression was *not* an exclusion. Rather, a psychiatric or psychological condition that impaired judgment was listed as being an exclusion. People could be depressed about dying, and they wouldn't be disqualified unless their condition was of psychotic proportions or the confusion was so severe that they could no longer make sound decisions about treatment.

I asked Barbara about the somewhat different approach of the Final Exit Network, and she expressed her opinion that the group "is so influenced by their libertarian philosophy that they feel, 'We just don't need those doctors. We would rather do something ourselves. Helium works. We don't mind the plastic bags. That is fine.'"

She contrasted this with C&C, the organization for which she has subsequently served as president, which is "dedicated to social reform and social justice to transform medicine and medical practice."

Barbara acknowledged: "It is difficult to change medical practice. Our goal is to change the power paradigm at the end of life so that it is undeniably clear that patients are in a position of deciding. It is their decision to make. That is our goal. I think this would be quite a revolutionary step for medicine—and a good one. Aid in dying happens to be the medical practice that is the point of the spear. It makes it happen. It makes it abundantly clear where the decision-making authority resides."

Barbara went on to wage two statewide campaigns and spent ten years defending Oregon's Death with Dignity Act (DWDA) in both the judicial and legislative arenas. She would help guide the crafting of the state of Washington's law. C&C and the Death with Dignity National Center[1] can take much of the credit for initiating campaigns to enact similar laws in other states.

I asked Barbara how Brittany intended to use the Oregon law, since it was drafted to avoid "suicide tourists." "They moved to Oregon in March or April," Barbara said, "and were there for a total of about eight months. During that time, she got a driver's license. She registered to vote. They established a home."

When Barbara went to visit Brittany, she assumed it would be in a rented house that was "as anonymous as a Marriott Suites." To the contrary, Dan and Brittany had found a comfortable home on top of a hill overlooking Portland that was situated close to the hospital. The couple had hired a moving van, transported their belongings, put up pictures on the wall, carefully arranged their own furniture, and brought their entire household, including the two dogs. When Barbara walked in, it looked like they had lived there for years. Brittany's mother and her stepfather had joined them, and while the middle-aged couple went back and forth to their own home, for the most part they remained with Brittany in Oregon. All of them, including visiting friends, like Sarah, had settled into the rented yellow house.

I inquired about how the organization helped Brittany, and mentioned my friend, the assisted-suicide opponent, Dr. Ira Byock, who had publicly critiqued C&C's involvement, suggesting that the dying woman was being manipulated. Barbara answered, "She didn't need any help. All the help Brittany wanted was amplification of her voice when she created the video tools. All we did was to arrange for the launch to be as impactful as possible, and to manage all the press inquiries. She didn't need help shaping her message or formulating a plan. . . . She was completely incapable of being manipulated.

You couldn't manipulate Brittany Maynard if you were the most fantastic manipulator in the world."

Brittany only approached C&C after she had already moved to Oregon, qualified for the DWDA, satisfied its every requirement, met the waiting period, and had the medication in hand. She was ready to speak up, and did not need anything from the organization except guidance about public relations. The organization helped to coordinate her relationship with *People* and launch the Brittany Maynard Fund.

Dan would write to me, "Brittany (and any terminally ill individual in her predicament) doesn't want to die, they want to live. . . . Brittany was simply taking the appropriate steps (in her case by moving to Oregon) in order to have the option of a gentle dying process should it become necessary for her. Left to run its course, the brain tumor would have ended Brittany's life horrifically. Brittany refused to accept that."

Brittany explained in one of her taped essays,[2] "I would not tell anyone else that he or she should choose death with dignity. My question is: Who has the right to tell me that I don't deserve this choice? That I deserve to suffer for weeks or months in tremendous amounts of physical and emotional pain? Why should anyone have the right to make that choice for me?"

In another tape aimed at elected officials, she described alternate means to hasten death, specifically palliative sedation—a practice that requires hospitalization and the administration of intravenous medications to place a person into a coma.[3] She understood that the coma was maintained until dehydration or infection would eventually cause the heart or breathing to cease. But Brittany rejected this method and preferred to rely on Oregon's aid-in-dying law, because: "I want to be sure my husband and mother are with me when I die. I want to leave this earth in my home, in the arms of my husband and my parents." The way that she chose would allow her to live her last months fully, "knowing I can leave this life with dignity allows me to focus on living."

In the CNN tape,[4] she continued this theme, saying:

Now that I've had the prescription filled and it's in my possession, I have experienced a tremendous sense of relief. And if I decide to change my mind about taking the medication, I will not take it.

Having this choice at the end of my life has become incredibly important. It has given me a sense of peace during a tumultuous time that otherwise would be dominated by fear, uncertainty and pain.

Now, I'm able to move forward in my remaining days or weeks I have on this beautiful Earth, to seek joy and love and to spend time traveling to outdoor wonders of nature with those I love. And I know that I have a safety net.

I plan to celebrate my husband's birthday on October 26 with him and our family. Unless my condition improves dramatically, I will look to pass soon thereafter.

I hope for the sake of my fellow American citizens that I'll never meet that this option is available to you. If you ever find yourself walking a mile in my shoes, I hope that you would at least be given the same choice and that no one tries to take it from you.

Brittany felt herself getting sicker each week, and she set a day in November to die, while reserving the right to change her mind. Brittany posted "A Video for All My Friends," in which she spoke from her bedroom. The recording included clips where she and Dan walk along forest trails while holding hands, setting a picnic table, and a close-up of Charlie, the Great Dane, sniffing the camera.[5] Brittany talked about the increasing frequency of seizures that were disrupting each day, and how she woke up from one of them seeing Dan's concerned face but being unable say his name. All the while her body was being transformed by the prescription medications taken to ameliorate the symptoms; she gained twenty-five pounds in three months and no longer wanted to look in a mirror or be photographed.

Sarah visited whenever she had a day or a weekend off from work. While the seizures were the most intolerable evidence of the cancer's progression, Brittany also suffered with bloating, acne, and bone pain in her legs. The last made it impossible for her to walk for days at a time.

In the videotape, Brittany tearfully wished that her mother wouldn't unduly grieve, and that Dan would be able to "move on" after her death and "become a father."

When she wasn't in the yellow house, Brittany spent the last months traveling to Alaska, British Columbia, and both Olympic and Yellowstone National Parks.[6] She and Dan took a helicopter ride through the Grand Canyon.

Her obituary would mention that "after being told by one doctor that 'she probably didn't even have weeks to be on her feet,' she was found climbing 10-mile trails along the ice fields of Alaska with her best friend in the sunshine months later."[7] Naturally, they were referring to Sarah, who had finally gone on her first trip with Brittany, and who appeared in photographs but declined to be named in the captions.

Sarah's description of Brittany's death is straightforward:

> The previous week, she was getting sicker and having some good days and some bad days. She brought together her three best friends, Dan, and her parents —everyone she loved. . . . We were living in the house, except for her mom and stepdad, who were staying at a hotel. . . . We would go for different walks every day. . . . It was hard at that point for her to walk a lot. We would take turns walking, supporting, and holding her hand. Then we would just make dinner together. . . .
>
> We made a really, really, nice breakfast for her the day that she died [on November 1]. On that morning, a friend had decorated the whole house with her favorite flowers, peonies. We just sat and laughed. We tried to tell stories and to not think about what was ahead. But we talked about it if she wanted, [let] her lean on us and vent, and just be there for her. The day that she died, we all went for a walk together after breakfast. Then we came back, and she said, "It's time."
>
> So, she got in bed and we all got kind of around her, and each took time one-on-one talking to her. Yes, that's

about it. I'm not sure how much of the intimacies of the day should be shared. It was special. It was really peaceful. It was beautiful, as far as death goes, and I have seen a lot of them. It was the most peaceful, beautiful death that I have ever been a part of. It was exactly what she wanted. She didn't suffer. She wasn't in pain and she got to be with everyone she loved. And when I die, I hope I am lucky enough to go the same way.

COWBOYS, MORMONS, AND SUNDANCE

Both Stan and Cody came from families in which religion is a source of strength but also a fount of great mystery and occasional bitter conflict. Stan's forebears were among the original group of Mormons who traveled west with Brigham Young. However, his paternal grandfather was a free-spirited cowboy who broke from the family creed, and his son—Stan's father—basically became an atheist. Stan's mother was not only a practicing Christian Scientist, but her relatives were leaders of the Christian Scientist Church—which is not very supportive of most medical practices. It is the Christian Scientists who occasionally face legal action for not providing their children with chemotherapy and other potentially life-saving treatments. According to Stan, Mary Baker Eddy, the church's founder, preached that reality is in your head and not physically important. The key is to think positive thoughts and to achieve spiritual dignity.

During Stan's childhood, his mother chided the family to avoid medical treatments and she counseled them to live and die naturally. By contrast, Stan's father was a scientist; he used to say, "that's a scientist with a small s," making it clear that he wasn't referring to Christian Scientists. When Stan's mother became terminally ill, Stan's father was determined to extend his wife's life as much as possible and benefit from more scientific practices. They needed to sort out their different beliefs. Gratifyingly, Stan's mother outlived her doctor's prognosis by a full decade.

Cody's father descended from a long line of Mormons, while her mother was Catholic. Stan describes both parents as having been intellectuals, as well as the black sheep of their respective families. The parents were married in London where her father was a Fulbright Scholar. He continued teaching and became a highly respected professor of economics. Cody's father rebelled from his Mormon roots, and his wife likewise abandoned most of her Catholic traditions.

Stan was a "forest service guy" hanging out at nearby bars when he met the seventeen-year-old Cody. They were wed when he was twenty-two-year-old student at Berkley and she had just turned nineteen. Cody was raised to believe that religion poses more problems than answers, and she became a Unitarian. Stan joined her in shunning most theological rituals but believed in the goodness of mankind, optimism about the future, and the importance of family and communal values.

Despite the academic accomplishments of their parents, Stan and Cody were the first generation to permanently leave the family farms. His ancestors had mainly settled in the Boise Valley of Idaho, while her family had ranches on both sides of the eastern Idaho and Montana border. Growing up on farms made an indelible mark on the couple, as they were raised around plenty of animals. Their families hunted wild game for the larder, and they raised and butchered cattle for meat. Although the ranchers took painstaking care of the herds and horses, animals have short life cycles and, growing up in a ranching family, one can't help but witness plenty of deaths. The local veterinarian was a frequent visitor, and domesticated animals and pets were regularly euthanized when suffering was apparent.

Stan and Cody were among the best educated in their extended families, and they relinquished certain career opportunities to pursue a highly intentional lifestyle. They became comparatively prosperous and able to extend financial assistance to friends and family who were in need. They were glad to assist numerous relatives with advice when struggling over college and career choices, and they offered themselves as a bridge between the farm and PhD communities.

Cody's organizational skills and the resources of their commodious Colonial house with its tranquil Japanese rose garden led her to become the mother figure for much of the extended family. Cody was well spoken and could give counsel and discuss sensitive issues with family members without trampling boundaries or sensibilities. She incorporated family traditions and regularly created new ones based more around food and seasonal changes than religion. These were what Stan called, "First Harvest kind of stuff—cutting asparagus, picking apples and strawberries, homemade ice cream, opening days for trout and salmon fishing." The homespun Curtis traditions formed the backbone of their communal activities and were extended to include a multitude of friends and neighbors.

Cody and her family would dispute any characterization of her final ten months as having been a sad or tragic time. The message she eagerly wished to convey was that this was a time for them all to remember what life is about and for each of them to live every day in as meaningful a way as possible. The Curtis family adamantly believed that her last months were more about living than about dying.

Like most of the people in Peter's documentary, Cody wanted the Seconal barbiturate to be easily available, but she simultaneously hoped she would never need to make use of it. She would have preferred to die from a fever. As she explained, "I'd rather just drift off. . . . I'd rather let nature take its course."

Cody did not ever reach the point of being bedbound. She was always entirely realistic and prepared that the going might be rough. But as her condition worsened, it also became increasingly unlikely she would be able to peacefully die without making use of the law's protocol.

Stan is convinced that Cody's reliance on the Death with Dignity Act option has had a lasting and positive impact on his family. Whether active or nonpracticing Mormons, Catholics,

Christian Scientists, Unitarians, or atheists, the Curtis clan has responded by becoming more accepting of the different ways that people choose to die. They will always continue to have doctrinaire disputes over a host of issues, but they have declared a moratorium when it comes to dying.

This became evident to Stan around the subsequent death of his mother, who succumbed despite the tender ministrations of her husband. In the past, his mother's Christian Scientist relatives might have snubbed Stan's father for violating their beliefs. Instead they communicated that they were aware and accepted the couple's arrangement around her terminal illness. Her relatives comforted the grieving spouse and behaved in a genuinely respectful and affectionate manner toward him.

While the Catholic Church continues to be the assisted-dying movement's greatest opponent, and six Canadian bishops have gone so far as to instruct their clergy to deny religious funerals to Catholics who make use of that country's legal option, there are other bishops who have adopted a more flexible approach.[1] The Church will continue struggling to reconcile its reverence for life, acceptance of suffering, veneration of martyrs, and evolving attitudes about how to respond to suicide.[2]

Some elements of Orthodox Judaism also object to *any* practice, let alone assisted dying, that accelerates death. The Satmar Bikur Cholim (a charitable group in a denomination of the ultraorthodox Chassidim) threatened a formal boycott against the New York University-Langone Hospital located on Manhattan's East Side. According to the Bikur Cholim director, the hospital today is "almost like a legal killing machine. . . . Our patients are in danger when they go there."[3]

The director said in an interview that "NYU Hospital's policies have changed and have become more difficult for the Jewish community. . . . We're very much pro-life and life being respected. Currently the hospital has initiated hospice and end-of-life care which goes against our community's halachic (legal) perspective. It comes up very often, weekly and sometimes daily where people call us with feeding tube issues or ventilator care."[4]

Rabbi Moshe Tendler, a dean at Yeshiva University, explained, "There is a major, major ethical challenge that has developed over the last decade. . . . The halacha [Jewish law] and the current practices in America were pretty well in line with each other. Now they're at variance. Under the guise of some kind of hospice care patients are being removed from active treatment and being allowed to die months in advance."[5]

While Judaic law is interpreted differently by Conservative and Reform Jews, at least this group of Orthodox Jews disapproves of any decision that falls short of maximally extending life.

In August, Stan and his children paid a visit to the farmstead cemetery in Idaho. While the primary purpose of the trip was to inter Cody's ashes and to erect a tombstone, they were also invited to participate in a wedding. According to Stan, they witnessed "the rodeo queen marrying the rodeo king." It was important for Thomas, Jill, and Stan to celebrate this event. Between their day at the cemetery and the wedding, they felt firmly connected with life, death, and their family's roots.

Cody Curtis was fifty-four years old when she died. As a couple, Stan and she had reached a life stage in which they were ready to embark on a novel adventure. "We never could have predicted it would involve a terminal illness," he told me. But he feels grateful to have been living in Oregon where Cody would have a choice and savor the precious remaining time. He is immensely proud of her surgeon for having had the "guts to stick with them."

Kate admits that she was initially hesitant about not only assisting them in the death but also taking a visible role in Peter's film project. She was concerned that any resultant publicity might inhibit her ability to care for patients who did not share these values. She feared being made a target by opponents of the movement. Kate said that it was intimidating "to come out of the closet," and she dreaded any possibility of notoriety.

Peter recognized her reluctance, and he began a campaign to win her over by emailing cute pictures of his own cats. The consummate "cat lady" was moved, and she gradually allowed his crew to film during Cody's office appointments. But she remained silent and off-camera.

However, things changed drastically in the week following Cody's death. Kate and her husband were relaxing at home and watching a show on public access cable television when they discovered that it featured an interview with one of her medical school professors. To their surprise, the academic explained to his audience that physicians involved with the Oregon act masquerade as caring doctors, do nothing but fill out prescriptions, and make their living entirely through this sordid activity. Kate, who was still in a profound state of awe by how Cody chose to end her life, "felt like what he was saying was so inaccurate that it was cruel." She decided that the other side of the story had to be told, and she immediately called up Peter and agreed to an on-camera interview.

At the Sundance premier, Kate accompanied Peter and the Curtis family. She had the surreal experience of seeing herself for the first time on a movie screen. There were empty seats at the initial showing. However, by the next performance, word had spread, enormous lines formed outside the theater, and the film played to a standing-room-only crowd. Kate found it impossible to watch the movie without weeping. Afterward, having dried her eyes, she accompanied the family in answering audience questions—all the while worrying that someone would stand up and accuse her of being a killer. She concluded that Cody and Peter had superbly accomplished their goals and it was nothing short of miraculous to have had a respectful public discourse on such a highly charged subject.

"This is a happily-ever-after movie of family love," is how Stan analyzed, "How to Die in Oregon." He was ecstatic recalling how his children received a standing ovation at the festival, and how pleased he was when the film received the year's Grand Jury Prize for Best Documentary.

Jeff Shannon, a movie critic, wrote that it is truly "a film that everyone (even and perhaps especially younger viewers, with parental supervision) should see, ponder, and openly discuss. It is a challenging yet beautiful film that many will start watching and not want to finish." [6] Shannon had been paralyzed for over thirty years following an accident, and he chose to share personal details about his life in the review, including his desire to determine for himself when his time had come, while knowing that these comments would "be hotly opposed in some religious, political and even disability-related circles."

Having had time to reflect upon and metabolize the events, Kate is confident that "It would have been very brutal to say to Cody, 'No, you're going to have to let your body deteriorate at its own pace. We're not going to help you.' It would have been harmful, because she was somebody who was so proud of the life she had led and created. She felt that she was just rotting away, and she didn't want to go that way. I don't think we should force anyone to go that way."

I think that were Cody still alive, she would chuckle to discover there are other kindred spirits following her example. For instance, Jane Catherine Lotter published a piece that began: "One of the few advantages of dying from Grade 3, Stage IIIC endometrial cancer, recurrent and metastasized to the liver and abdomen, is that you have time to write your own obituary. (The other advantages are no longer bothering with sunscreen and no longer worrying about your cholesterol.)"[7]

After the cancer recurred, sixty-year-old Lotter, a wife and mother of two adult children, made a conscious decision to be joyful, rather than sad about dying, and to accept that which she could not change. She wrote, "Amazingly, this outlook worked for me. (Well, you know, most of the time.)"

Like Cody, Lotter fully understood that knowing and loving her family and friends were the key ingredients for a successful existence. She made use of Washington State's Death with Dignity Act and died peacefully at home, surrounded by her beloveds. Lotter wrote in the obituary, "I was given the gift of life, and now I have to give it back. This is hard. But I was a lucky woman."

In Oregon, Dr. Kate Morris would subsequently participate in one more death with dignity. This involved an eighty-eight-year-old patient of hers who was diagnosed with metastatic stomach cancer. Surgery would have been ultimately futile and fraught with complications. The patient had undergone the death of a daughter two years before from ovarian cancer, and she was resolute about what she wanted and what she did not want. Kate describes her as having been a plucky woman with strong opinions, especially on political subjects, who each day wrote personal letters to the president, her senators, and congressmen informing them of her views. Once again, Kate was present at the bedside when her patient drank the lethal dose of Seconal.

On Halloween of 2010 (coincidentally, Cody's birthday), Kate left Portland for a new position at the University of New Mexico in Albuquerque. This did not alter her advocacy for death with dignity. She promptly got in touch with C&C, which along with the American Civil Liberties Union of New Mexico wanted to challenge the state's law against assisted suicide. In 2012, she became one of the doctor plaintiffs in a lawsuit filed in district court. The statute on the books made it a fourth-degree felony to help someone take his or her life, and Kate's suit argued that the current law shouldn't apply to a licensed physician providing aid to a dying person who was mentally competent. The suit also claimed that the state law was overly vague and violated the state's constitution. Over the next several years, the case slowly meandered its way through the various courts before failing to come to the desired resolution.

Kate currently has a clinical and research practice as an associate professor in the Department of Surgery at the University of Oklahoma Health Sciences Center, where she primarily works with patients who have gastrointestinal malignancies. In her biosketch, she has chosen to quote an E. E. Cummings poem that concludes, "I'd rather learn from one bird how to sing than teach 10,000 stars how not to dance."[8] Like much of the poet's compositions, the line is subject to widely different interpretations, but I think it is about positively reaching out and learning lessons from one person at a time rather than instructing a large group. Unquestionably, the experience with Cody has left an indelible impression upon the sensitive surgeon.

PART IV

My phone rang and it was Paul Spiers, the Hercules-loving activist. Paul was in a poetry-reading mood.

"Do you know the poet Paul Hostovsky?" he asked.

"Never heard of him," I replied

Spiers said he was especially fond of Hostovsky's "Tree Poem" and began to recite:

It wasn't that he wanted to take his life.
He wanted to take his death
into his own hands. There was
a difference, he knew, though he couldn't
articulate it. More speculative than suicidal,
more curious than depressed,
more interested than not,
he didn't want to talk to a therapist.
He wanted to talk to Walt Whitman.
He wanted to talk to his best friend from
kindergarten, who'd moved away
on the cusp of first grade, and he never
saw him again. He wanted to climb a tree
and sit up there all alone in the top branches

watching it absorb the carbon dioxide.
He had a bit of the tree in him himself.
He had similar aspirations
and spent much of his time in the branching
ramifications in his head. But because his children
would never live it down, he climbed
down from the tree in the car in the garage
every time, and walked back into his life with a few
leaves and twigs still sticking to his head.[1]

"Hostovsky," Paul said, "is a poet who earns his living as a sign language interpreter at the Massachusetts Commission for the Deaf and Hard of Hearing. Although the character in his poem struggles to articulate the subtleties of suicide and death-hastening actions, I love the way his opening words convey the distinctions."

As I learned a couple of years later, Hostovsky himself was diagnosed with non-Hodgkin's follicular lymphoma and was told by his doctor, "If you're going to get cancer, this is the one to get—you'll probably get hit by a bus before you die of this thing." Nevertheless, it got the young man thinking about doctors, about cancer, about suffering and, as he told me, "about taking my life or taking my death into my own hands." It was from these musings that the first two lines of the poem emerged.

29

୨୦

WE HAVE CHOICES

One year after Brittany Maynard's death, Dan Diaz and Compassion & Choices (C&C) released another videotape containing unused segments from the original film, along with comments by Barbara Coombs Lee.[1]

In it, Barbara said: "Brittany's video appeared on People. com first thing in the morning on October 6, 2014. By that afternoon, it broke all the records. Over 400,000 people came to Brittany's website and took action. By the time she died, a little over three weeks later, over one hundred million people worldwide knew her and knew her cause."[2]

Brittany's thirtieth birthday would have been on November 19, 2014.

According to Lee: "Brittany came on the scene and set in motion a chain of events that passed an aid-in-dying bill through the California legislature less than one year after her death. We had been [repeatedly and unsuccessfully] trying to do that since 1991."

That "chain of events" had plenty of kinks, however, including considerable uncertainty about whether California's bill would ever actually be enacted. It had originally stalled in the

Assembly Health Care Committee.[3] Nonetheless, in mid-August 2015, the End of Life Option Act was resurrected by Assembly-woman Susan Eggman, a former hospice social worker.[4]

Even after its passage, many remained unsure whether Governor Jerry Brown, a former Jesuit seminary student, would sign the bill.[5] Brown himself had survived multiple brushes with cancer, and he experienced the deaths of a number of family members. The governor sought input from doctors, a Catholic bishop, and several advocates for the disabled. He considered the views of retired South African archbishop Desmond Tutu, who had spoken up in favor of assisted dying during the contentious debate in the House of Lords. Tutu had more recently declared, "I believe in the sanctity of life, and that death is part of life."[6] Brittany and Governor Brown talked by phone three days before her death, and he would later speak with her husband and her mother.

"In the end," Brown said, "I was left to reflect on what I would want in the face of my own death. I do not know what I would do if I were dying in prolonged and excruciating pain. I am certain, however, that it would be a comfort to be able to consider the options afforded by this bill. And I wouldn't deny that right to others."[7]

And, with that, Governor Jerry Brown signed the End of Life Options Act into law on October 15, 2015. While in 2018 a court challenge temporarily halted its implementation, further judicial decisions reinstated it later that year.

Among the first Californians to take advantage of the new law was Betsy Davis, a forty-one-year-old artist suffering from Lou Gehrig's Disease.[8] Like Brittany, she summoned her friends and family for a final goodbye celebration. In the invitation that she slowly typed on her iPad, Davis complimented her guests. She wrote: "These circumstances are unlike any party you have attended before, requiring emotional stamina, centeredness, and openness."

There was only one rule: "Do not cry in front of me," Davis requested.

Davis's sister explained, "She turned death into a reason to celebrate, and she was there to enjoy the party."

I think that Brittany, Cody, and the people who preceded them and fought for this legal option would have been pleased. California is the most populous state in the United States, with a population larger than that of Canada. Overnight with the passage of California's act, the number of Americans living in states where medical aid in dying was legal nearly quadrupled—from thirteen million to more than fifty million. In 2014, before Brittany became known to the public, aid-in-dying bills were pending in just four states. In succeeding years, however, similar laws were to be enacted in Colorado, the District of Columbia, and Hawaii and, according to a 2018 report from the Death with Dignity National Center, aid-in-dying bills were considered in *half* of the nation's state legislatures.[9] In addition, the most recent Gallup poll found that 72 percent of Americans believed doctors should be able to help terminally ill patients die, and 65 percent supported that view even when the poll question included the more emotionally charged words, "commit suicide."[10]

I was greatly saddened to read Paul Spiers's obituary in the *Boston Globe*. It began: "On September 11, 2013, Dr. Paul Spiers passed peacefully in his sleep, now free to soar above the wheels that grounded his brilliant and unencumbered mind."[11]

His sister, Blue, told me that like many paraplegic men, he eventually developed a skin ulcer and infection. This led to multiple surgical procedures and months of hospitalizations before he died in his sleep—presumably from heart failure.

When he was thrown from his horse, Paul's body was irreparably changed, but he relished the unexpected opportunities that followed the accident. In a moving tribute following his death, Peg Sandeen, executive director of the Death with Dignity National Center, wrote:

> Paul spoke clearly and without reservation in support of Death with Dignity laws. He was deeply instrumental in [the November 2012] Massachusetts ballot initiative campaign which introduced the idea of Death with Dignity to Bay Staters and elevated the discussion about end-of-life care options throughout New England. Eager to help

the effort any way he could, Paul was one of the original petitioners to bring the initiative before the voters, and he didn't stop there. Throughout the lead-up to election day, Paul participated in public debates and spoke prominently at events throughout the state.[12]

Peg politely refrained from mentioning Paul's often unruly sense of humor and habit of proudly referring to himself as "the Movement's crip." He was a quirky, lifelong Grateful Dead fan, who undeniably brought a unique zest to all his relationships. *Hercules*, the Disney movie, was one of his and Blue's favorite childhood cartoons, and I think in some ways he modeled himself into an amalgam of its hero and the joke-cracking sidekick.

I'm sorry that he didn't live to read the words of Presidential Medal of Freedom winner, Stephen Hawking, who noted after the death of Brittany Maynard that, "If you have a terminal illness, and are in great pain, I think you should have the right to end your life. . . . It is discrimination against the disabled to deny them the right . . . that able-bodied people have."[13] The celebrated physicist died in 2018 after fifty-five years enduring a variant of Amyotrophic Lateral Sclerosis (ALS).

Paul would have enjoyed a piece by Sara Myers and Dustin Hankinson, who wrote: "As two individuals who also live with significant physical disabilities, ALS and Duchenne muscular dystrophy, we could not agree with [Stephen Hawking] more. . . . Recent state polls show a strong majority of voters living with disabilities support death with dignity in Connecticut (65 percent), Massachusetts (74 percent) and New Jersey (63 percent), and support for the bill is nearly identical for all voters in these three states. Like others, we want the freedom to enjoy life. This freedom should include the full range of options at the end of life, including hospice, palliative care and aid in dying."[14]

Like me, Paul would have been struck by the official announcement prior to Barbara Bush's death, in which a spokesman notified the media: "Following a recent series of hospitalizations, and after consulting her family and doctors, Mrs. Bush, now age 92, has decided not to seek additional medical treatment and will instead focus on comfort care."[15] It is a testament to our society's evolving position on end-of-life matters that this wife of a president and mother of another president could choose to forestall efforts that might have prolonged her life.[16] I am confident that if her death had taken place a decade or so ago, the public would have read only about her "valiant battle" to stay alive.

Later that same year, Senator John McCain issued a similar statement about discontinuing further efforts at curative therapy.[17] In the not-to-distant past, his diagnosis of a glioblastoma might have possibly been concealed, and at the end we would have only heard about his "brave fight" and other combat metaphors reflecting a steadfast desire to stay alive at any cost. The media certainly would have not reported that McCain, a genuine war hero, decided to convene a weekly Friday meeting with staff, family, and close friends to work through the details of his services of remembrance. Rather than becoming overwhelmed by the imminence of death, the senator took time to identify the themes he wished to be covered in the funeral orations. He selected and extended personal invitations to speakers (Presidents Bush and Obama, Senators Lieberman and Biden, etc.), and made explicit who would *not* be invited (Governor Sarah Palin and President Trump).[18] The resulting five-day event demonstrated how a public icon can accept and stage-manage his own death.

Paul would have been ecstatic in December of 2017 when the Massachusetts Medical Society conducted an internal poll and found that its doctors had shifted in their opinion about assisted dying. According to the *Boston Globe*, 60 percent of the physician respondents supported the notion of prescribing a lethal dose of medication to patients with terminal illnesses who were seeking to die.[19] In response, the medical society broke with its traditional opposition and shifted to a neutral stance. This was a major victory for advocates from the Bay State, because both Colorado and California went on to approve similar bills only after their medical societies similarly adopted neutral positions. In doing so, Massachusetts became the tenth American Medical Association chapter to allow its physicians to follow a course that comports with their consciences and to not be bound by an oath from the fifth century BC that most doctors no longer even intone upon graduating. These developments have prompted the American Medical Association to begin the laborious process of reconsidering its Code of Medical Ethics.[20] Quite unexpectedly, in 2018, the AMA House of Delegates rejected the Council on Ethical and Judicial Affairs recommendation to remain opposed, and by a margin of 56 to 44 percent voted instead that they continue studying this issue. I am cautiously hopeful about the future, although this is an exceedingly conservative organization.[21]

In the last few years, six Massachusetts municipalities, including my small but progressive city of Northampton, approved nonbinding resolutions asking the state to pass an act affirming "a terminally ill patient's right to compassionate aid in dying."[22] I can only imagine that if Paul had been present when the resolution was passed at the Northampton City Hall, he would have been zipping around the room in his wheelchair and enthusiastically giving "high-fives" to each of the assembled councilmembers.

30

LAST THOUGHTS

I would like to conclude by expressing some of my thoughts, observations, and opinions regarding this complex and thorny subject. These are certainly not offered as a recommendation to anyone, and they should not even be taken as being my final word concerning life-limiting decisions. During the years that I've been considering the subject, my thinking has evolved about several of the issues. I'm confident that this process will continue.

Today's death-with-dignity activists largely accept that at least in the short term all North American protocols continue to be limited to people who are imminently dying. While this accommodates to current political realities, I hope the criteria will soon change, for two reasons. First, I am not nearly as frightened of dying from an aggressive cancer as of being tortured by the relentless symptoms accompanying a neurodegenerative condition, such as a progressive dementia. Second, there are numerous people with cancer and other conditions who suffer from constant pain that is only relieved with the help of opiate medications, but either the medication or further involvement of brain disease "robs them of the capacity for consent before they realize what's happened."[1] In both instances, current laws effectively bar these individuals from receiving aid in dying or compel them to hasten death earlier than they might prefer.[2]

When I began this writing project, I hadn't realized the extent of my fear concerning the neurodegenerative disorders, until it was brought to the surface by Beth Weinstein's narrative and the challenges presented by Alzheimer's disease. In addition, only after I spoke with Gillian Bennett's daughter did I come to appreciate the unnecessary cruelty of forcing people to hurriedly hasten their deaths out of concern that they would lose capacity.

Gary Rodin, a psychiatrist and palliative medicine physician at Toronto's University Health Network, has cautiously spoken up in favor of broadening the legislation around advance requests.[3] "I think we should be able to legalize substitute decision-making," he said, explaining that there is a growing consensus in the Canadian medical community that the law should be amended. "As we've developed frameworks which have a lot of safeguards in them, I think we've seen that this protective clause has had an unintended effect of depriving some people of their rights."

Rodin is part of a quiet but concerted push to bring the right-to-die debates to a new frontier, and this includes similar efforts in Quebec and in the state of Oregon. Despite pushback from within the American movement, involving such admirable groups as C&C and the Death with Dignity National Center, Rep. Mitch Greenlick (D), chair of Oregon's House Committee on Health Care, intends to expand that state's act to dementia patients by stripping from it all stipulations about terminal time limits.[4]

Like Greenlick and Rodin, I don't want people who are suffering from neurodegenerative diseases like Parkinson's or Alzheimer's to be automatically excluded from aid in dying. I think there are workarounds for individuals who are fearful of cognitive impairments that could involve the use of health care proxies and carefully written advance directives, perhaps supplemented with online videotaped apps. Twenty-four years later, Oregon's original criteria seems to me to be unduly restrictive.

A Canadian editorial states: "Maybe it's time to take a small, second step. At the very least, the law should allow for earlier consent. People facing the end of their lives should not have to give up any more time than necessary."[5]

Derek Humphry, the Tolkien wizard of the right-to-die movement, has recently stated, "It's time to update and improve [the American laws], chiefly to give adults with serious degenerative illness the chance to qualify for relief. And to strengthen the Advance Directives (Living Wills as they were known). Let's be progressive, not stuck in the past."[6]

My personal hope is that this book will serve to encourage us to talk further about broadening inclusion measures and cautiously liberalizing future laws. Medical aid in dying should be linked to irremediable suffering and not solely to the imminence of death. It should be available to those individuals who have had a consistent and unwavering desire for it. People should have the right to insist on controlling the end of their lives when life as they know it—when the identity that they have proudly forged—has already ceased to exist.

Paradoxically, when I began this project, I also had no idea as to the extent that those who self-identify as having disabilities—including men and women who suffered traumas and accommodated to radically changed identities—would influence my thinking. I want to recognize the concerns of disability activists, while appreciating that there is a chasm separating the able-bodied and relatively healthy from those who are not. I can at least attempt to imagine what it is like to be dependent on a delicate structure of social supports or clunky mechanical devices, such as a wheelchair, and I can try to grasp the concept that what legislators provide they can also remove. Preserving and improving the Americans with Disability Act and having access to comprehensive health care are obvious priorities for disability activists, and assisted dying is only a tertiary issue for most of them. However, I can observe the rise of nationalism, white supremacy, anti-Semitism, and anti-immigration sentiments and believe that terrible things are possible. Similarly, I can understand how some disability activists fear that aid-in-dying legislation is only the first step toward the resurrection of a modern version of eugenics. But my alarm over all of these matters is lessened by the conviction that we are a nation of well-meaning citizens whose basic principles are good, generous, and solid.

I have also come to more fully realize that although we are individuals—and each of us has our own terminal care preferences—we are also social animals embedded in families and groups with responsibilities toward others. I believe that our autonomous individual wishes should be accorded priority; however, we must also attend to the repercussions of our decisions upon loved ones and community. Ideally, but not always, we can achieve consensus within families through ongoing, frank, and honest communication. If we arrive at a decision to accelerate dying, then this must require as detailed a plan as is possible. If there is no consensus, then the family group needs to make more of an effort to hear what the person is going through and to better grasp why they want to get off the train. We may yet choose *not* to assist them, even if we respect and love them. But if we persist in obstructing their persistent wishes, then I suspect that in most cases this represents a failure of empathy on our part.

I have been a palliative medicine practitioner and researcher for decades, which is why I appreciate the subspecialty's enormous strengths as well as its limitations. Promoters sometimes airbrush the truth. Spokespersons for palliative medicine may be blindly optimistic. They proclaim that there's always something to be done—which is true—although it may not make a desired difference. Pain and most other forms of suffering can be ameliorated, but the use of analgesics may result in intolerable impairment of cognition. Furthermore, treatments that result in institutionalization or confinement to bed may be similarly unacceptable. Most people who opt for assisted dying in the United States have been receiving excellent palliative care. However, it doesn't always satisfactorily manage their suffering. Sometimes, we just can't cure the underlying disease, and sometimes we can't fix the symptoms. And sometimes, people simply run out of patience coping with illness. I think it is incumbent upon us to hear and accept an individual's determination that they've had enough.

Despite my wish to alter the criteria regarding the imminence of death and patient capacity for assisted dying, I feel that we should persist in hesitating when people have primary psychiatric disorders. This is, admittedly, a bias based on having spent my clinical career conducting literally thousands of psychiatric consultations related to the aftermath of suicide attempts and suicidal ideation. Put simply, I do *not* hold that people with major psychiatric disorders or those who have a history of making suicide attempts when physically healthy should qualify for aid in dying. I understand that a person who has a severe psychological condition such as schizophrenia or recurrent bipolar affective disorder may be resistant to available psychosocial and pharmacological treatments and may spend many decades suffering. In the future, I may change my opinion and come to accept their right to access end-of-life protocols; however, I don't feel that way presently.

My current belief is predicated on repeated experiences with individuals whose underlying psychiatric disorders eventually did respond or whose concomitant suicidal thoughts proved to be transitory. I have also seen far too many people with personality and character disorders talk about wanting to die but behave in a way more consistent with a powerful need to express rage through injuring themselves and secondarily frustrating and hurting others who care about them. They may have extensively made use of the word "suicide," but they were not primarily motivated to die. I agree with Derek Humphry that offering assistance in dying to such individuals is a mistake that will inevitably lead to regret.

In this book, I have not hidden where my sympathies lie. I can't help but admire those who demand to take control at a moment when people are usually most helpless and dependent on others. I have the utmost admiration for those who can summon their remaining energy to assemble friends and family and celebrate life immediately before dying. Their honesty and clarity are inspiring. I am simply in awe of the loved ones who help them, and this encompasses the right-to-die activists who take part in the achievement of final requests.

I did not have an opportunity to meet Brittany Maynard or Cody Curtis, other than through their online postings and videotaped interviews. The two women left a trove of recordings that reveal their common resilience, delicate beauty, wry sense of humor, and fierce determination. I am convinced they are moral exemplars, defined in the book *Some Do Care* as being individuals who display "widely shared ideas of what it means to be a highly moral person."[7] The authors clarified that they were not referring to saints who led unblemished lives, but rather "dedicated persons who, through their sustained commitment and talents, labor to make the world a better place." I am impressed that these two women knew with enviable certainty just how they wanted to spend their remaining time—promoting the death-with-dignity movement. I greatly admire their heroism, although both would have vigorously denied that they were especially courageous. As best as I can surmise, their actual fears of dying were largely set aside because each was consumed with a conviction that people ought to be able to speak up and have their individualized terminal care preferences honored. Although both women were by nature exceedingly private, they nevertheless chose to reveal their stories to the public. And I find that absolutely amazing!

Then there is the question of "What would I, Lew Cohen, do tomorrow if I decided it was my time for assisted dying?"

Presuming that I sought out and received the best available medical care and yet continued to either suffer or to face a dismal prognosis, my first thought would be to hold a series of meetings with my family. Wife, sons, nieces, nephews, and the other members of the clan are all aware of my basic stance on issues of aid in dying, but a specific situation mandates precise consideration and conversation. A careful discussion with an attorney and a review of financial matters would also be on my to-do list.

Several years ago, I raised this subject with my primary care physician and, although couched abstractly, I still recall feeling exquisitely uncomfortable. At the time, I realized that unlike

Sigmund Freud and Max Schur, I didn't have a clue as to his personal beliefs. Was he an observant Catholic, political conservative, or a fervent supporter of the sanctity of life? Our patient-doctor relationship had previously left no room to enlighten myself on such topics. I experienced considerable relief when he said that he would be responsive to requests to hasten my death. But since we both live in Massachusetts, which still doesn't condone aid-in-dying practices, I am not sure that I can fully trust his assurance. Faced with an actual situation and accompanied by my wife, I would want to meet with him again and determine his position when the question is no longer theoretical.

I would also not hesitate to take advantage of my own medical license—or that of friends (I'm thinking of you, Mike and Rich)—to acquire the latest recommended lethal cocktail. However, I would prefer to see empirical evidence, and not just anecdotes, concerning its efficacy, rapidity, and absence of side effects—and these are exceedingly difficult to attain. More research needs to be performed.

Otherwise, this leaves me with helium (almost impossible to obtain in sufficiently pure form) and nitrogen (a bit more clunky to acquire and use). I am grateful that Derek continues to sponsor NuTech's efforts to discover easier and more efficacious techniques.

I would consider three additional possibilities. The first would be to follow in Brittany's footsteps and take up residency— presuming I had the time and resources—in a state that has a legal protocol. These locales are not especially interested in attracting "suicide tourists," but this can hopefully be sorted out, as residency does not appear to be an insurmountable barrier.

Residence is a legally amorphous concept. Vermont, which is just up the road from me, does not specify how residency may be established, while any one of the following suffice for the state of California: possession of a driver's license or other identification issued by the state, registration to vote, evidence that the person owns or leases property—even a self-storage locker—or filing of a California tax return for the most recent tax year.

An alternative possibility is to seek membership in the Final Exit Network and then appeal for help from its plucky volunteers. I am still amazed at the combination of personality characteristics that allow someone to undergo the training and then travel to a stranger's home to provide the necessary information and emotional support for a facilitated death. I'm glad that the organization continues to function despite its legal travails; Larry Egbert, its former medical director, was one of the most remarkable human beings I have ever encountered.

The last possibility involves flying to Switzerland and seeking out the resources of Dignitas or a similar organization, such as the Eternal SPIRIT Foundation.[8] Medical aid in dying has been tolerated in Switzerland since 1942, provided that the person assisting has no selfish motive. One must self-administer the lethal drug and retain decision-making capacity. On average, the amount of time required between the first contact with Dignitas or any of the other Swiss sources of assisted dying is roughly three to six months. It is *not* a simple option for Americans, but one that many Europeans rely upon.

My personal goal has been well described by Faye Girsh: a peaceful, gentle, quick, and certain death. When it happens, I would like to be with my loved ones and have Mozart's Requiem Mass in D minor (K. 626), the ultimate death-inspired piece of music, playing in the background (contact me if you're interested in discussing other suitable music!).

One final thought? Death has been described as part of the connective tissue that binds mankind across time and culture and place. Humans engage in rites, explanatory narratives, mythological stories, and acts of transcendence that offer the promise of fortitude and consolation when we cross the bridge to our deaths. My sincerest hope is that we will persist in trying to help each other with dignity, respect, and compassion on all the stages of this journey.

NOTES

Part I

1. Ovid, *The Metamorphoses*, trans. A. S. Kline (Poetry in Translation, 2000), IX:159–210, https://www.poetryintranslation.com/PITBR/Latin/Metamorph9.php.

2. Sophocles, *Women of Trachis*, trans. George Theodoridis (Houghton Mifflin, 1966), https://www.poetryintranslation.com/theodoridisg womenoftrachis.php.

3. Aroop Mangalik, *Dealing with Doctors, Denial, and Death: A Guide to Living Well with Serious Illness* (London: Rowman & Littlefield, 2017).

4. Herman Feifer, *The Meaning of Death* (New York: Blakiston Division, McGraw-Hill, 1959), xiii.

5. Pamela Druckerman, "To Live and Die in Paris," *New York Times*, August 19, 2018, p. 9.

6. Sarah Lyall, "The Last Thing Mom Asked," *New York Times*, August 31, 2018, last accessed September 2, 2018, https://www.nytimes .com/2018/08/31/sunday-review/mother-death-euthanasia.html.

7. Andrew Solomon, "A Death of One's Own," *Andrew Solomon* (Blog), May 22, 1995, accessed September 1, 2018, http://andrewsolomon .com/articles/a-death-of-ones-own/.

Chapter 1

1. Lewis M. Cohen, "Deaths with Dignity," *Slate*, June 6, 2013, accessed September 1, 2018, https://slate.com/technology/2013/06/

death-with-dignity-joint-suicide-of-rear-adm-chester-nimitz-jr-and-joan-nimitz.html.

2. Sara Rimer, "With Suicide, an Admiral Keeps Command until the End," *New York Times*, January 12, 2002, accessed September 1, 2018, https://www.nytimes.com/2002/01/12/us/with-suicide-an-admiral-keeps-command-until-the-end.html.

3. Ibid.

4. "Chester Nimitz Jr.," *Wikipedia*, last modified August 31, 2018, accessed September 1, 2018, https://en.wikipedia.org/wiki/Chester_Nimitz_Jr.

5. Brayton Harris, *Admiral Nimitz: The Commander of the Pacific Ocean Theater* (New York: St. Martin's Press, 2012); Walter R. Borneman, *The Admirals: Nimitz, Halsey, Leahy, and King—the Five-Star Admirals Who Won the War at Sea* (New York: Little, Brown and Co., 2012).

6. Philip Delves Broughton, "Family Backs Suicide Pact of Admiral and His Wife," *Telegraph*, January 14, 2002, accessed September 1, 2018, https://www.telegraph.co.uk/news/worldnews/northamerica/usa/1381463/Family-backs-suicide-pact-of-admiral-and-his-wife.html.

Chapter 2

1. Atif Kukaswadia, "History of Epidemiology: Jonas Salk and the Eradication of Polio," *Public Health Perspectives*, June 4, 2013, accessed September 2, 2018, https://blogs.plos.org/publichealth/2013/06/04/history-of-epidemiology-jonas-salk-and-the-eradication-of-polio/.

2. Margalit Fox, "Adrienne Asch, Bioethicist and Pioneer in Disability Studies, Dies at 67," *New York Times*, November 23, 2013, accessed September 2, 2018, https://www.nytimes.com/2013/11/23/nyregion/adrienne-asch-bioethicist-and-pioneer-in-disability-studies-dies-at-67.html.

3. Lewis Mitchel Cohen, *No Good Deed: A Story of Medicine, Murder Accusations, and the Debate over How We Die* (New York: Harper Collins, 2010).

4. Jan A. Witkowski, *The Road to Discovery: A Short History of Cold Spring Harbor Laboratory* (Woodbury, NY: Cold Spring Harbor Laboratory Press, 2015).

5. Cohen, *No Good Deed*, 9.

6. Ibid., 10.

7. Stephen M. Silverman, "President Bush Responds to Schiavo Death," *People*, March 31, 2005, accessed September 2, 2018, https://people.com/celebrity/president-bush-responds-to-schiavo-death/.

8. Andrew Solomon, "A Death of One's Own" *Andrew Solomon* (Blog), September 1, 2018, http://andrewsolomon.com/articles/a-death-of-ones-own/.

Chapter 3

1. Diane Rehm, *On My Own* (New York: Alfred A. Knopf, Inc., 2016), 7.

2. Lindsey Bever, "The Apparent Murder-Suicide of a Death-with-Dignity Advocate and His Ailing Wife," *Washington Post*, April 22, 2016, accessed September 2, 2018, https://www.washingtonpost.com/news/morning-mix/wp/2016/04/22/its-horrific-the-apparent-murder-suicide-of-a-right-to-die-advocate-and-his-ailing-wife/?noredirect=on&utm_term=.c4a22ce06aee.

3. Wesley Robinson, "Husband Gets House Arrest for Aiding Wife's Suicide by Putting Pills in Her Pudding," *Penn Live*, November 14, 2017, accessed September 2, 2018, https://www.pennlive.com/news/2017/11/husband_gets_house_arrest_for.html.

4. Tom Knapp, "'Fair and Appropriate': Manor Twp. Man Will Serve up to 23 Months in House Arrest for Aiding Wife's Suicide," *Lancaster Online*, November 13, 2017, accessed September 2, 2018, https://lancasteronline.com/news/local/fair-and-appropriate-manor-twp-man-will-serve-up-to/article_ae782910-c8a7-11e7-b863-07a7c5a114da.html.

5. Tom Knapp, "Manor Twp. Woman at Heart of Assisted Suicide Case Dies; Funds Raised for Husband," *Lancaster Online*, January 30, 2017, accessed September 2, 2018, https://lancasteronline.com/news/local/manor-twp-woman-at-heart-of-assisted-suicide-case-dies/article_2644509c-e72e-11e6-8da5-571bf27a5c2e.html.

6. Ibid.

7. "62-Year-Old Marine Veteran Shoots, Kills Wife with Dementia," *USMC Life*, April 1, 2017, accessed September 2, 2018, http://www.usmclife.com/2017/04/62-year-old-marine-veteran-shoots-kills-wife-dementia/.

8. Christine Pelisek, "Florida Murder Suspect Claims Wife Asked Him to Kill Her—to Spare Her from Dementia," *People*, March 29, 2017, accessed September 2, 2018, https://people.com/crime/florida-man-murder-wife-save-her-dementia/.

9. Gary Stein, "Florida Must Allow Death with Dignity: Opinion," *(South Florida) SunSentinel*, March 29, 2017, accessed September 2, 2018, http://www.sun-sentinel.com/opinion/todays-buzz/sfl-florida-must-allow-death-with-dignity-opinion-20170329-story.html.

10. Ibid.

11. Linda Marx," The Agony Did Not End for Roswell Gilbert, Who Killed His Wife to Give Her Peace," *People*, January 12, 1987, http://people.com/archive/the-agony-did-not-end-for-roswell-gilbert-who-killed-his-wife-to-give-her-peace-vol-27-no-2/.

12. Ibid.

13. Ibid.

14. The Associated Press, "Roswell Gilbert, 85, Who Killed His Ill Wife and Went to Prison," *New York Times*, September 8, 1994, accessed September 3, 2018, http://www.nytimes.com/1994/09/08/obituaries/roswell-gilbert-85-who-killed-his-ill-wife-and-went-to-prison.html.

15. Barbara Walsh, "Loneliness, Age Imprison Freed Roswell Gilbert," *(South Florida) SunSentinel*, August 4, 1991, accessed September 3, 2018, http://articles.sun-sentinel.com/1991-08-04/news/9101290438_1_sea-ranch-lakes-roswell-gilbert-gilbert-s.

16. Ibid.

17. Mary C. Williams. "Roswell Gilbert Dies at 85, *(South Florida) SunSentinel*, September 7, 1994, accessed January 4, 2018, http://articles.sun-sentinel.com/1994-09-07/news/9409070117_1_gilbert-s-clemency-sea-ranch-lakes-roswell-gilbert.

18. Ibid.

Chapter 4

1. Sigmund Freud, *The Interpretation of Dreams: The Complete and Definitive Text*, trans. James Strachey (New York: Basic Books, 2010).

2. Max Schur, *Freud: Living and Dying* (New York: International Universities Press, 1972).

3. Jack D. McCue and Lewis Mitchel Cohen, "Freud's Physician-Assisted Death," *Archives of Internal Medicine* 159 (1999): 1521–25.

4. Lewis Cohen, "How Sigmund Freud Wanted to Die," *Atlantic*, September 23, 2014, accessed Sept 3, 2018, https://www.theatlantic.com/health/archive/2014/09/how-sigmund-freud-wanted-to-die/380322/.

5. Ibid.

6. Felix Deutsch, "Reflections on Freud's One Hundredth Birthday," *Psychosomatic Medicine* 8, (1965): 279–83.

7. Ibid.

8. Ernest Jones, *The Life and Work of Sigmund Freud, Volume 3, The Last Phase 1919–1939* (New York: Basic Books, Inc, 1957), 90–96.

9. "Hippocratic Oath," *Wikipedia*, last modified August 22, 2018, accessed September 4, 2018, https://en.wikipedia.org/wiki/Hippocratic_Oath.

10. Helene Deutsch, *Confrontations with Myself: An Epilogue* (New York: W.W. Norton & Company, 1973).

11. Deutsch, "Reflections on Freud's One Hundredth Birthday."

12. Ronald Williams Clark, *Freud, the Man and the Cause* (New York: Random House, 1980), 439.

13. Joseph Popper-Lynkeus, *Das Recht zu leben und Die Pflicht zu sterben—Sozialphilosophische Betrachtungen anknüpfend an die Bedeutung Voltaires für die neuere Zeit*. Vienna, Leipzig: R. Löwit Verlag, 1924.

14. Peter Gay, *Freud: A Life for Our Time* (London: W.W. Norton & Company, 2006), 410–20.

15. Deutsch, "Reflections on Freud's One Hundredth Birthday"; R. W. Clark, *Freud: The Man and the Cause* (New York, Random House, 1980), 439.

16. Schur, *Freud: Living and Dying*, 412, 450.

17. Scott Wilson, "Dying for a Smoke: Freudian Addiction and the Joy of Consumption," *Angelaki* 7, no. 2 (2010): 161–73, doi: 10.1080/0969725022000046242; Deutsch, "Reflections on Freud's One Hundredth Birthday."

18. Robert A. Caro, "The Transition: Lyndon Johnson and the Events in Dallas," *New Yorker*, April 2, 2012, https://www.newyorker.com/magazine/2012/04/02/the-transition.

19. Elisabeth Kübler Ross, *On Death and Dying* (New York: Simon and Schuster, 1969).

20. Peter Tyson, "The Hippocratic Oath Today," *NOVA*, March 27, 2001, https://www.pbs.org/wgbh/nova/body/hippocratic-oath-today.html.

21. Ibid.

22. Ramin Walter Parsa-Parsi, "The Revised Declaration of Geneva: A Modern-Day Physician's Pledge," *Journal of the American Medical Association* 318, no. 20 (2017): 1971–72.

23. P. C. Hebert, B. Hoffmaster, K. C. Glass, and P. A. Singer, "Bioethics for Clinicians: 7. Truth Telling," *Canadian Medical Association Journal* 156 (1997): 225–28.

Chapter 5

1. "Chester Nimitz Jr., Navy Admiral, 86," *New York Times*, January 8, 2002, accessed October 28, 2012, http://www.nytimes.com/2002/01/08/us/chester-nimitz-jr-navy-admiral-86.html; Sara Rimer, "With Suicide, an Admiral Keeps Command until the End," *New York Times*, January 12, 2002, accessed September 1, 2018, https://www.nytimes.com/2002/01/12/us/with-suicide-an-admiral-keeps-command-until-the-end.html.

2. Meera Balasubramaniam, "Rational Suicide in Elderly Adults: A Clinician's Perspective," *Journal of the American Geriatrics Society*, March 2, 2018, https://doi.org/10.1111/jgs.15263; Liz Dzeng and Steve Pantilat, "Social Causes of Rational Suicide in Older Adults," *Journal of the American Geriatrics Society*, March 2, 2018, https://doi.org/10.1111/jgs.15290.

3. Rimer, "With Suicide."

4. Paul Span, "In Elderly Hands, Firearms Can Be Even Deadlier." *New York Times*, May 29, 2018, D5.

5. Patrick J. Buchanan, "The Sad Suicide of Admiral Nimitz," January 18, 2002, accessed October 28, 2012, http://www.wnd.com/2002/01/12433/.

6. Ibid.

7. Ibid.

8. W. Carol Cleigh, "Bigotry in the BDTD (Better Dead Than Disabled) Movement," Not Dead Yet, December 28, 2017, accessed April 5, 2018, http://notdeadyet.org/tag/nonvoluntary-euthanasia.

9. A. D. Weisman, and T. P. Hackett, "Predilection to Death: Death and Dying as a Psychiatric Problem," *Psychosomatic Medicine* 23 (1961): 232–56.

10. Ibid.; N. H. Cassem, "The Dying Patient," in *Massachusetts General Hospital: Handbook of General Hospital Psychiatry*, ed. T. P. Hackett and N. H. Cassem (St. Louis: C.V. Mosby Company, 1978), 390–98.

11. Lexi Salazar, "Daughter: Parents' Suicide Highlights a Need for Assisted Suicide," *Cape Cod Times*, October 19, 2012.

12. Atul Gawande, *Being Mortal: Medicine and What Matters in the End* (New York: Metropolitan Books/Henry Holt & Company, 2014).

Chapter 7

1. "Beth Weinstein," *Hartford Courant* (Hartford, CT), February 3, 2012, accessed January 5, 2018, https://www.legacy.com/obituaries/hartfordcourant/obituary.aspx?page=lifestory&pid=155751056.

2. Thomas L. Friedman, "Call Your Mother," *The New York Times* (New York, NY), May 11, 2008, accessed June 5, 2018, https://www.nytimes.com/2008/05/11/opinion/11friedman.html.

3. Jane Gross, "At AIDS Epicenter, Seeking Swift, Sure Death," *New York Times*, June 20, 1993, http://www.nytimes.com/1993/06/20/us/at-aids-epicenter-seeking-swift-sure-death.html.

4. Ibid.

5. Ibid.

6. Ibid.

7. Sarah Varney, "A Racial Gap in Attitudes toward Hospice Care," *New York Times*, August 21, 2015, accessed June 15, 2018, https://www.nytimes.com/2015/08/25/health/a-racial-gap-in-attitudes-toward-hospice-care.html.

8. Ibid.

9. Ibid.

10. Liz Kowalczyk, "Color Line Persists, in Sickness as in Health," *Boston Globe*, December 12, 2017, accessed June 5, 2018, https:apps.bostonglobe.com/spotlight/boston-racism-image-reality/series/hospitals/.

11. Junaid Nabi, "'No One Was Listening to Us.' Lessons from the Jahi McMath Case," *The Hastings Center*, April 4, 2018, https://www.thehastingscenter.org/no-one-listening-us-lessons-jahi-mcmath-case/.

12. "Pneumocystis Pneumonia—Los Angeles," *Morbidity and Mortality Weekly Report* 30, no. 21 (June 5, 1981): 250–52, http://www.jstor.org/stable/23295554.

13. Lisa Genova, *Still Alice* (Bloomington, IN: iUniverse, 2007).

14. Gillian Bennett, "Goodbye & Good Luck!," *Dead at Noon*, August 18, 2014, last accessed January 6, 2018, http://deadatnoon.com/index.html.

15. Denise Ryan, "Dead at Noon: B.C. Woman Ends Her Life Rather Than Suffer Indignity of Dementia (with video)," *Vancouver Sun*, January 14, 2015, http://www.vancouversun.com/health/Dead+noon+woman+ends+life+rather+than+suffer+indignity+dementia+with+video/10132068/story.html.

16. Ibid.

17. Paul T. Menzel and Bonnie Steinbock, "Advance Directives, Dementia, and Physician-Assisted Death," *Journal of Law, Medicine & Ethics* 4, no. 2 (June 6, 2013): 484–500, http://onlinelibrary.wiley.com/doi/10.1111/jlme.12057/abstract.

18. Ryan, "Dead at Noon."

19. "Ontario Man with Dementia on Crusade to Plan His Own Death: Ron Posno Wants a Medically Assisted Death, but the Law Does Not Allow Advance Directives," CBC Radio, September 29, 2018, https://www.cbc.ca/radio/thesundayedition/the-sunday-edition-september-30-2018-1.4841264/ontario-man-with-dementia-on-crusade-to-plan-his-own-death-1.4841267.

20. Ibid.

21. Irene Tuffrey-Wijne, Leopold Curfs, Ilora Finlay, and Sheila Hollins, "Euthanasia and Assisted Suicide for People with an Intellectual Disability and/or Autism Spectrum Disorder: An Examination of Nine Relevant Euthanasia Cases in the Netherlands (2012–2016)," *BMC Medical Ethics* 19, no. 1 (March 5, 2018): 17, doi: 10.1186/s12910-018-0257-6.

22. Ministerie Van Volksgezondheid, "Code of Practice," *Regional Euthanasia Review Committees*, January 5, 2017, accessed April 14, 2018, https://english.euthanasiecommissie.nl/the-committees/code-of-practice.

23. Ibid.

24. Norman L. Cantor, "Bill of Health," *Harvard Law*, last accessed June 5, 2018, http://blogs.harvard.edu/billofhealth/2017/04/20/changing-the-paradigm-of-advance-directives/.

25. Mike Bassett, "Judicious Feeding Options at the End of Life," *Today's Geriatric Medicine*, last accessed April 2, 2018, http://www.todaysgeriatricmedicine.com/news/ex_020218.shtml.

26. Ibid.

27. JoNel Aleccia, "New 'Instructions' Could Let Dementia Patients Refuse Spoon-Feeding," *Kaiser Health News*, November 3, 2017, https://khn.org/news/new-instructions-could-let-dementia-patients -refuse-spoon-feeding/

28. Jane E. Brody, "Alzheimer's? Your Paperwork May Not Be in Order," *New York Times*, April 30, 2018, https://www.nytimes com/2018/04/30/well/live/an-advance-directive-for-patients-with -dementia.html.

29. "About the Advance Directive for Receiving Oral Food and Fluids in Dementia," accessed March 30, 2018, https://urldefense. proofpoint.com/v2/url?u=http-3A__files.constantcontact.com_ 6d73ca9c401_cf8128dc-2D8e90-2D46a9-2Db6c7-2D4f90ed611c4a .pdf-3Fver-3D1522287407000&d=DwICAg&c=BLF1codk7gr ETTA02F6JwR5DiXMTPyNdcZpbXT_1iEc&r=Y32Jdti78y5qGXYtr HBEB7WASefzL5gZfv7Q1V4dHlY&m=R7At1nzy7vn_yPp3v7zgy bKrswfThJ8Ym3UH5-VOZD4&s=cbfFkaxxc2cVlJKAjZiAJql7IrwTh ScxGqAwexsLf5k&e=.

30. Elisabetta Povoledo, "Italy to Allow Living Wills and the Refusal of End-of-Life Care," *New York Times*, December 14, 2017, accessed June 8, 2018, https://www.nytimes.com/2017/12/14/world/europe/italy -living-will-end-of-life-right-to-die-assisted-suicide.html.

31. "Institute on HealthCare Directives," LinkedIn, https://www .linkedin.com/company/institute-on-healthcare-directives/.

32. Maya Salam, "Consent in the Digital Age: Can Apps Solve a Very Human Problem?" *New York Times*, March 2, 2018, https://www .nytimes.com/2018/03/02/technology/consent-apps.html.

33. We-Consent App Suite by ISCE.edu, http://we-consent.org/.

34. "Get Explicit about Sexual Consent," LegalFling, https://legal fling.io/.

35. Salam, "Consent in the Digital Age."

36. Lewis Mitchel Cohen, *No Good Deed: A Story of Medicine, Murder Accusations, and the Debate Over How We Die* (New York: Harper Collins, 2010).

37. Paula Span, "A Debate over 'Rational Suicide,'" *New York Times*, August 31, 2018, accessed December 10, 2018, https://www.nytimes .com/2018/08/31/health/suicide-elderly.html.

Chapter 8

1. Ernest Jones, *The Life and Work of Sigmund Freud, 1919–1939, Volume 3, The Last Phase* (New-York: Basic Books, 1957), xii–xiii; Peter Gay, *Freud: A Life for Our Time* (London: Anchor Books, 1989).

2. Peter Schur, "The Freud-Schur Connection" (presentation, Vienna Psychoanalytic Association, Vienna, February 1994).

3. Ibid.

4. Stephen M. Wittenberg and Lewis M. Cohen, "Max Schur, M.D., 1897–1969: Images in Psychiatry," *American Journal of Psychiatry* 159, no. 2 (February 2002): 216, https://ajp.psychiatryonline.org/doi/pdf/10.1176/appi.ajp.159.2.216.

5. Peter Gay, *Freud: A Life for Our Time* (London: Anchor Books, 1989).

6. Max Schur, *Freud: Living and Dying* (London: International Universities Press, 1972).

7. Ibid., 408.

8. Ibid., 445.

9. Gay, *Freud: A Life for Our Time*.

10. Jack D. McCue and Lewis Mitchel Cohen, "Freud's Physician-Assisted Death," *Archives of Internal Medicine* 159 (1999): 1521–25.

11. Jones, *The Life and Work of Sigmund Freud*, 219–24.

12. Schur, *Freud: Living and Dying*, 495.

13. Jones, *The Life and Work of Sigmund Freud*.

14. Schur, *Freud: Living and Dying*, 498.

Chapter 9

1. "Aid in Dying: History and Background for Students, Activists and Professionals," Compassion and Choices, accessed January 9, 2018, https://www.compassionandchoices.org/wp-content/uploads/2016/02/Aid-in-Dying-History-and-Background.pdf.

2. "Patients' Rights to Self-Determination at the End of Life," American Public Health Association, October 8, 2008, accessed April 26, 2018, https://www.apha.org/policies-and-advocacy/public-health-policy-statements/policy-database/2014/07/29/13/28/patients-rights-to-self-determination-at-the-end-of-life; Peter Ubel, "A Debate on Death with Dignity," *Forbes*, September 11, 2013, accessed September 9, 2018, https://www.forbes.com/sites/peterubel/2013/09/11/a-debate-on-death-with-dignity/#2469e1866a0e.

3. American Association of Suicidology, "Statement of the American Association of Suicidology: "'Suicide' Is Not the Same as 'Physician Aid in Dying,'" news release, October 30, 2017, Suicidology, accessed April 26, 2018, http://www.suicidology.org/Portals/14/docs/Press Release/AAS PAD Statement Approved 10.30.17 ed 10-30-17.pdf; William Dwight and John Berkowitz, "A Different Perspective on 'Death with Dignity' Bill (Guest Viewpoint)," *Masslive*, December 1, 2017, http://www.masslive.com/opinion/index.ssf/2017/12/a_different_view_about_death_w.html.

4. Thomas Szasz, *Fatal Illness: The Ethics and Politics of Suicide* (Syracuse, NY: Syracuse University Press, 2002); Thomas Stephen Szasz, *Suicide Prohibition: The Shame of Medicine* (Syracuse, NY: Syracuse University Press, 2011), 10–12.

5. S. H. Wanzer, D. D. Federman, S. J. Adelstein, et al., "The Physician's Responsibility toward Hopelessly Ill Patients: A Second Look." *New England Journal of Medicine* 320 (1989): 844–49.

6. Szasz, *Suicide Prohibition*, 10–12.

7. David J. Garrow, "Letting the Public Decide about Assisted Suicide," *New York Times*, June 29, 1997, accessed June 5, 2018, https://www.nytimes.com/1997/06/29/weekinreview/letting-the-public-decide-about-assisted-suicide.html.

8. Ibid.

9. Laura A. Petrillo et al., "How California Prepared for Implementation of Physician-Assisted Death: A Primer," *American Journal of Public Health* 107, no. 6 (June 2017), doi:10.2105/ajph.2017.303755.

10. Neil M. Gorsuch, *The Future of Assisted Suicide and Euthanasia* (Princeton, NJ: Princeton University Press, 2009), 4–5.

11. Ibid., 153.

12. Derek Hawkins, "Neil Gorsuch Wrote the Book on Assisted Suicide. Here's What He Said," *Washington Post*, February 1, 2017, accessed July 14, 2018, https://www.washingtonpost.com/news/morning-mix/wp/2017/02/01/neil-gorsuch-wrote-the-book-on-assisted-suicide-heres-what-he-said/?utm_term=.cf7787eca948.

13. Desmond Tutu, "Archbishop Desmond Tutu: When My Time Comes, I Want the Option of an Assisted Death," *Washington Post*, October 6, 2016, accessed June 5, 2018, https://www.washingtonpost.com/opinions/global-opinions/archbishop-desmond-tutu-when-my-time-comes-i-want-the-option-of-an-assisted-death/2016/10/06/97c804f2-8a81-11e6-b24f-a7f89eb68887_story.html?utm_term=.e79b644c7a61.

14. Lewis M. Cohen, "Stephen Hawking and Desmond Tutu Just Endorsed Assisted Suicide," *Slate*, August 11, 2014, accessed May 23, 2018, http://www.slate.com/articles/health_and_science/medical_examiner/2014/08/assisted_suicide_debate_in_united_kingdom_house_of_lords_on_death_with_dignity.html.

15. Tutu, "Archbishop Desmond Tutu: When My Time Comes."

16. Ibid.

17. Frank Newport, "Public Historically Supports a Terminally Ill Patient's Right to Die," Gallup.com, October 30, 2003, accessed January 10, 2018, http://news.gallup.com/poll/9607/public-historically-supports-terminally-ill-patients-right-die.aspx.

18. Jade Wood and Justin McCarthy, "Majority of Americans Remain Supportive of Euthanasia," Gallup.com, June 12, 2017, accessed January 10, 2018, http://news.gallup.com/poll/211928/majority-americans-remain-supportive-euthanasia.aspx.

19. Ibid.

20. Dennis Thompson, "Most Americans Agree with Right-to-Die Movement," *Consumer HealthDay*, December 5, 2014, accessed January 10, 2018, https://consumer.healthday.com/mental-health-information-25/behavior-health-news-56/most-americans-agree-with-right-to-die-movement-694268.html.

21. Ibid.

22. Bill Briggs, "Most U.S. Doctors Now Support Aid in Dying: Survey," NBC News, December 16, 2014, accessed January 10, 2018, https://www.nbcnews.com/health/health-news/most-u-s-doctors-now-support-aid-dying-survey-n269691.

23. Ibid.

24. Celia Seupel Watson, "The Job to End All Others," *New York Times*, June 13, 2011, accessed March 3, 2018, https://newoldage.blogs.nytimes.com/2011/06/13/the-job-to-end-all-others/.

25. National Alliance for Caregiving, *Caregiving in the U.S. 2009* (Bethesda, MD: Author, 2009), https://www.caregiving.org/data/Caregiving_in_the_US_2009_full_report.pdf.

26. Susan Jacoby, "Real Life Among the Old Old," *New York Times*, December 30, 2010, accessed June 5, 2018, https://www.nytimes.com/2010/12/31/opinion/31jacoby.html.

27. Michael Wolff, "A Life Worth Ending," *New York*, May 20, 2012, accessed May 23, 2018, http://nymag.com/news/features/parent-health-care-2012-5/.

28. Paul Anka, "My Way," Metrolyrics, http://www.metrolyrics.com/my-way-lyrics-frank-sinatra.html.

29. "My Way," Wikipedia, September 14, 2018, https://en.wikipedia.org/wiki/My_Way#cite_note-24.

30. David Ward and Lucy Ward, "My Way Tops Funeral Charts," *Guardian*, November 17, 2005, https://www.theguardian.com/uk/2005/nov/17/arts.artsnews1.

Chapter 10

1. Ernest Jones, *The Life and Work of Sigmund Freud, 1919–1939, Volume 3, The Last Phase* (New York: Basic Books, 1957).

2. Ibid.

3. Anonymous, "How a Nazi Saved Sigmund Freud," *Jewish Chronicle*, January 8, 2010, accessed August 4, 2018, https://www.thejc.com/lifestyle/features/how-a-nazi-saved-sigmund-freud-1.13679.

4. Ibid.

5. Jones, *The Life and Work of Sigmund Freud. 1919-1939, Volume 3*, 240.

6. Ibid., 244.

7. Ibid., 245.

8. Max Schur, *Freud: Living and Dying* (London: International Universities Press, 1972).

9. Jones, *The Life and Work of Sigmund Freud, 1919-1939, Volume 3*, 95.

10. Ibid., 246; Schur, *Freud: Living and Dying*, 529.

11. Roy Lacoursiere, "Freud's Death: Historical Truth and Biographical Fictions," *American Imago* 65, no. 1 (2008): doi:10.1353/aim.0.0003.

12. Jones, *The Life and Work of Sigmund Freud, 1919-1939, Volume 3*, 246.

13. "Freud Family," Wikipedia, July 22, 2018, https://en.wikipedia.org/wiki/Freud_family; "Sigmund Freud and the Holocaust," Holocaust Research Project, accessed April 30, 2018, http://www.holocaustresearchproject.org/ghettos/freud.html.

14. "Freud Family," Wikipedia, July 22, 2018, https://en.wikipedia.org/wiki/Freud_family; "Sigmund Freud and the Holocaust," Holocaust Research Project, accessed April 30, 2018, http://www.holocaustresearchproject.org/ghettos/freud.html.

15. Schur, *Freud: Living and Dying*, 2.

16. Martin S. Bergmann, "Platonic Love, Transference Love, and Love in Real Life," in *The Origins and Organization of Unconscious Conflict: The Selected Works of Martin S. Bergmann* (New York: Routledge, 2017).

17. Peter Schur, "The Freud-Schur Connection" (presentation, Vienna Psychoanalytic Association, Vienna, Austria, February 1994).

18. Jack D. McCue and Lewis M. Cohen, "Freud's Physician-Assisted Death," *Archives of Internal Medicine* 159, no. 14 (July 26, 1999): 1521–55, doi:10.1001/archinte.159.14.1521.

19. P. C. Herbert et al., "Bioethics for Clinicians: 7. Truth Telling," *Canadian Medical Association Journal* 156, no. 2 (January 15, 1997).

20. McCue and Cohen, "Freud's Physician-Assisted Death."

21. Schur, *Freud: Living and Dying*, 174.

22. Jones, *The Life and Work of Sigmund Freud, 1919-1939, Volume 3*, 246–47.

Chapter 11

1. Mike Lynch, "New Alzheimer's Association Report Reveals Sharp Increases in Alzheimer's Prevalence, Deaths and Cost of Care," Alzheimer's Association, May 30, 2018, accessed June 9, 2018, https://www.alz.org/news/2018/new_alzheimer_s_association_report_reveals_sharp_i.

2. Gina Kolata, "Trump Passed a Cognitive Exam. What Does That Really Mean?" *New York Times*, January 19, 2018, https://www.nytimes.com/2018/01/19/health/trump-cognitive-screening-dementia.html.

3. "Facts and Figures," Alzheimer's Association, accessed June 5, 2018, https://www.alz.org/alzheimers-dementia/facts-figures.

4. Michael D. Hurd et al., "Monetary Costs of Dementia in the United States," *New England Journal of Medicine*, April 4, 2013, accessed June 5, 2018, https://www.nejm.org/doi/full/10.1056/NEJMsa1204629.

5. "Treatment Horizon," Alzheimer's Association, accessed June 5, 2018, https://www.alz.org/research/science/alzheimers_treatment_horizon.asp.

6. Pauline Anderson, "Finally, a Winner for Alzheimer's? Anti-amyloid Shows Promise," *Medscape*, July 26, 2018, accessed July 27, 2018, https://www.medscape.com/viewarticle/899841?nlid=124071_3901&src=wnl_newsalrt_180726_MSCPEDIT&uac=262098PY&impID=1695330&faf=1.

7. Benedict Carey, "The First Step toward a Personal Memory Maker?" *New York Times*, February 12, 2018, https://www.nytimes.com/2018/02/12/health/memory-dementia-brain-implants.html?rref=collection/byline/benedict-carey&action=click&contentCollection=undefined®ion=stream&module=stream_unit&version=latest&contentPlacement=14&pgtype=collection.

8. Laura Kelly, "Older Adults Overprescribed Dementia Medication at High Cost: Study," *Washington Times*, August 21, 2018, accessed August 27, 2018, https://www.washingtontimes.com/news/2018/aug/21/older-adults-overprescribed-dementia-medication/.

9. Jeanne Erdmann, "At 100, My Mom Had Dementia and Needed Hospice Care. Getting It Was Nearly Impossible," *Washington Post*, May 5, 2018, accessed May 5, 2018, https://www.washingtonpost.com/national/health-science/at-100-my-mom-had-dementia-and-needed-hospice-care-getting-it-was-nearly-impossible/2018/05/04/c6b7efdc-4724-11e8-8b5a-3b1697adcc2a_story.html?utm_term=.d96d6f45f799.

10. Brett Molina, "Bill Gates Unveils $100M Plan to Fight Alzheimer's, Dementia," *USA Today*, November 13, 2017, accessed April 2, 2018, https://www.usatoday.com/story/tech/news/2017/11/13/bill-gates-made-big-investment-fight-alzheimers/857721001/.

11. Alice Park, "Baby Boomers: Not the 'Healthiest Generation,'" *Time*, February 5, 2013, accessed January 6, 2018, http://healthland.time.com/2013/02/05/baby-boomers-not-the-healthiest-generation/.

12. Dana E. King et al., "The Status of Baby Boomers Health in the United States," *JAMA Internal Medicine* 173, no. 5 (2013): doi:10.1001/jamainternmed.2013.2006.

13. "What Is Unbearable?" *Economist*, August 4, 2016, https://www.economist.com/news/science-and-technology/21703359-some-data-about-emotional-issue-what-unbearable; Emily B. Rubin, Anna E.

Buehler, and Scott D. Halpern, "States Worse Than Death among Hospitalized Patients with Serious Illnesses," *JAMA Internal Medicine* 176, no. 10 (2016): doi:10.1001/jamainternmed.2016.4362.

14. Katie Roiphe, *Violet Hour: Great Writers at the End* (New York: Dial Press, 2016).

15. Ibid.

16. Polly Toynbee, "The Writer Katharine Whitehorn Would Rather Die Than Live Like This," *Guardian*, May 29, 2018, accessed June 14, 2018, https://www.theguardian.com/commentisfree/2018/may/29/assissted-dying-katharine-whitehorn-alzheimers.

17. "How the Oregon DWD Law Should Be Modified," *Org.opn.lists. right-to-die Digest* 25, no. 52 (June 27, 2018).

18. René Bruemmer, "Québec Election: CAQ Pledges $5 Million for Alzheimer's Research," *Montreal Gazette*, September 17, 2018, accessed September 19, 2018, https://montrealgazette.com/news/local-news/quebec-election-caq-pledges-5-million-for-alzheimers-research.

Chapter 12

1. Derek Humphry, *Good Life, Good Death: The Memoir of a Right to Die Pioneer* (New York: Carrel Books, 2017).

2. Richard N. Côté, *In Search of Gentle Death: The Fight for Your Right to Die with Dignity* (Mt. Pleasant, SC: Corinthian Books, 2012).

3. Humphry, *Good Life, Good Death*.

4. Derek Humphrey, *Jean's Way* (Junction City, OR: Norris Lane Press, 2003).

5. Côté, *In Search of Gentle Death*.

Chapter 13

1. Neal Nicol and Harry L. Wylie, *Between the Dying and the Dead: Dr. Jack Kevorkian, the Assisted Suicide Machine and the Battle to Legalize Euthanasia* (Madison: University of Wisconsin Press, 2006).

2. Jack Lessenberry, "Death Becomes Him," PBS *Frontline*, from *Vanity Fair*, July 1994, accessed September 26, 2018, https://www.pbs.org/wgbh/pages/frontline/kevorkian/aboutk/vanityfair.html.

3. Jennifer Latson, "Jack Kevorkian Doctor Death Trial: He Wanted to Be Tried for Murder," *Time*, March 26, 2015, accessed January 31, 2018, http://time.com/3748245/kevorkian-trial-history/.

4. Derek Humphry, *Good Life, Good Death: The Memoir of a Right to Die Pioneer* (New York: Carrel Books, 2017), 233–39.

5. Nicol and Wylie, *Between the Dying and the Dead*, 2.

6. Ibid.

7. Humphry, *Good Life, Good Death*, 239.

8. Stephen Garrard Post, *The Moral Challenge of Alzheimer Disease: Ethical Issues from Diagnosis to Dying* (Baltimore: Johns Hopkins University Press, 2002).

9. J. Roberts and C. Kjellstrand, "Jack Kevorkian: A Medical Hero," *British Medical Journal* 313, no. 7051 (June 8, 1996), https://www.ncbi.nlm.nih.gov/pmc/articles/PMC2351178/.

10. Steven N. Drake, "The All-Too-Familiar Story," *Ragged Edge*, no. 2, 2001, accessed September 26, 2018, http://www.raggededge magazine.com/0301/0301ft5.htm.

11. Jack Lessenberry, "Dr. Death Gets Out of Prison," *Detroit Metro Times*, December 20, 2006, accessed July 1, 2018, https://www.metro-times.com/detroit/dr-death-gets-out-of-prison/Content?oid=2186216.

12. "The Kevorkian Verdict," PBS, *Frontline*, aired May 14, 1996, accessed August 2, 2018, https://www.pbs.org/wgbh/pages/frontline/kevorkian/kevorkianscript.html.

13. "Dr. Jack Kevorkian's *60 Minutes* Interview," *60 Minutes Overtime*, June 4, 2011, https://www.cbsnews.com/news/dr-jack-kevorkians-60-minutes-interview.

14. Keith Schneiderjune, "Dr. Jack Kevorkian Dies at 83, a Doctor Who Helped End Lives," *New York Times*, June 3, 2011, accessed July 2, 2018, https://www.nytimes.com/2011/06/04/us/04kevorkian.html.

15. Sarah Hulett, "Jack Kevorkian, Assisted Suicide Advocate, Dies at 83," NPR, June 3, 2011, accessed September 28, 2018, https://www.npr.org/2011/06/03/136917033/jack-kevorkian-assisted-suicide-advocate-dies-at-83?t=1538130986884.

16. Lessenberry, "Dr. Death Gets Out of Prison."

Chapter 14

1. Robert D. McFadden, "Karen Ann Quinlan, 31, Dies; Focus of '76 Right to Die Case," *New York Times*, June 12, 1985, accessed April 26, 2018, https://www.nytimes.com/1985/06/12/nyregion/karen-ann-quinlan-31-dies-focus-of-76-right-to-die-case.html.

2. Ibid.

3. Tamar Lewin, "Nancy Cruzan Dies, Outlived by a Debate over the Right to Die," *New York Times*, December 27, 1990, accessed April 27,

2018, https://www.nytimes.com/1990/12/27/us/nancy-cruzan-dies
-outlived-by-a-debate-over-the-right-to-die.html.

4. William H. Colby, *Long Goodbye: The Deaths of Nancy Cruzan* (Carlsbad, CA: Hay House, 2002).

5. Lewin, "Nancy Cruzan Dies."

6. *"Whose Life Is It Anyway?* (play)," Wikipedia, April 7, 2018, accessed September 26, 2018, https://en.wikipedia.org/wiki/Whose_Life_Is_It_Anyway?_(play).

7. *"Whose Life Is It Anyway?* (film)," Wikipedia, May 30, 2018, accessed September 26, 2018, https://en.wikipedia.org/wiki/Whose_Life_Is_It_Anyway?_(film).

8. Richard N. Côté, *In Search of Gentle Death: The Fight for Your Right to Die with Dignity* (Mt. Pleasant, SC: Corinthian Books, 2012).

9. Derek Humphry, *Let Me Die Before I Wake: Hemlock's Book of Self-Deliverance for the Dying* (New York: Dell Publishing, 1984).

10. Derek Humphry, *Final Exit: The Practicalities of Self-Deliverance and Assisted Suicide for the Dying* (New York: Dell Publishing, 1991).

11. *"Final Exit,"* Wikipedia, September 1, 2018, accessed July 1, 2018, https://en.wikipedia.org/wiki/Final_Exit.

12. G. Garry Abrams, "A Bitter Legacy: Angry Accusations Abound after the Suicide of Hemlock Society Co-founder Ann Humphry," *Los Angeles Times*, October 23, 1991, http://articles.latimes.com/1991-10-23/news/vw-283_1_ann-humphry/3.

13. Trip Gabriel, "A Fight to the Death," *New York Times*, December 8, 1991, https://www.nytimes.com/1991/12/08/magazine/a-fight-to-the-death.html.

14. Ann Wickett, *Double Exit: When Aging Couples Commit Suicide Together* (Eugene, OR: Hemlock Society, 1989).

15. Ibid.

16. Gabriel, "A Fight to the Death."

17. Ibid.

18. Ibid.

19. Ibid.

20. Ibid.

Chapter 15

1. Neal Nicol and Harry Wylie, *Between the Dying and the Dead: Dr. Jack Kevorkian, the Assisted Suicide Machine and the Battle to Legalize Euthanasia* (Madison: University of Wisconsin Press, 2006).

2. Ibid.

3. Ibid., 39.

4. Ibid., 58.

5. Ibid., 63.

6. *"You Don't Know Jack* (film)," Wikipedia, September 4, 2018, https://en.wikipedia.org/wiki/You_Don't_Know_Jack_(film).

7. Jeff Kowalsky, "America's 'Doctor Death,' Jack Kevorkian Dies at 83," *Yahoo! News*, June 3, 2011, https://sg.news.yahoo.com/news/assisted-suicide-advocate-kevorkian-dies-us-hospital-142417059.html?guccounter=1.

8. Keith Schneider, "Dr. Jack Kevorkian Dies at 83: A Doctor Who Helped End Lives," *New York Times*, June 3, 2011, accessed April 23, 2018, https://www.nytimes.com/2011/06/04/us/04kevorkian.html.

9. Zoe FitzGerald Carter, "The Poignant Irony of Dr. Kevorkian's Death," *Salon*, September 25, 2011, accessed April 23, 2018, https://www.salon.com/2011/06/04/kevorkian_death_reaction/.

10. Ibid.

11. Timothy E. Quill, "On Trial—How We Die," *Baltimore Sun*, September 28, 1993, http://articles.baltimoresun.com/1993-09-28/news/1993271203_1_kevorkian-dying-patients-medical-and-legal.

12. "The Kevorkian Verdict," PBS *Frontline*, aired May 14, 1996, accessed August 2, 2018, https://www.pbs.org/wgbh/pages/frontline/kevorkian/kevorkianscript.html.

13. William Breitbart, Personal Communication.

14. Charlie Breitrose, "Watertown's Armenian Museum Will Keep 4 of Kevorkian's Paintings, Give Up the Rest," *Stone Mountain-Lithonia (Georgia) Patch*, October 5, 2012, https://patch.com/massachusetts/watertown/watertown-s-armenian-museum-will-keep-4-of-kevorkian-6ccc90b6c4.

15. Ibid.

16. "Kevorkian's Papers Donated to UM Historical Library," *Detroit News*, October 13, 2015, accessed January 32, 2018, http://www.detroitnews.com/story/news/local/michigan/2015/10/13/kevorkians-papers-donated-um-historical-library/73863100/.

17. Andrew Solomon, "On My Mother, and Dr. Kevorkian," *New Yorker*, June 20, 2017, https://www.newyorker.com/news/news-desk/on-my-mother-and-dr-kevorkian.

18. "Kevorkian Interviewed on *60 Minutes*," UPI, May 19, 1996, accessed October 5, 2018, https://www.upi.com/Archives/1996/05/19/Kevorkian-interviewed-on-60-Minutes/9648832478400/.

19. Andy Rooney and Jack Kevorkian, *60 Minutes* interview, produced by Robert R. Forte and Jane Jaffin, May 19, 1996, accessed October 5, 2018, https://www.youtube.com/watch?v=ozwoYhxdbTQ.

Chapter 16

1. "*Monty Python and the Holy Grail*," Wikipedia, September 17, 2018, last accessed April 30, 2018, https://en.wikipedia.org/wiki/Monty_Python_and_the_Holy_Grail.

2. Ibid.

3. "Not Dead Yet," Wikipedia, June 7, 2018, last accessed April 29, 2018, https://en.wikipedia.org/wiki/Not_Dead_Yet.

4. Mike Ludwig, "Disability Activists Crash Congress to Stop a Bill That Would Undermine Their Civil Rights," Truthout, February 16, 2018, last accessed April 29, 2018, http://www.truth-out.org/news/item/43570-disability-activists-crash-congress-to-stop-a-bill-that-would-undermine-their-civil-rights; Anita Cameron, "ADAPT and Not Dead Yet: In Solidarity. Not Dead Yet News & Commentary," Not Dead Yet, August 11, 2018, last accessed September 22, 2018, http://notdeadyet.org/.

5. "Not Dead Yet—Staff," Not Dead Yet, 2018, last accessed April 30, 2018, http://notdeadyet.org/about/staff.

6. John B. Kelly, "A Battle Waged in Boston: Right to Die vs. Will to Live," *Ragged Edge*, September 3, 2000, last accessed April 30, 2018, http://www.raggededgemagazine.com/extra/ndykellyoped.htm.

7. Access Living, March 11, 2008, last accessed April 30, 2018, https://www.accessliving.org/k.

8. Little People of America, last accessed April 30, 2018. http://www.lpaonline.org/.

9. Steve Reinberg, "Sen. Kennedy Up and Walking after Brain Tumor Surgery," ABC News, June 4, 2008, last accessed July 1, 2018, https://abcnews.go.com/Health/Healthday/sen-kennedy-walking-brain-tumor-surgery/story?id=4990884.

10. "Disability Groups Opposed to Assisted Suicide Laws," Not Dead Yet, last accessed July 2, 2018, http://notdeadyet.org/disability-groups-opposed-to-assisted-suicide-laws.

11. Daniel P. Sulmasy, "An Open Letter to Norman Cantor Regarding Dementia and Physician-Assisted Suicide," *Hastings Center Report* 48, no. 4 (August 16, 2018): doi:10.1002/hast.868.

12. Ibid.

13. Stephen Drake, "Meet Our New Regional Director, John Kelly," Not Dead Yet, November 6, 2013, last accessed July 2, 2018, http://notdeadyet.org/2013/11/meet-our-new-regional-director-john-kelly.html.

14. Ibid.

15. Ibid.

16. "John Kelly Gives His Take on the NDY Protest of the World Federation Conference," Not Dead Yet, September 24, 2014, last accessed July 2, 2018, http://notdeadyet.org/2014/09/john-kelly-gives-his-take-on-the-ndy-protest-of-the-world-federation-conference.html.

17. Ibid.

18. W. Erickson, C. Lee, and S. Von Schrader, *2016 Disability Status Report: United States* (Ithaca, NY: Yang-Tan Institute on Employment and Disability, Cornell University, 2018).

19. Dhruv Khullar, "Who Will Care for the Caregivers?" *New York Times*, January 19, 2017, last accessed July 2, 2018, https://www.nytimes.com/2017/01/19/upshot/who-will-care-for-the-caregivers.html.

20. Rachel Aviv, "What Does It Mean to Die?" *New Yorker*, February 5, 2018, last accessed July 1, 2018, https://www.newyorker.com/magazine/2018/02/05/what-does-it-mean-to-die; Samantha Schmidt, "Jahi McMath, the Calif. Girl in Life-Support Controversy, Is Now Dead," *Washington Post*, June 29, 2018, last accessed June 30, 2018, https://www.washingtonpost.com/news/morning-mix/wp/2018/06/29/jahi-mcmath-the-calif-girl-declared-brain-dead-4-years-ago-is-taken-off-life-support/?noredirect=on&utm_term=.a8d277be9f5a.

21. Schmidt, "Jahi McMath."

22. Ibid.

23. Aviv, "What Does It Mean to Die?"

24. Ibid.

25. Joseph P. Shapiro, *No Pity: People with Disabilities Forging a New Civil Rights Movement* (New York: Three Rivers Press, 1993), 74–75; Chuck Oldham and Rhonda Carpenter, *Equal Access, Equal Opportunity: 25th Anniversary of the Americans with Disabilities Act* (Tampa, FL: Faircount Media Group, 2015), 48–57.

26. "John Kelly Gives His Take."

27. Ibid.

Chapter 17

1. The World Federation of Right to Die Societies, last accessed April 30, 2018, https://www.worldrtd.net/.

2. Justin Wm. Moyer, "Meet the Terminal Cancer Patient Who Stumped Hillary Clinton on Death with Dignity at CNN's Town Hall," *Washington Post*, February 4, 2016, last accessed April 29, 2018, https://www.washingtonpost.com/news/morning-mix/wp/2016/02/04/meet-the-cancer-patient-who-challenged-clinton-about-death-with-dignity-on-cnn/?utm_term=.f37227d6026c.

3. Tone Stockenström, "Is Dying a Pro-Choice Issue? The Right-to-Die Movement Gains National Attention." *Humanist*, December 22, 2014, accessed April 28, 2018, https://thehumanist.com/magazine/january-february-2015/features/is-dying-a-pro-choice-issue.

4. Lewis M. Cohen, "Dignified Debate," *Slate*, August 11, 2014, https://slate.com/technology/2014/08/assisted-suicide-debate-in-united-kingdom-house-of-lords-on-death-with-dignity.html.

5. Ibid.

6. Desmond Tutu, "Desmond Tutu: Revere the Sanctity of Life but Not at All Costs," *Ottawa Citizen*, October 12, 2014, last accessed April 28, 2018, http://ottawacitizen.com/news/national/desmond -tutu-revere-the-sanctity-of-life-but-not-at-all-costs.

7. Stockenström, "Is Dying a Pro-Choice Issue?"

8. Ibid.

9. Richard N. Côté, *In Search of Gentle Death: The Fight for Your Right to Die with Dignity* (Mt. Pleasant, SC: Corinthian Books, 2012).

10. Manuel Roig-Franzia, "After the Death of Jack Kevorkian, a New Public Face of American Assisted Suicide," *Washington Post*, January 19, 2012, last accessed April 28, 2018, https://www.washingtonpost.com/ lifestyle/magazine/after-the-death-of-jack-kevorkian-a-new-public -face-of-american-assisted-suicide/2011/12/23/gIQAXhtkAQ_story .html?utm_term=.e9e2b1e13cd8.

11. Address of His Holiness Pope Francis to Participants in the Commemorative Conference of the Italian Catholic Physicians' Association on the Occasion of Its 70th Anniversary of Foundation," Vatican, November 15, 2014, last accessed April 28, 2018, https://w2.vatican .va/content/francesco/en/speeches/2014/november/documents/ papa-francesco_20141115_medici-cattolici-italiani.html.

12. David Itzkoff, *Robin* (New York: Henry Holt & Company, 2018), 424–27.

13. Stockenström, "Is Dying a Pro-Choice Issue?"

14. Mary Johnson, "Right to Life, Fight to Die: The Elizabeth Bouvia Saga," *Ragged Edge*, last accessed April 28, 2018 (first published 1984 in *Disability Rag*), http://www.raggededgemagazine.com/archive/ bouvia.htm.

15. Ibid.

16. "A Brief History of Not Dead Yet," Not Dead Yet, last accessed April 28, 2018, http://notdeadyet.org/about/a-brief-history-of-not -dead-yet.

Chapter 18

1. Andrew Solomon, "A Death of One's Own," *New Yorker*, May 22, 1995, accessed July 1, 2018, https://www.newyorker.com/ magazine/1995/05/22/a-death-of-ones-own.

Chapter 19

1. C. Blanke, M. LeBlanc, D. Hershman, L. Ellis, and F. Meyskens, "Characterizing 18 Years of the Death With Dignity Act in Oregon," *JAMA Oncology* 3, no. 10 (2017): 1403–6, last accessed June 10, 2017, doi:10.1001/jamaoncol.2017.0243.

2. Lynne Terry, "Study: Oregon Patients Using Physician-Assisted Suicide Steadily Increase," *Oregonian/OregonLive*, April 6, 2017, last accessed June 10, 2018, http://www.oregonlive.com/health/index.ssf/2017/04/study_oregon_patients_using_ph.html.

3. Catherine Offord, "Accessing Drugs for Medical Aid-in-Dying," *Scientist*, August 17, 2017, last accessed June 10, 2018, https://www.the-scientist.com/?articles.view/articleNo/49879/title/Accessing-Drugs-for-Medical-Aid-in-Dying/.

4. Roxanne Nelson, "When Dying Becomes Unaffordable," *Medscape Medical News*, November 9, 2017, last accessed June 10, 2018, https://www.medscape.com/viewarticle/888271#vp_1; "Dilemmas in Aid in Dying: Podcast with Bernie Lo," interview with Alex Smith, *GeriPal*, podcast, July 13, 2018, https://www.geripal.org/2018/07/dilemmas-in-aid-in-dying-podcast-with.html.

5. Offord, "Accessing Drugs for Medical Aid-in-Dying."

6. Ibid.; Nelson, "When Dying Becomes Unaffordable."

7. JoNel Aleccia, "Death with Dignity Doctors Thwart Drugmaker's Price Hike with New Medication," *Seattle Times*, April 2, 2016, last accessed June 10, 2018, https://www.seattletimes.com/seattle-news/health/death-with-dignity-doctors-thwart-steep-price-hike-for-lethal-drug/.

8. Ibid.

9. Nelson, "When Dying Becomes Unaffordable."

10. Ibid.

11. Ibid.

12. "NuTech," Exit International, https://exitinternational.net/nutech/.

13. Ibid.

14. "Nutech—Self-Deliverance New Technology—Report from ERGO," Final Exit, http://www.finalexit.org/ergo_nutech_new_technology.html.

15. Winston Ross, "Suicide Kits: The 91-Year-Old Woman Selling Instant Death on the Internet," *Daily Beast*, April 27, 2011, last accessed July 31, 2018, https://www.thedailybeast.com/suicide-kits-the-91-year-old-woman-selling-instant-death-on-the-internet.

16. ERGO, "New Ideas for Self-Deliverance Displayed at NuTech Conference," *Assisted-Dying* (Blog), December 23, 2017, last accessed June 12, 2018, http://assisted-dying.org/blog/2017/12/23/new-ideas-for-self-deliverance-displayed-at-nutech-conference/.

17. Mitch Smith, "Potent Opioid with Deadly Track Record Gets Put to a New Use," *New York Times*, August 15, 2018. A10.

18. Denise Grady and Jan Hoffman, "States Turn to an Unproven Method of Execution: Nitrogen Gas," *New York Times*, May 8, 2018, https://www.nytimes.com/2018/05/07/health/death-penalty-nitrogen-executions.html.

19. Ibid.

20. Tom McNichol, "Death by Nitrogen: Will This New Method of Execution Save the Death Penalty?" *Slate*, May 22, 2014, last accessed June 10, 2018, http://www.slate.com/articles/news_and_politics/jurisprudence/2014/05/death_by_nitrogen_gas_will_the_new_method_of_execution_save_the_death_penalty.html.

21. Grady and Hoffman, "States Turn to an Unproven Method of Execution."

22. "Controversial Euthanasia Proponent Releases 3D Printing Blueprints for Assisted Suicide Pod," *International Business Times UK*, November 29, 2017, last accessed June 10, 2018, https://www.ibtimes.co.uk/new-suicide-pod-humans-comes-built-coffin-1649284.

23. Ibid.

24. Nicole Goodkind, "Meet the Elon Musk of Assisted Suicide, Whose Machine Lets You Kill Yourself Anywhere," *Newsweek*, December 1, 2017, last accessed June 11, 2018, http://www.newsweek.com/elon-musk-assisted-suicide-machine-727874.

Chapter 20

1. Ryan J. Reilly and Julia Craven, "Lawyers Go After 'Dank and Dangerous' Conditions at Aging Baltimore Jail," *Huffington Post*, June 2, 2015, last accessed July 21, 2018, https://www.huffingtonpost.com/2015/06/02/baltimore-jail-lawsuit_n_7493962.html.

2. Justin Fenton, "2 in Aided-Suicide Case Won't Fight Extradition," *Baltimore Sun*, February 28, 2009, last accessed July 21, 2018, http://articles.baltimoresun.com/2009-02-28/news/0902270130_1_final-exit-egbert-suicide.

3. Sarah Kliff, "Lawrence Egbert: Assisted Suicide's New Face," *Newsweek*, March 14, 2010, last accessed June 4, 2018, http://www.newsweek.com/lawrence-egbert-assisted-suicides-new-face-69677.

4. Michael Majchrowicz, "The Volunteers Who Help People End Their Own Lives," *Atlantic*, July 6, 2016, last accessed June 3, 2018, https://www.theatlantic.com/health/archive/2016/07/the-volunteers-who-help-people-end-their-own-lives/489602/.

5. Daniel Bates, "My Life, My Death, My Choice: Fury over Roadside Billboards That 'Advocate Suicide,'" *Daily Mail Online*, July 16, 2010, last accessed June 4, 2018, http://www.dailymail.co.uk/news/article-1295354/My-life-death-choice-Fury-roadside-billboards-advocate-suicide.html#ixzz5HNr4Aixy.

6. Courtney Hutchison, "Euthanasia Billboards, Books Fight for Death on Your Own Terms," ABC News, July 19, 2010, last accessed June 4, 2018, https://abcnews.go.com/Health/MindMoodNews/billboards-advertise-death-terms/story?id=11164242.

7. Steve Strunsky, "National Campaign Guiding Ill Adults to End Lives Advertises on Hillside Billboard," *NJ.com*, July 14, 2010, last accessed June 4, 2018, http://www.nj.com/news/index.ssf/2010/07/national_campaign_guiding_ill.html.

8. Majchrowicz, "The Volunteers Who Help People End Their Own Lives."

9. Wesley J. Smith, "My Take On, "My Life, My Death, My Choice," *First Things*, August 5, 2010, last accessed June 5, 2018, https://www.firstthings.com/blogs/firstthoughts/2010/08/my-take-on -my-life-my-death-my-choice-fen-billboards.

10. Georgia Bureau of Investigation documents provided by Robert Rivas.

11. Greg Bluestein, "4 Members of Assisted Suicide Group Are Arrested," *San Diego Union-Tribune*, February 26, 2009, last accessed July 22, 2018, http://www.sandiegouniontribune.com/sdut-assisted -suicide-ring-022609-2009feb26-story.html.

12. Charles Bethea, "Final Exit," *Atlanta Magazine*, March 1, 2010, last accessed June 5, 2018, http://www.atlantamagazine.com/great-reads/final-exit-network/.

13. Sarah Kliff, "Lawrence Egbert: Assisted Suicide's New Face," *Newsweek*, March 14, 2010, last accessed June 4, 2018, http://www.newsweek.com/lawrence-egbert-assisted-suicides-new-face-69677.

14. Bethea, "Final Exit."

15. Bluestein, "4 Members of Assisted Suicide Group Are Arrested."

16. Richard Fausset, "Assisted Suicide Back in Spotlight after Georgia Arrest," *Seattle Times*, March 1, 2009, last accessed July 22, 2018, https://www.seattletimes.com/seattle-news/health/assisted-suicide -back-in-spotlight-after-georgia-arrest/.

17. Robbie Brown, "Arrests Draw New Attention to Assisted Suicide," *New York Times*, March 10, 2009, last accessed July 22, 2018, https://archive.nytimes.com/www.nytimes.com/2009/03/11/us/11suicide.html; "Who Should Be Able to Seek Assisted Suicide?," NPR, *Talk of the Nation*, March 9, 2009.

18. "The Suicide Plan," PBS, *Frontline*, November 13, 2012, last accessed August 1, 2018, https://www.pbs.org/wgbh/frontline/film/suicide-plan/.

19. "Who Should Be Able to Seek Assisted Suicide?"

Chapter 21

1. Charles Bethea, "Final Exit," *Atlanta Magazine*, March 1, 2010, last accessed June 5, 2018, http://www.atlantamagazine.com/great-reads/final-exit-network/.

2. Jaime Joyce, "Kill Me Now: The Troubled Life and Complicated Death of Jana Van Voorhis," *BuzzFeed*, December 27, 2013, last accessed

June 3, 2018, https://www.buzzfeed.com/jaimejoyce/kill-me-now-the
-troubled-life-and-complicated-death-of-jana?utm_term=.yvw2YBqyy#
.tr0lzMoLL.

3. Ibid.

4. Justin Fenton, "Baltimore Doctor Helps the Ill Commit Suicide:
Dr. Lawrence Egbert Has Been Dubbed 'The New Doctor Death,'" *Baltimore Sun*, May 21, 2011, last accessed July 22, 2018, http://articles
.baltimoresun.com/2011-05-21/news/bs-md-right-to-die-20110520_1_
final-exit-network-assisted-suicide-baltimore-doctor.

5. Michael Majchrowicz, "The Volunteers Who Help People
End Their Own Lives," *Atlantic*, July 6, 2016, last accessed June
3, 2018, https://www.theatlantic.com/health/archive/2016/07/
the-volunteers-who-help-people-end-their-own-lives/489602/.

6. Joyce, "Kill Me Now."

7. "Group on Trial, Accused of Aiding Minnesota Woman's Suicide," CBS Minnesota, May 10, 2015, last accessed July 22, 2018,
https://minnesota.cbslocal.com/2015/05/10/group-on-trial-accused
-of-aiding-minnesota-womans-suicide/.

8. Associated Press, "Right-to-die Group Gave Doreen Dunn
Instructions on How to Kill Herself," *Daily Mail*, May 14, 2015, last
accessed July 22, 2018, http://www.dailymail.co.uk/news/article
-3081067/Right-die-group-gave-woman-blueprint-instructions-kill
-say-prosecution-landmark-case-transform-legislation.html.

9. Jessie Van Berkel, "Final Exit Network Fined $30,000 for Assist-
ing Apple Valley Woman's Suicide" *(Minneapolis) Star Tribune*, August
24, 2015, last accessed July 22, 2018, http://www.startribune.com/
final-exit-network-fined-30-000-for-assisting-apple-valley-woman-s
-suicide/322700141/.

10. Ibid.

11. Majchrowicz, "The Volunteers."

12. "Final Exit Network Appeals Minnesota Conviction to U.S.
Supreme Court," *PR Newswire*, July 9, 2013, last accessed July 22, 2018,
https://www.prnewswire.com/news-releases/final-exit-network
-appeals-minnesota-conviction-to-us-supreme-court-300477092.html.

13. Che Guevara, "Socialism and Man in Cuba," Marxists, March
12, 1965, accessed July 22, 2018 (First published as "From Algiers, for
Marcha: The Cuban Revolution Today"), https://www.marxists.org/
archive/guevara/1965/03/man-socialism.htm.

14. David Brooks, "What Moral Heroes Are Made Of," *New York
Times*, May 22, 2018, A25; Anne Colby and William Damon, *Some Do
Care: Contemporary Lives of Moral Commitment* (New York: Free Press,
1992).

Part III

1. Sophocles, *Philoktetes*, Poetry in Translation, last accessed January 30, 2018, http://www.poetryintranslation.com/PITBR/Greek/Philoctetes.php.

Chapter 22

1. Cody Curtis, "My Story," How We Die, last accessed July 4, 2018, http://www.how-we-die.org/howwedie/story?sid=10.

Chapter 23

1. Nicole Weisensee Egan, "Terminally Ill 29-Year-Old Woman: Why I'm Choosing to Die on My Own Terms," *People*, October 24, 2016, last accessed July 16, 2018, https://people.com/celebrity/terminally-ill-29-year-old-woman-why-im-choosing-to-die-on-my-own-terms/.
2. CompassionChoices, "The Brittany Maynard Story," YouTube Video, 6:30, October 6, 2014, last accessed July 14, 2018, https://www.youtube.com/watch?v=yPfe3rCcUeQ; CompassionChoices, "A Video for All My Friends," YouTube Video, 5:58, October 29, 2014, last accessed July 14, 2018, https://www.youtube.com/watch?v=1lHXHUZb2QI.
3. Brandon Griggs, "Dying Young: Why Brittany Maynard's Story Resonates," CNN, October 14, 2014, accessed July 7, 2018, https://www.cnn.com/2014/10/08/living/death-dignity-brittany-maynard/index.html; Brittany Maynard, "My Right to Death with Dignity at 29," CNN, November 2, 2014, last accessed July 12, 2018, http://www.cnn.com/2014/10/07/opinion/maynard-assisted-suicide-cancer-dignity/index.html.
4. CompassionChoices, "Brittany Maynard Legislative Testimony," YouTube Video, 6:33, March 31, 2015, last accessed July 14, 2018, https://www.youtube.com/watch?v=Mi8AP_EhM94.
5. CompassionChoices, "Brittany Maynard's Legacy: One Year Later," YouTube Video, 6:21, October 5, 2015, last accessed July 7, 2018, https://www.youtube.com/watch?v=uzp0tp8Fzio.
6. "Brittany Maynard's Official Obituary from Her Family," KTLA, November 2, 2014, last accessed July 14, 2018, https://ktla.com/2014/11/02/official-obituary-from-family-of-brittany-maynard/.
7. Ashley E. McGuire, "Brittany Maynard and the Trouble with Suicide," *Acculturated*, October 23, 2014, last accessed July 15, 2018, https://acculturated.com/brittany-maynard-and-the-trouble-with-suicide/.

Chapter 24

1. David Rieff, *Swimming in a Sea of Death: A Son's Memoir* (New York: Simon & Schuster, 2008); Katie Roiphe, "Without Metaphor," *New York Times*, February 3, 2008, last accessed July 4, 2018, https://www.nytimes.com/2008/02/03/books/review/Roiphe-t.html.

2. Cody Curtis, "My Story," How We Die, last accessed July 4, 2018, http://www.how-we-die.org/howwedie/story?sid=10.

3. Ibid.

4. Public Health Division, Center for Health Statistics, *Oregon Death with Dignity Act: 2017 Data Summary*, report, February 9, 2018, last accessed July 4, 2018, https://www.oregon.gov/oha/PH/PROVIDER PARTNERRESOURCES/EVALUATIONRESEARCH/DEATHWITH DIGNITYACT/Documents/year20.pdf.

5. Katrina Hedberg and Craig New, "Oregon's Death with Dignity Act: 20 Years of Experience to Inform the Debate," *Annals of Internal Medicine* 167, no. 8 (October 17, 2017): 579–83, doi:10.7326/m17-2300.

6. Bernard Lo, "Beyond Legalization: Dilemmas Physicians Confront Regarding Aid in Dying," *New England Journal of Medicine* 378, no. 22 (May 31, 2018): 2060–62, doi:10.1056/nejmp1802218.

7. Hedberg and New, "Oregon's Death with Dignity Act."

8. E. J. Emanuel et al., "Attitudes and Practices of Euthanasia and Physician-Assisted Suicide in the United States, Canada, and Europe," *Journal of the American Medical Association* 316, no. 1 (July 5, 2016): 79–90, doi:10.1001/jama.2016.8499.

9. Lo, "Beyond Legalization."

10. Brooks Barnes, "Unflinching End-of-Life Moments," *New York Times*, January 24, 2011, accessed September 24, 2018, https://www.nytimes.com/2011/01/25/movies/25sundance.html.

Chapter 25

1. Brandon Griggs, "Dying Young: Why Brittany Maynard's Story Resonates," CNN, October 14, 2014, accessed July 7, 2018, https://www.cnn.com/2014/10/08/living/death-dignity-brittany-maynard/index.html; Deborah Ziegler, *Wild and Precious Life* (New York: Atria Books, 2016).

2. Brittany Maynard, "My Right to Death with Dignity at 29," CNN, November 2, 2014, accessed July 12, 2018, http://www.cnn.com/2014/10/07/opinion/maynard-assisted-suicide-cancer-dignity/index.html.

3. Ibid.

4. Ibid.

5. Linda Ganzini et al, "Physicians' Experiences with the Oregon Death with Dignity Act," *New England Journal of Medicine* 342 (2000): 557–63, doi: 10.1056/NEJM200002243420806.

6. Ibid.

7. L. Ganzini et al., "Oregon Physicians' Perceptions of Patients Who Request Assisted Suicide and Their Families," *Journal of Palliative Medicine* 6, no. 3 (2003): 381–90, doi: 10.1089/109662103322144691.

8. Oregon Health Authority, "Death with Dignity Act Annual Reports," 2018, last accessed July 21, 2018, https://www.oregon.gov/oha/PH/PROVIDERPARTNERRESOURCES/EVALUATION-RESEARCH/DEATHWITHDIGNITYACT/Pages/ar-index.aspx.

9. L. Ganzini et al., "Oregonians' Reasons for Requesting Physician Aid in Dying," *Archives of Internal Medicine* 169, no. 5 (2009): 489–92, doi: 10.1001/archinternmed.2008.579.

10. Ganzini et al., "Physicians' Experiences with the Oregon Death with Dignity Act."

11. Ganzini et al., "Oregon Physicians' Attitudes about and Experiences with End-of-Life Care since Passage of the Oregon Death with Dignity Act," *Journal of the American Medical Association* 285, no. 18 (2001): 2363–69, https://www.ncbi.nlm.nih.gov/pubmed/11343484.

12. Ganzini et al., "Physicians' Experiences."

13. L. Ganzini et al., "Attitudes of Oregon Psychiatrists toward Physician-Assisted Suicide," *American Journal of Psychiatry* 153, no. 11 (1996): 1469–75, doi: 10.1176/ajp.153.11.1469; D. S. Fenn and L. Ganzini, "Attitudes of Oregon Psychologists toward Physician-Assisted Suicide and the Oregon Death with Dignity Act," *Professional Psychology: Research and Practice* 30, no. 3 (1999): 235–44, https://www.ncbi.nlm.nih.gov/pubmed/14626273.

14. B. Carlson et al., "Oregon Hospice Chaplains' Experiences with Patients Requesting Physician-Assisted Suicide," *Journal of Palliative Medicine* 8, no. 6 (2005): 1160–66, doi: 10.1089/jpm.2005.8.1160; Linda Ganzini, "Experiences of Oregon Nurses and Social Workers with Hospice Patients Who Requested Assistance with Suicide," *New England Journal of Medicine* 347, (2002): 582–88, doi: 10.1056/NEJMsa020562; L. L. Miller et al., "Attitudes and Experiences of Oregon Hospice Nurses and Social Workers Regarding Assisted Suicide," *Palliative Medicine* 18, no. 8 (2004): 685–91, doi: 10.1191/0269216304pm961oa.

15. Linda Ganzini, Elizabeth R. Goy, and Steven K. Dobscha, "Prevalence of Depression and Anxiety in Patients Requesting Physicians' Aid in Dying: Cross Sectional Survey," *British Medical Journal* 337, (2008): a1682, doi: https://doi.org/10.1136/bmj.a1682.

16. L. M. Cohen et al., "Psychiatric Evaluation of Death-Hastening Requests: Lessons from Dialysis Discontinuation," *Psychosomatics* 41, no. 3 (2000): 195–203, doi: 10.1176/appi.psy.41.3.195.

17. Linda Ganzini, Elizabeth R. Goy, and Steven K. Dobscha, "Why Oregon Patients Request Assisted Death: Family Members' Views," *Journal of General Internal Medicine* 23, no. 2 (2008): 154–57, doi: 10.1007/ s11606-007-0476-x; L. Ganzini et al., "Mental Health Outcomes of Family Members of Oregonians Who Request Physician Aid in Dying," *Journal of Pain and Symptom Management* 38, no. 6 (2009): 807–15, doi: 10.1016/j.jpainsymman.2009.04.026.

Chapter 26

1. Cody Curtis, "Dealing with Body Image Change," The Cholangiocarcinoma Foundation, November 6, 2009, last accessed July 5, 2018, https://cholangiocarcinoma.org/db/topic/dealing-with-body-image -change/.
2. Ibid.

Chapter 27

1. "Death with Dignity National Center," https://www.deathwith dignity.org.
2. Brittany Maynard, "My Right to Death with Dignity at 29," CNN, November 2, 2014, last accessed July 12, 2018, http://www.cnn .com/2014/10/07/opinion/maynard-assisted-suicide-cancer-dignity/ index.html.
3. CompassionChoices, "Brittany Maynard Legislative Testimony," YouTube Video, 6:33, March 31, 2015, last accessed July 14, 2018, https:// www.youtube.com/watch?v=Mi8AP_EhM94.
4. Brittany Maynard, "My Right to Death with Dignity at 29," CNN, November 02, 2014, last accessed July 12, 2018, http://www.cnn .com/2014/10/07/opinion/maynard-assisted-suicide-cancer-dignity/ index.html.
5. CompassionChoices, "A Video for All My Friends," YouTube Video, 5:58, October 29, 2014, last accessed July 14, 2018, https://www .youtube.com/watch?v=1lHXH0Zb2QI.
6. Nicole Weisensee Egan, "Terminally Ill Woman Brittany Maynard Has Ended Her Own Life," *People*, May 9, 2017, last accessed July 12, 2018, https://people.com/celebrity/terminally-ill -woman-brittany-maynard-has-ended-her-own-life/.
7. "Brittany Maynard's Official Obituary from Her Family," KTLA, November 2, 2014, last accessed July 14, 2018, https://ktla .com/2014/11/02/official-obituary-from-family-of-brittany-maynard/.

Chapter 28

1. Geordan Omand, "Catholic Leaders Divided over Funerals in Assisted Death Cases," *Vancouver (BC) Globe and Mail*, updated April 3, 2017, https://www.theglobeandmail.com/news/british-columbia/catholic-leaders-divided-over-assisted-death-funerals/article32312534/.

2. Bruno Chenu et al., *The Book of Christian Martyrs* (New York: Crossroad Publishing Company, 1990), vii.

3. Debra Nussbaum Cohen, "Hasidic Volunteers, Kicked Out of a Major NY Hospital, Blame a Clash over Medical Ethics," *Jewish Telegraphic Agency*, May 22, 2018.

4. Ibid.

5. Ibid.

6. Jeff Shannon, "'How to Die in Oregon': It's Personal," *The Demanders* (blog), May 26, 2011, last accessed September 22, 2018, https://www.rogerebert.com/demanders/how-to-die-in-oregon-its-personal.

7. Jane Catherine Lotter, "Jane Catherine Lotter," *Seattle Times*, August 3, 2013, last accessed May 19, 2018, http://www.legacy.com/obituaries/seattletimes/obituary.aspx?n=jane-catherine-lotter&pid=166098479.

8. E. E. Cummings, "you shall above all things be glad and young," in *Selected Poems*, introduction and commentary by Richard S. Kennedy (New York: W.W. Norton, 2007), 67.

Part IV

1. Paul Hostovsky, "Tree Poem," *A Little in Love a Lot* (Mint Hill, NC: Main Street Rag, 2011).

Chapter 29

1. Compassion & Choices, "Brittany Maynard's Legacy: One Year Later," YouTube Video, 6:21, October 5, 2015, last accessed July 7, 2018, https://www.youtube.com/watch?v=uzp0tp8Fzio.

2. Ibid.

3. Kelly Davis, "What I Learned Helping My Sister Use California's New Law to End Her Life," *Voice of San Diego*, August 9, 2016, last accessed May 14, 2018, https://docs.google.com/document/d/1gvclLSDIyI6XGMQK93fRBvuqA2yiWcOCtqrrNeKYE1I/edit.

4. Nicholas Filipas, "Eggman Introduces Aid-in-Dying Bill," *(Stockton, CA) Record*, August 18, 2015, last accessed May 14, 2018, https://www.recordnet.com/article/20150818/NEWS/150819711.

5. Patrick McGreevy, "After Struggling, Jerry Brown Makes Assisted Suicide Legal in California," *Los Angeles Times*, October 5, 2015, last accessed May 14, 2018, http://www.latimes.com/local/political/la-me-pc-gov-brown-end-of-life-bill-20151005-story.html.

6. Christopher Torchia, "Tutu Urges Regulated Euthanasia after Campaigner's Arrest," *Associated Press News*, September 21, 2018, last accessed September 23, 2018, https://apnews.com/2c2dd0bd948b4ac0bc31dc75402362db.

7. Ibid.

8. Lindsey Bever, "A Terminally Ill Woman Had One Rule at Her End-of-Life Party: No Crying," *Washington Post*, August 16, 2016, last accessed May 14, 2018, www.washingtonpost.com/news/inspired-life/wp/2016/08/16/a-terminally-ill-woman-had-one-rule-at-her-end-of-life-party-no-crying/?utm_term=.e7aa82479f.

9. Peg Sandeen, "State of the Death with Dignity Movement in 2018," Death with Dignity National Center, July 14, 2018, last accessed July 16, 2018, https://www.deathwithdignity.org/news/2018/07/state-of-death-with-dignity-movement-2018/.

10. Megan Brenan, "Americans' Strong Support for Euthanasia Persists," *Gallup News*, May 31, 2018, last accessed May 31, 2018, https://news.gallup.com/poll/235145/americans-strong-support-euthanasia-persists.aspx.

11. "Paul Spiers, PhD, Obituary," *Boston Globe*, September 13, 2013, last accessed July 15, 2018, http://www.legacy.com/obituaries/bostonglobe/obituary.aspx?n=paul-spiers&pid=167005930&fhid=9261.

12. Peg Sandeen, personal communication, December 20, 2018.

13. Brooks Hays, "Stephen Hawking Supports Parliament's Assisted Dying Bill," United Press International, July 16, 2014, last accessed April 26, 2018, https://www.upi.com/Science_News/2014/07/16/Stephen-Hawking-supports-Parliaments-Assisted-Dying-Bill/8941405547351/.

14. Sara Myers and Dustin Hankinson, "People Living with Disabilities Support Death with Dignity," *Missoulian*, July 25, 2014, last accessed July 14, 2018, https://missoulian.com/news/opinion/columnists/people-living-with-disabilities-support-death-with-dignity/article_ab4a1cea-1409-11e4-a3cf-001a4bcf887a.html.

15. Peter Baker, "Barbara Bush, Gravely Ill, Opts to Halt Treatment," *New York Times*, April 15, 2018, last accessed July 14, 2018, https://www.nytimes.com/2018/04/15/us/politics/barbara-bush-ill.html.

16. Anne Moyer, "Does How We Talk about Cancer Matter?," *Psychology Today*, October 19, 2016, last accessed August 23, 2018, https://www.psychologytoday.com/us/blog/beyond-treatment/201610/does-how-we-talk-about-cancer-matter.

17. Jacob Passy, "John McCain Is a War Hero—but Think Twice before Saying He's 'Battling' Cancer," *Market Watch*, August 25, 2018, last accessed August 27, 2018, https://www.marketwatch.com/story/john-mccain-is-a-war-hero-but-think-twice-before-saying-hes-battling -cancer-2017-07-21.

18. Sarah Lyall, "The Last Thing Mom Asked," *New York Times*, August 31, 2018, last accessed September 2, 2018, https://www .nytimes.com/2018/08/31/sunday-review/mother-death-euthanasia .html.

19. Laura Crimaldi, "Massachusetts Medical Society Ends Opposition to Physician-Assisted Suicide, Adopts Neutral Stance," *Boston Globe*, December 2, 2017, last accessed July 14, 2018, https://www .bostonglobe.com/metro/2017/12/02/massachusetts-medical-society -decide-whether-doctors-should-help-dying-end-their-lives/GtVH 8TuY1IebcMmltEoy4M/story.html; "Our Opinion: MMS Takes Key Step on Death with Dignity," *Berkshire Eagle*, December 4, 2017, last accessed July 14, 2018, https://www.berkshireeagle.com/stories/ our-opinion-mna-takes-key-stepon-death-with-dignity,526186.

20. Lindsey Bever, "The American Medical Association Has Long Opposed Assisted Suicide. Is That About to Change?," *Washington Post*, June 10, 2018, https://www.washingtonpost.com/news/ to-your-health/wp/2018/06/10/the-american-medical-association -has-long-opposed-assisted-suicide-is-that-about-to-change/?utm_ term=.93e896f575b3; Ronald W. Pies, "Will the AMA Heed Its Own Ethics Council Regarding Assisted Suicide?," *Psychiatric Times* 35, no 7 (2018), accessed May 31, 2018, http://www.psychiatrictimes.com/ couch-crisis/will-ama-heed-its-own-ethics-council-regarding-assisted -suicide?rememberme=1&elq_mid=1595&elq_cid=860745.

21. Lindsey Bever, "American Medical Association to Keep Reviewing Its Opposition to Assisted Death," *Washington Post*, June 11, 2018, https://www.washingtonpost.com/news/to-your-health/ wp/2018/06/11/american-medical-association-to-keep-reviewing -its-opposition-to-assisted-death/?utm_term=.80721d5ecb17.

22. Cynthia McCormick, "Falmouth Backs Death with Dignity," *Cape Cod Times*, July 10, 2018, last accessed July 16, 2018, http://www.capecod times.com/news/20180710/falmouth-backs-death-with-dignity.

Chapter 30

1. "Editorial: It May Be Time for a Cautious Second Step in Assisted Dying Legislation," *(Halifax, NS) Chronicle Herald*, September 27, 2018, https://www.thechronicleherald.ca/opinion/editorials/editorial

-it-may-be-time-for-a-cautious-second-step-in-assisted-dying-legisla-tion-245015/.

2. Josh Bloom, Henry I. Miller, "Assisted Suicide for Alzheimer's Patients Raises Incredibly Difficult Issues," December 2, 2018, Fox News, last accessed December 10, 2018, https://www.foxnews.com/opinion/assisted-suicide-for-alzheimers-patients-raises-incredibly-difficult-issues.

3. "Ontario Man with Dementia on Crusade to Plan His Own Death," CBC Radio, September 29, 2018, last accessed December 10, 2018, https://www.cbc.ca/radio/thesundayedition/the-sunday-edition-september-30-2018-1.4841264/ontario-man-with-dementia-on-crusade-to-plan-his-own-death-1.4841267.

4. Rob Kuznia, "In Oregon, Pushing to Give Patients with Degen-erative Diseases the Right to Die," March 11, 2018, *Washington Post*, last accessed December 10, 2018, https://www.washingtonpost.com/national/in-oregon-pushing-to-give-patients-with-degenerative-diseases-the-right-to-die/2018/03/11/3b6a2362-230e-11e8-94da-ebf9d112159c_story.html?noredirect=on&utm_term=.35d87795ed9c.

5. "Editorial: It May Be Time."

6. Derek Humphry, "Opinion: Time to Improve the Oregon-Style Death with Dignity Law," *Right-to-Die Digest*, November 4, 2018, Right-to-die-requests@lists, last accessed December 10, 2018, https://out-look.bhs.org/owa/?bO=1#path=/mail.

7. David Brooks, "What Moral Heroes Are Made Of," *New York Times*, May 21, 2018, A25; Anne Colby and William Damon, *Some Do Care* (New York: Free Press, 1992).

8. Samuel Blouin, "'Suicide Tourism' and Understanding the Swiss Model of the Right to Die," *The Conversation*, May 23, 2018, accessed July 25, 2018, http://theconversation.com/suicide-tourism-and-understanding-the-swiss-model-of-the-right-to-die-96698.

AUTHOR'S NOTES AND ACKNOWLEDGMENTS

Dignified Ending began with Dr. Martin Raff's invitation for me to join his think tank, and soon afterward, I called up the ever-generous Peg Sandeen, the executive director of the Death with Dignity National Center. It was she who suggested that I come to Oregon and meet Derek Humphry. He is, indeed, the wizard of assisted dying, and both Derek and Peg kindly provided introductions to many of the other people, including Faye Girsh, George Eighmey, Stan Curtis, and filmmaker Peter Richardson. Barbara Coombs Lee represented another branching point for my convenience sample of interview subjects, and it was she who offered me a firsthand account of the movement's history in the United States, as well as opportunities to speak with the family and friends of Brittany Maynard. Writing this book over the past seven years, I have sat down with between two hundred and three hundred people—proponents and opponents—to hear their perspectives about this complex topic. Some of those interviews were edited out of the final manuscript, but all of them influenced my thinking.

Many of these individuals allowed me to record their words. They understood that this was to be a nonfiction work and each

agreed to the disclosure of their names. In these pages, I have
taken the liberty of using forenames of the people who told me
their stories. Otherwise, surnames alone are relied upon in the
text for identification purposes, except in a few instances where
forenames were needed to distinguish individuals from family
members.

Although I regularly fact-checked, interviewed multiple
participants to obtain different perspectives of the same events,
and submitted a few requests using the Freedom of Information
Act, errors have undoubtedly slipped into the book. I sincerely
apologize for these and would like to hear about and correct
them. Any mistakes are my responsibility alone. In only three
instances did I intentionally conceal a few identifying features.

According to the writer Cormac McCarthy, "The ugly fact is
books are made out of books. The novel depends for its life on
the novels that have been written." So, too, a nonfiction book
like this one could only have been written because it was preceded by *Being Mortal, How We Die, Tuesdays with Morrie,* and *On
Death and Dying.*

I regularly follow the *New York Times* and didn't hesitate to
dip into Wikipedia, *Salon,* the *Economist,* and other bountiful
sources of information. My apologies if I inadvertently neglected
to acknowledge any contributors to the book. *The Writer's Alma-
nac* has been an entertaining source of poetry for me over the
years.

Although my interview with Betsy Nimitz Van Dorn provided key details about her father's death, I am indebted to Sara
Rimer's article in the *New York Times,* "With Suicide, an Admiral Keeps Command until the End." Neil McCormick's piece in
the *Telegraph,* "Paul Anka: One Song the Sex Pistols Won't Be
Singing," was invaluable in comprehending the origin of "My
Way." While Anka was not necessarily talking about hastening
death, I believe he captured some of the essential personality
characteristics that often drives these decisions. Likewise, there
is a piece in the *Economist* titled, "Doctors Should Be Allowed
to Help the Suffering and Terminally Ill to Die When They
Choose," which was exceedingly stimulating. Sarah Kliff and

Arian Campo-Flores wrote a fine piece about Larry Egbert that was posted on *Newsweek*'s website. The kindest biography ever written about Jack Kevorkian is *Between the Dying and the Dead* by Neal Nicol and Harry Wylie. While Lennard J. Davis lost me in some of the details of political wrangling, *Enabling Acts* is a passionate account of the Americans with Disabilities Act. Although Richard Côté died way too soon after publishing *In Search of Gentle Death*, it is the best history of the right-to-die movement from a proponent's perspective. Lastly, while I devoted considerable space to describing Derek Humphry's story, his autobiography, *Good Life, Good Death*, and the self-deliverance handbook, *Final Exit*, are required reading.

One cannot write about death and dying without being connected to a source of love and life, and that has always been my family. My wife, Professor Joan Berzoff, tolerated my obsessive researching and writing with impressive affection and forbearance. Joan has been a never-ending fount of encouragement. This book would not have been completed without her patience and sage advice, but also her firmness in reminding me about life's priorities. She is a skilled author by her own right, and she is my eternal mate. This book is dedicated to her.

My sons have been always curious about the project's twists and turns; Baltimore Councilman Zeke Cohen was especially helpful in offering me a politician's view of the material, while Jake Cohen not only accompanied me to visit Derek Humphry but also alerted me to Larry Egbert's original indictment. My two daughters-in-law are still probably puzzled about why I would immerse myself in this subject, but they consistently offered thoughtful observations and managed to appear mildly bemused by my accounts.

Likewise, I appreciate the support extended by various friends and extended family, for example, the Grunberger and Tider clans, Bob and Cynthia Shilkret, Rorry Zahourek and Jay Holzman, Marilyn August, Booker and Reverend Janet Bush, Richard Meyer, and others, who frequently sent me emails with relevant links and then were (almost) always willing to let me drone on about some aspect of the book that caught my fancy. Thanks to Professor Sarah Olsen of Amherst College for her expertise about Heracles. Dr. Ben Liptzin was my longtime chairman, and along with Drs. Ed Lowenstein, Andy Billings, and Marcia Angell offered valuable thoughts on this subject.

Seth Shulman is well deserving of his own paragraph of acknowledgment. He is a superb science writer and editor but also a real mensch. Seth would energetically deny that he coauthored this book, and I won't pin that responsibility on him. But he sure did much more than read through different iterations of the manuscript and point out where I was going wrong. Seth was my guru, and he is one of the most talented and modest men that I have ever had the good fortune to meet. His contribution to my writing is immeasurable.

I owe considerable thanks to the consummate professionals from Rowman & Littlefield, and especially senior editor Suzanne Starzick. Jemma Stephenson from Smith College provided invaluable assistance with the references.

I am deeply obliged to Baystate Medical Center, which throughout my career has generously provided the necessities of academic life: professional colleagues of the highest order, material support, and the freedom to split my time between clinical and academic activities. The thoughts and opinions expressed in this book do not reflect my association with Baystate and are strictly my own. My secretary/administrator, June Plasse, has been always exuberant and helpful in a thousand practical ways, while Drs. Jay Kilpatrick and Steven Fischel, and Stephen Luipold, APRN, kept the psychiatric consultation service functioning when I was unavailable during writing sabbaticals.

Grateful acknowledgment is made for permission to quote from the following sources:

My thanks to George Theodoridis for his translation of Sophocles's *The Women of Trachis*, and *Philoktetes*, and also to Adam Kline, whose father is the translator of Ovid's *Metamorphoses*.

I am in debt to the poet, Paul Hostovsky, for permission to reprint "Tree Poem," and to the family of Gillian Bennett for extensively reprinting her online letter.

Permission was acquired from Grove Atlantic to reprint Raymond Carver's "What the Doctor Said," from *A New Path to the Waterfall*, copyright 1989.

I can only try to humbly express my special appreciation of the Bogliasco Foundation and the Rockefeller Foundation for their inestimable contributions to this project. Winston Churchill's publishers understood that he would never fulfill his contractual obligations unless they sent him on a writing "vacation." As book deadlines approached (or passed), the publishers would arrange for the former prime minister to go to exotic locales where he could work without the interruptions and responsibilities of quotidian life. Churchill, Clementine, their friends, and an entourage of literary researchers and assistants would be provided with villas in the south of France, Capri, and other seaside locales. And it was in those gorgeous places, well stocked with the finest food, the best whiskey, port, claret, and an ample supply of cigars that the man who said, "History will be kind to me for I intend to write it," completed his monumental books.

I am no Churchill, but the Bogliasco Fellowship and Rockefeller's Bellagio Residency offer a few lucky people a Churchillian experience, and my wife and I are eternally grateful for the opportunity to have joined their vibrant communities of artists, poets, authors, and musicians (cigars were not provided). I have no words to adequately express my thanks to these foundations or to my fellow residents.

BIBLIOGRAPHY

The following articles previously appeared in online publications or medical journals and were the foundation for several stories in this book:

Cohen, Lewis M. "Dignified Debate." *Slate*, August 11, 2014, accessed September 28, 2015. https://slate.com/technology/2014/08/assisted-suicide-debate-in-united-kingdom-house-of-lords-on-death-with-dignity.html.

Cohen, Lewis M. "How Rear Adm. Chester Nimitz Jr. and Joan Nimitz Chose to Die." *Slate*, June 6, 2013, accessed September 28, 2015. http://www.slate.com/articles/health_and_science/medical_examiner/2013/06/death_with_dignity_joint_suicide_of_rear_adm_chester_nimitz_jr_and_joan.html.

Cohen, Lewis M. "How Sigmund Freud Wanted to Die." *Atlantic*, September 23, 2014, accessed September 28, 2015. http://www.theatlantic.com/health/archive/2014/09/how-sigmund-freud-wanted-to-die/380322/.

Cohen, Lewis M. "Massachusetts Vote May Change How the Nation Dies: Why It Matters That Death with Dignity Is Poised to Become the New Norm." *Slate*, October 29, 2012, accessed September 28, 2015. http://www.slate.com/articles/health_and_science/medical_examiner/2012/10/massachusetts_death_with_dignity_2012_kevorkian_and_humphry_started_the.html.

McCue, Jack D., and Lewis M. Cohen. "Freud's Physician-Assisted Death." *Archives of Internal Medicine* 159, no. 14 (July 26, 1999). doi:10.1001/archinte.159.14.1521.

Books

Albom, Mitch. *Tuesdays with Morrie*. New York: Doubleday, 1997.

Cohen, Lewis Mitchel. *No Good Deed: A Story of Medicine, Murder Accusations, and the Debate Over How We Die*. New York: Harper Collins, 2010.

Colby, Anne, and William Damon. *Some Do Care: Contemporary Lives of Moral Commitment*. New York: Free Press, 1992.

Colby, William H. *Long Goodbye: The Deaths of Nancy Cruzan*. Carlsbad, CA: Hay House, 2002.

Côté, Richard N. *In Search of Gentle Death: The Fight for Your Right to Die with Dignity*. Mt. Pleasant, SC: Corinthian Books, 2012.

Feifer, Herman. *The Meaning of Death*. New York: Blakiston Division, McGraw-Hill, 1959.

Gawande, Atul. *Being Mortal: Medicine and What Matters in the End*. New York: Metropolitan Books/Henry Holt & Company, 2014.

Gay, Peter. *Freud: A Life for Our Time*. London: W.W. Norton & Company, 2006.

Gorsuch, Neil M. *The Future of Assisted Suicide and Euthanasia*. Princeton, NJ: Princeton University Press, 2009.

Harris, Brayton. *Admiral Nimitz: The Commander of the Pacific Ocean Theater*. New York: St. Martin's Press, 2012.

Humphry, Derek. *Jean's Way*. Junction City, OR: Norris Lane Press, 2003.

Humphry, Derek. *Final Exit: The Practicalities of Self-Deliverance and Assisted Suicide for the Dying*. New York: Dell Publishing, 1991.

Humphry, Derek. *Good Life, Good Death: The Memoir of a Right to Die Pioneer*. New York, NY: Carrel Books, 2017.

Kalanithi, Paul. *When Breath Becomes Air*. New York: Random House, 2016.

Kübler-Ross, Elisabeth. *On Death and Dying*. New York: Simon and Schuster, 1969.

Mangalik, Aroop. *Dealing with Doctors, Denial, and Death: A Guide to Living Well with Serious Illness*. Lanham, MD: Rowman & Littlefield, 2017.

Nicol, Neal, and Harry L. Wylie. *Between the Dying and the Dead: Dr. Jack Kevorkian, the Assisted Suicide Machine and the Battle to Legalize Euthanasia*. Madison: University of Wisconsin Press, 2006.

Rehm, Diane. *On My Own*. New York: Alfred A. Knopf, Inc., 2016.

Roiphe, Katie. *Violet Hour: Great Writers at the End*. New York: Dial Press, 2016.

Schur, Max. *Freud: Living and Dying*. New York: International Universities Press, 1972.

Szasz, Thomas. *Fatal Illness: The Ethics and Politics of Suicide*. Syracuse, NY: Syracuse University Press, 2002.

Szasz, Thomas Stephen. *Suicide Prohibition: The Shame of Medicine*. Syracuse, NY: Syracuse University Press, 2011.

Warraich, Haider. *Modern Death: How Medicine Changed the End of Life*. New York: St. Martin's Press, 2017.

Articles

American Association of Suicidology. "Statement of the American Association of Suicidology: "Suicide" Is Not the Same as 'Physician Aid in Dying.'" October 30, 2017, accessed April 26, 2018. http://www.suicidology.org/Portals/14/docs/Press Release/AAS PAD Statement Approved 10.30.17 ed 10-30-17.pdf.

Balasubramaniam, Meera. "Rational Suicide in Elderly Adults: A Clinician's Perspective." *Journal of the American Geriatrics Society*, March 2, 2018. https://doi.org/10.1111/jgs.15263.

Bassett, Mike. "Judicious Feeding Options at the End of Life." Today's Geriatric Medicine, last accessed April 2, 2018. http://www.todaysgeriatricmedicine.com/news/ex_020218.shtml.

Bever, Lindsey. "The Apparent Murder-Suicide of a Death-with-Dignity Advocate and his Ailing Wife." *Washington Post*, April 22, 2016, accessed September 2, 2018. https://www.washingtonpost.com/news/morning-mix/wp/2016/04/22/its-horrific-the-apparent-murder-suicide-of-a-right-to-die-advocate-and-his-ailing-wife/?noredirect=on&utm_term=.c4a22ce06aee.

Brody, Jane E. "Alzheimer's? Your Paperwork May Not Be in Order." *New York Times*, April 30, 2018. https://www.nytimes.com/2018/04/30/well/live/an-advance-directive-for-patients-with-dementia.html.

Brooks, David. "What Moral Heroes Are Made Of." *New York Times*, May 22, 2018, A25.

Buchanan, Patrick J. "The Sad Suicide of Admiral Nimitz." WND, January 18, 2002, accessed October 28, 2012. http://www.wnd.com/2002/01/12433/.

Carter, Zoe FitzGerald. "The Poignant Irony of Dr. Kevorkian's Death." *Salon*, September 25, 2011, accessed April 23, 2018. https://www.salon.com/2011/06/04/kevorkian_death_reaction/.

Deutsch, Felix. "Reflections on Freud's One Hundredth Birthday." *Psychosomatic Medicine* 8, (1965): 279–83.

Drake, Steven N. "The All-Too-Familiar Story." *Ragged Edge*, 2001, accessed September 26, 2018. http://www.raggededgemagazine .com/0301/0301ft5.htm.

Druckerman, Pamela. "To Live and Die in Paris." *New York Times*, August 19, 2018, p. 9.

Dzeng, Liz, and Steve Pantilat. "Social Causes of Rational Suicide in Older Adults." *Journal of the American Geriatrics Society*, March 2, 2018. https://doi.org/10.1111/jgs.15290.

Economist. "What Is Unbearable?" August 4, 2016. https://www.econ-omist.com/news/science-and-technology/21703359-some-data -about-emotional-issue-what-unbearable.

Egan, Nicole Weisensee. "Terminally Ill 29-Year-Old Woman: Why I'm Choosing to Die on My Own Terms." *People*, October 24, 2016, last accessed July 16, 2018. https://people.com/celebrity/terminally -ill-29-year-old-woman-why-im-choosing-to-die-on-my-own -terms/.

Erdmann, Jeanne. "At 100, My Mom Had Dementia and Needed Hospice Care. Getting It Was Nearly Impossible." *Washing-ton Post*, May 5, 2018, accessed May 05, 2018. https://www .washingtonpost.com/national/health-science/at-100-my-mom -had-dementia-and-needed-hospice-care-getting-it-was-nearly -impossible/2018/05/04/c6b7efdc-4724-11e8-8b5a-3b1697adcc2a_ story.html?utm_term=.d96d6f45f799.

Friedman, Thomas L. "Call Your Mother." *New York Times*, May 11, 2008, accessed June 5, 2018. https://www.nytimes.com/2008/05/11/ opinion/11friedman.html.

Ganzini, Linda, et al. "Physicians' Experiences with the Oregon Death with Dignity Act." *New England Journal of Medicine* 342, (2000): 557–63. doi. 10.1056/NEJM200002243420806.

Gross, Jane. "At AIDS Epicenter, Seeking Swift, Sure Death." *New York Times*, June 20, 1993. http://www.nytimes.com/1993/06/20/us/ at-aids-epicenter-seeking-swift-sure-death.html.

Hedberg, Katrina, and Craig New. "Oregon's Death with Dignity Act: 20 Years of Experience to Inform the Debate." *Annals of Internal Med-icine* 167, no. 8 (October 17, 2017): 579–83. doi:10.7326/m17-2300.

Jacoby, Susan. "Real Life among the Old." *New York Times*, Decem-ber 30, 2010, accessed June 5, 2018. https://www.nytimes.com/ 2010/12/31/opinion/31jacoby.html.

Kelly, Laura. "Older Adults Overprescribed Dementia Medication at High Cost: Study." *Washington Times*, August 21, 2018, accessed August 27, 2018. https://www.washingtontimes.com/news/ 2018/aug/21/older-adults-overprescribed-dementia-medication/.

Kliff, Sarah. "Lawrence Egbert: Assisted Suicide's New Face." *Newsweek*, March 14, 2010, last accessed June 4, 2018. http://www.newsweek.com/lawrence-egbert-assisted-suicides-new-face-69677.

Kowalczyk, Liz. "Color Line Persists, in Sickness as in Health." *Boston Globe*, December 12, 2017, accessed June 5, 2018. https:apps.bostonglobe.com/spotlight/boston-racism-image-reality/series/hospitals/.

Lessenberry, Jack. "Dr. Death Gets Out of Prison." *Detroit Metro Times*, December 20, 2006, accessed July 1, 2018. https://www.metrotimes.com/detroit/dr-death-gets-out-of-prison/Content?oid=2186216.

Lewin, Tamar. "Nancy Cruzan Dies, Outlived by a Debate over the Right to Die." *New York Times*, December 27, 1990, accessed April 27, 2018. https://www.nytimes.com/1990/12/27/us/nancy-cruzan-dies-outlived-by-a-debate-over-the-right-to-die.html.

Lyall, Sarah. "Could I Kill My Mother?" *New York Times*, August 31, 2018, last accessed September 2, 2018. https://www.nytimes.com/2018/08/31/sunday-review/mother-death-euthanasia.html.

Majchrowicz, Michael. "The Volunteers Who Help People End Their Own Lives." *Atlantic*, July 6, 2016, last accessed June 3, 2018. https://www.theatlantic.com/health/archive/2016/07/the-volunteers-who-help-people-end-their-own-lives/489602/.

Marx, Linda. "The Agony Did Not End for Roswell Gilbert, Who Killed His Wife to Give Her Peace." *People*, January 12, 1987, accessed September 2, 2018. http://people.com/archive/the-agony-did-not-end-for-roswell-gilbert-who-killed-his-wife-to-give-her-peace-vol-27-no-2/.

McFadden, Robert D. "Karen Ann Quinlan, 31, Dies; Focus of '76 Right to Die Case." *New York Times*, June 12, 1985, accessed April 26, 2018. https://www.nytimes.com/1985/06/12/nyregion/karen-ann-quinlan-31-dies-focus-of-76-right-to-die-case.html.

Menzel, Paul T., and Bonnie Steinbock. "Advance Directives, Dementia, and Physician-Assisted Death." *Journal of Law, Medicine & Ethics* 4, no 2 (June 6, 2013): 484–500. http://onlinelibrary.wiley.com/doi/10.1111/jlme.12057/abstract.

Nabi, Junaid. "'No One Was Listening to Us': Lessons from the Jahi McMath Case." The Hastings Center, April 4, 2018. https://www.thehastingscenter.org/no-one-listening-us-lessons-jahi-mcmath-case/.

Nelson, Roxanne. "When Dying Becomes Unaffordable." *Medscape Medical News*, November 9, 2017, last accessed June 10, 2018. https://www.medscape.com/viewarticle/888271#vp_1.

Offord, Catherine. "Accessing Drugs for Medical Aid-in-Dying." *Scientist*, August 17, 2017, last accessed June 10, 2018. https://

www.the-scientist.com/?articles.view/articleNo/49879/title/Accessing-Drugs-for-Medical-Aid-in-Dying/.

Pelisek, Christine. "Florida Murder Suspect Claims Wife Asked Him to Kill Her— to Spare Her from Dementia." *People*, March 29, 2017, accessed September 2, 2018. https://people.com/crime/florida-man-murder-wife-save-her-dementia/.

Rimer, Sara. "With Suicide, an Admiral Keeps Command until the End." *New York Times*, January 12, 2002, accessed September 1, 2018. https://www.nytimes.com/2002/01/12/us/with-suicide-an-admiral-keeps-command-until-the-end.html.

Rubin, Emily B., Anna E. Buehler, and Scott D. Halpern. "States Worse Than Death among Hospitalized Patients with Serious Illnesses." *JAMA Internal Medicine* 176, no. 10 (2016). doi:10.1001/jamainternmed.2016.4362.

Ryan, Denise. "Dead at Noon: B.C. Woman Ends Her Life Rather Than Suffer Indignity of Dementia (with video)." *Vancouver Sun*, January 14, 2015. http://www.vancouversun.com/health/Dead+noon+woman+ends+life+rather+than+suffer+indignity+dementia+with+video/10132068/story.html.

Salam, Maya. "Consent in the Digital Age: Can Apps Solve a Very Human Problem?" *New York Times*, March 2, 2018. https://www.nytimes.com/2018/03/02/technology/consent-apps.html.

Schwarz, Judith. "A New Way to Handle Dementia Care." Baystate Health, March 30, 2018. https://outlook.bhs.org/OWA/#path=/mail.

Solomon, Andrew. "A Death of One's Own" *Andrew Solomon* (Blog), May 22, 1995, accessed September 1, 2018. http://andrewsolomon.com/articles/a-death-of-ones-own/.

Solomon, Andrew. "On My Mother, and Dr. Kevorkian." *New Yorker*, June 20, 2017, https://www.newyorker.com/news/news-desk/on-my-mother-and-dr-kevorkian.

Tutu, Desmond. "Archbishop Desmond Tutu: When My Time Comes, I Want the Option of an Assisted Death." *Washington Post*, October 6, 2016, accessed June 5, 2018. https://www.washingtonpost.com/opinions/global-opinions/archbishop-desmond-tutu-when-my-time-comes-i-want-the-option-of-an-assisted-death/2016/10/06/97c804f2-8a81-11e6-b24f-a7f89eb68887_story.html?utm_term=.e79b644c7a61.

Varney, Sarah. "A Racial Gap in Attitudes toward Hospice Care." *New York Times*, August 21, 2015, accessed June 15, 2018. https://www.nytimes.com/2015/08/25/health/a-racial-gap-in-attitudes-toward-hospice-care.html.

Wanzer, S. H., D. D. Federman, S. J. Adelstein, et al. The Physician's Responsibility toward Hopelessly Ill Patients: A Second Look. *New England Journal of Medicine* 320 (1989): 844–49.

Watson, Celia Seupel. "The Job to End All Others." *New York Times*, June 13, 2011, accessed March 3, 2018. https://newoldage.blogs.nytimes.com/2011/06/13/the-job-to-end-all-others/.

Weisman, A. D., and T. P. Hackett. "Predilection to Death: Death and Dying as a Psychiatric Problem." *Psychosomatic Medicine* 23 (1961): 232–56.

Wolff, Michael. "A Life Worth Ending." *New York*, May 20, 2012, accessed May 23, 2018. http://nymag.com/ncws/features/parent-health-care-2012-5/.

INDEX

and data on, 263–67; socioeconomic class and, 164–65;
suffering and, 30–31, 34–36,
86; Supreme Court on, 87–88,
217, 225–26; synonyms, 25;
terminology issues and, 25,
85–87; in United Kingdom,
88–89, 108, 120; Weinstein
and, 29–32, 63–64, 69. *See also*
death with dignity; *specific
topics*
"At AIDS Epicenter, Seeking
Swift, Sure Death" (Gross),
64–65, 314n3
Austen, Jane, 21–22
Austria, 81–83
automobile exhaust asphyxiation, 65
Aviv, Rachel, 167

baby boomers, 88, 90, 103–6
barbiturates, 65, 144, 180, 183–84,
188–89, 196–99, 251–54,
271–74
Barfield, Ellen, 175, 209–10
Battle of Midway, 10
Battle of the Coral Sea, 10
Because They're Black (Humphry,
D.), 115
bedbound, 96, 134–35
Being Mortal (Gawande), 51
beliefs, 8, 10–11, 19, 149–50. *See
also* religion
Belli, Laura, 174
Benight, Philip M., 32–33
Benight, Rebecca, 32–33
Bennett, Gillian, 70–74, 108, 302
Bethea, Charles, 215
Beychok, Irving, 55–56, 57
Billboard Project, 211–12
Black Coalition on AIDS, 66–69
Blanke, Charles, 196–97

Blehr, Claire, 216–17
blindness, 20
Bonaparte, Marie, 80, 96, 98, 99
Boston Globe, 143
Boston Medical Center, 67
Bouvia, Elizabeth, 177–78
brain, 21; damage, 134–35; death,
166–67
Breitbart, William, 150
Brown, Jerry, 296
Brunswick, Ruth, 79
Buchanan, Patrick J., 48–49
Bush, Barbara, 298–99
Bush, George H. W., 168
Bush, George W., 23

California: End of Life Options
Act in, 296–97; law in, 134,
178–79, 197, 295–97, 299–300;
living will in, 134
Camay, Ray, 256
Canada: Act Respecting End of
Life Care in, 174; Alzheimer
Society of Canada, 74; dementia in, 109; euthanasia in,
199–200; law in, 74, 109, 174,
199, 302–3; Valeant Pharmaceuticals in, 197
cancer, 139–41, 193–94, 291–92,
294; of Celmer, J., 215–16;
Curtis, C., and, 233–40,
249–53, 255–58, 269–73;
Freud S., and, 40–46, 80–81,
82, 96–98; Humphry, J., and,
115–17; of Kennedy, 160–61;
Lotter and, 291; Maynard
and, 241–44, 259–63; McCain
and, 299; patient-physician
relationships and, 41–46; of
"The Woman," 180–84, 187–90
Cantor, Norman L., 75
"Capital Crawl," 168

Caplan, Arthur, 90, 150
caregiving: in assisted living
 facilities, 30–32, 34, 64, 91,
 106; employment and, 91;
 family and, 91, 166; marriage
 and, 91; palliative care, 21,
 23–24, 86, 304–5. *See also*
 dementia
Caring Friends: assisted suicide
 and, 180–84, 187–90, 191–92,
 194–96, 279; death-acceleration
 and, 181–90; FEN compared to,
 210–12; founding of, 179–80;
 Girsh and, 179–80, 195–96;
 Goodwin and, 219; *Hemlock
 Society* and, 179–80, 182–83,
 210; Humphry, D., and, 179–80;
 MacDonald and, 181–90,
 191–92, 194–96, 201; "The
 Woman" and, 180–84, 187–90
Carter, Brian, 136
Carter, Michelle, 225
Carter, Zoe Fitzgerald, 149
Catholicism, 86–87, 134, 139, 174,
 176, 212, 287–88
causation, of death, 225–26
C&C. *See* Compassion & Choices
celebrity support, 88
cells, 92
Celmer, John, 207–8, 214–17,
 223–24
Celmer, Sue, 215
Centers for Disease Control and
 Prevention, 48; Morbidity and
 Mortality Weekly Report by,
 67–68
Cherkasky, Andrew D., 78
chloral hydrate, 199
Christian Scientists, 285–88
civil rights, 11, 27–28; disability
 rights movement and, 156–69;
 dying and, 51

Clinton, Hillary, 172–73
Code of Medical Ethics, 299–300
cognition: assisted suicide and,
 166–67; death and, 21, 26;
 dementia and, 104. *See also*
 dementia; mental health
Cohen, Lewis Mitchel, 163–64;
 on assisted suicide, 301–8; *No
 Good Deed* by, 21
Colby, Anne, 306, 340n7
Colby, William H., 134–35
Cold Spring Harbor Laboratory,
 19–24, 53–54
Coleman, Diane, 156–58, 169
Colorado, 297, 299–300
Compassion & Choices (C&C):
 Curtis, C., and, 252, 255; Diaz
 and, 242, 295; *Hemlock Society*
 and, 50–51, 195–96; Maynard
 and, 280–81
consent: advance directives and,
 77–78; sex and, 77–78, 316n32;
 We-Consent and, 77
"Consent in the Digital Age"
 (Salam), 77–78, 316n32
Conti, Tom, 136
Cooper, Jessica, 131
Côté, Richard, 119, 138, 174–75
Council of Braga, 86
Council on Ethical and Judicial
 Affairs, 300
countertransference, 41
Crocker, Gretchen, 144
Cruzan, Joe, 135
Cruzan, Nancy, 134–35, 136
culture, 23
Cummings, E. E., 292
Curtis, Cody: assisted suicide
 and, 237–40, 249–53, 255–58,
 269–75, 286–87, 289–91, 306;
 background on, 237–38;
 cancer and, 233–40, 249–53,

ABOUT THE AUTHOR

Lewis Mitchel Cohen, MD, is a professor of psychiatry at the University of Massachusetts Medical School–Baystate and a clinical professor at Tufts University School of Medicine. He has been a contributor to *The Atlantic*, *Slate*, and *Huffington Post* and is the author of a nonfiction book, *No Good Deed: A Story of Medicine, Murder Accusations, and the Debate Over How We Die* (2010). The recipient of a Guggenheim Fellowship for Medicine and Health, two Rockefeller Foundation Bellagio Residency awards, and a Bogliasco Fellowship for the Arts and Humanities, he is an active palliative medicine researcher who has written more than one hundred academic publications relating to the integration of bioethics, nephrology, and psychiatry.